SIGNS & SYMPTOMS
IN EMERGENCY MEDICINE

Literature-Based Guide to Emergent Conditions

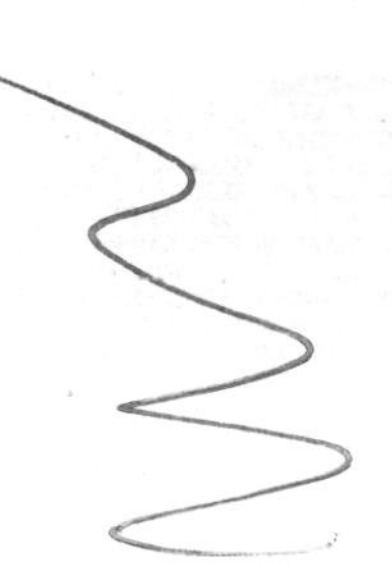

Editors

SCOTT R. VOTEY, MD
Associate Professor of Medicine/Emergency Medicine
UCLA School of Medicine;
Co-Director, UCLA Medical Center/Olive View–UCLA Medical Center
Combined Emergency Medicine Residency, Los Angeles, California

P. GREGG GREENOUGH, MD, MPH
School of Public Health
Johns Hopkins University
School of Hygiene and Public Health
Baltimore, Maryland

Consulting Editors

Jerome R. Hoffman, MD, MA
Professor of Medicine/Emergency Medicine
UCLA School of Medicine
UCLA Emergency Medicine Center, Los Angeles, California

Richard M. Schwartzenstein, MD
Clinical Director, Division of Pulmonary and Critical Care
Department of Medicine, Beth Israel Deaconess Medical Center;
Instructor of Medicine, Harvard Medical School
Boston, Massachusetts

Michael I. Zucker, MD
Professor of Radiological Sciences
Chief, Trauma and Emergency Radiology
Faculty Emergency Medicine Center
UCLA Medical Center, Los Angeles, California

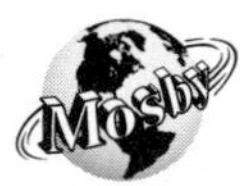

Visit our website at **www.mosby.com**

SIGNS & SYMPTOMS IN EMERGENCY MEDICINE

Literature-Based Guide to Emergent Conditions

Editor-in-Chief

MARK A. DAVIS, MD, MS
Director, Center for International Emergency Medicine
Harvard Medical School;
Director, Curriculum Development
Department of Emergency Medicine
Beth Israel Deaconess Medical Center
Boston, Massachusetts

Editors

SCOTT R. VOTEY, MD
P. GREGG GREENOUGH, MD, MPH

Consulting Editors

Jerome R. Hoffman, MD, MA
Richard M. Schwartzenstein, MD
Michael I. Zucker, MD

With World Wide Web Reference and Decision Support
www.signsandsymptoms.com

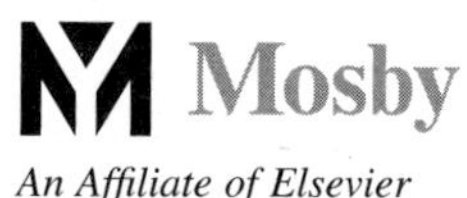

An Affiliate of Elsevier

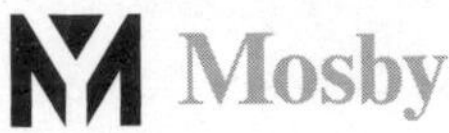

An Affiliate of Elsevier

Publisher: Richard Furn
Senior Managing Editor: Kathy Falk
Developmental Editor: Kristen Volkmann
Project Manager: Patricia Tannian
Production Editor: John Casey
Senior Composition Specialist: Joan Herron
Design Manager: Gail Morey Hudson
Manufacturing Manager: Don Carlisle
Cover Design: Teresa Breckwoldt
Cover photographs courtesy Tom Conlin, Bruce Wahl,
and Anthony J. Mancini.

Mosby, Inc.
11830 Westline Industrial Drive
St. Louis, Missouri 63146

ISBN 0-323-00211-0

03 04 05 06 / 9 8 7 6 5

Contributors

Beverly Bauman, MD, FAAP
Associate Director, Pediatric Emergency Medicine
Legacy Emanuel and Children's Hospital;
Clinical Instructor of Emergency Medicine
Oregon Health Sciences University
Portland, Oregon

Jeremy Brown, MD
Associate in Medicine, Division of Emergency Medicine
Beth Israel Deaconess Medical Center;
Instructor of Medicine, Harvard Medical School
Boston, Massachusetts

Michael J. Burns, MD
Director, Section of Toxicology, Department of Emergency Medicine
Beth Israel Deaconess Medical Center;
Instructor of Medicine, Harvard Medical School
Boston, Massachusetts

Victor A. Candioty, MD
Attending Physician, Emergency Department
Saint John's Health Center, Santa Monica, California;
Clinical Faculty, UCLA Medical Center
Los Angeles, California

Elizabeth Char, MD
Attending Physician, Department of Surgery
Division of Emergency Medicine
Queens Medical Center
Honolulu, Hawaii

Richelle Cooper, MD
Clinical Instructor and Research Fellow
Department of Medicine/Emergency Medicine
UCLA School of Medicine
Los Angeles, California

Hilarie Cranmer, MD
Resident Physician, Department of Emergency Medicine
Brigham & Women's Hospital
Boston, Massachusetts

Gerianne Dudley, MD
Senior Resident, UCLA Emergency Medicine Center
Los Angeles, California

Pamela Dyne, MD, FACEP
Assistant Professor of Medicine/Emergency Medicine
UCLA School of Medicine, Los Angeles, California;
Co-Director, UCLA Medical Center/Olive View–UCLA Medical Center Combined Emergency Medicine Residency
Sylmar, California

Jonathan A. Edlow, MD
Acting Chief, Division of Emergency Medicine
Beth Israel Deaconess Medical Center;
Instructor of Medicine, Harvard Medical School
Boston, Massachusetts

Joseph S. Englanoff, MD
Visiting Assistant Clinical Professor of Medicine/Emergency Medicine
UCLA School of Medicine, UCLA Emergency Medicine Center
Los Angeles, California

Stephen Epstein, MD, MPP
Associate in Medicine, Division of Emergency Medicine
Beth Israel Deaconess Medical Center;
Instructor of Medicine, Harvard Medical School
Boston, Massachusetts

Steven Go, MD, FACEP
Assistant Professor of Emergency Medicine
Director of Emergency Medicine Student Education
University of Missouri–Kansas City School of Medicine
Department of Emergency Medicine
Truman Medical Center-West
Kansas City, Missouri

Thomas Graham, MD
Assistant Professor of Medicine/Emergency Medicine
UCLA School of Medicine
UCLA Emergency Medicine Center
Los Angeles, California

Myles Greenberg, MD
Assistant Clinical Director, Department of Emergency Medicine
Beth Israel Deaconess Medical Center;
Instructor of Medicine, Harvard Medical School
Boston, Massachusetts

Daniel Grossman, MD, FACEP
Visiting Assistant Professor of Medicine/Emergency Medicine
UCLA School of Medicine
Los Angeles, California;
Physician, Saint John's Emergency Medicine Center
Santa Monica, California

John Halamka, MD
Executive Director, CareGroup Center for Quality and Value
Beth Israel Deaconess Medical Center;
Instructor of Medicine, Harvard Medical School
Boston, Massachusetts

Mel E. Herbert, MD
Assistant Professor of Medicine, UCLA School of Medicine
Assistant Professor of Nursing, UCLA School of Nursing
Los Angeles, California;
Department of Emergency Medicine
Olive View–ULCA Medical Center
Sylmar, California

Michelle Krueger, MD
Assistant Clinical Professor, Department of Emergency Medicine
University of California San Diego
San Diego, California

Mary L. Lanctot, BS, RN, CEN
Staff Nurse, Department of Emergency Medicine
Olive View–UCLA Medical Center
Sylmar, California

Kenneth R. Lawrence, BS, PharmD
Manager, Clinical Pharmacy Services
Beth Israel Deaconess Medical Center
Boston, Massachusetts

Eric Legome, MD
Attending Physician, Department of Emergency Medicine
Massachusetts General Hospital;
Instructor of Medicine, Harvard Medical School
Boston, Massachusetts

Resa Lewiss, MD
Harvard Affiliated Emergency Medicine Residency Program
Boston, Massachusetts

Julian G. Lis, MD
Fellow, International Emergency Medicine
Department of Emergency Medicine, Johns Hopkins University
Baltimore, Maryland

Mark Louden, MD
Attending Emergency Medicine Physician
Wake Medical Center
Raleigh, North Carolina

Laura Macnow, MD
Senior Resident, Harvard Affiliated Emergency Medicine Residency Program, Department of Emergency Medicine
Brigham & Women's Hospital
Boston, Massachusetts

Frances McCabe, MD
Emergency Physician/Flight Surgeon for the Chairman of the Joint Chiefs of Staff
United States Air Force Flight Medicine Clinic, The Pentagon
Washington, DC

Lynne McCullough, MD
Clinical Instructor of Emergency Medicine
UCLA School of Medicine
UCLA Emergency Medicine Center
Los Angeles, California

Maureen McCollough, MD, MPH
Assistant Professor of Medicine/Emergency Medicine
UCLA School of Medicine
Olive View–UCLA Medical Center
Sylmar, California

Brian Miura, MD
Visiting Assistant Professor of Medicine/Emergency Medicine
UCLA School of Medicine
Los Angeles, California;
Attending Physician, Emergency Medicine
Torrance Memorial Medical Center
Torrance, California

Richard Oh, MD
Attending Physician, Emergency Medicine
Kaiser Hospital
Santa Clara, California

Samuel Ong, MD
Visiting Assistant Professor of Medicine/Emergency Medicine
UCLA School of Medicine
Olive View–UCLA Medical Center
Sylmar, California

Neal Peeples, MD
Attending Physician, Department of Emergency Medicine
Washington Hospital Center and Children's National Medical Center
Washington, DC

Jolie Hall Pfahler, MD
Physician, Department of Emergency Medicine
UCLA Medical Center
Los Angeles, California

Charles Pozner, MD
Director, Section on Emergency Medical Services
Department of Emergency Medicine
Beth Israel Deaconess Medical Center;
Instructor of Medicine, Harvard Medical School
Boston, Massachusetts

Virginia M. Ribeiro, MD
Associate in Medicine, Division of Emergency Medicine
Beth Israel Deaconess Medical Center;
Instructor of Medicine, Harvard Medical School
Boston, Massachusetts;
Attending Physician, Department of Emergency Medicine
South Shore Hospital
Weymouth, Massachusetts

Vena Ricketts, MD, FACEP
Associate Professor of Medicine/Emergency Medicine
UCLA School of Medicine
Los Angeles, California;
Department of Emergency Medicine
Olive View–ULCA Medical Center
Sylmar, California

Scott Rodi, MD
Attending Physician, Emergency Medicine
Kaiser Hospital
San Rafael, California

Carolyn Sachs, MD
Assistant Professor of Medicine/Emergency Medicine
UCLA School of Medicine
UCLA Emergency Medicine Center
Los Angeles, California

Eric Salk, MD
Attending Physician, Emergency Department
Charlotte Hungerford Hospital
Torrington, Connecticut

Eric Savitsky, MD
Assistant Professor of Medicine/Emergency Medicine
UCLA School of Medicine
UCLA Emergency Medicine Center
Los Angeles, California

Richard Sonner, MD
Director of Pediatric Emergency Services
Attending Physician in Emergency Medicine
Torrance Memorial Medical Center
Torrance, California;
Visiting Assistant Professor of Medicine/Emergency Medicine
UCLA School of Medicine
Los Angeles, California

Atilla Uner, MD
Emergency Medical Services Fellow
UCLA Emergency Medicine Center
Los Angeles, California

Jorge Vournas, MD
Senior Resident
UCLA Emergency Medicine Center
Los Angeles, California

Michael Weitz, MD, FACEP
Assistant Professor of Medicine/Emergency Medicine
UCLA School of Medicine;
Attending Physician, Department of Emergency Medicine
Olive View–UCLA Medical Center
Sylmar, California;
Associate Director of Emergency Services
Saint John's Health Center
Santa Monica, California

John Wong, MD
Attending Physician, Department of Emergency Medicine
Sacred Heart Medical Center
Eugene, Oregon

To

SIGALIT, ERIC, MICHAEL

RUTH and JOE

Preface

Patients come to the emergency department (ED) with symptoms, not diagnoses. Emergency physicians must worry about patients' symptoms representing a serious disease before making a diagnosis of a common and more benign condition. Migraine is not diagnosed without consideration of subarachnoid hemorrhage, nor is spontaneous abortion diagnosed before evaluation for ectopic pregnancy.

This pocket-text provides a symptom-based approach to emergency department patient care based on current literature. It is designed to be used in the ED and to serve as a study guide of many emergent conditions. It is not a "cookbook" for patient care, nor does it provide a comprehensive differential diagnosis of disease. The text focuses the physician's attention on many conditions that must be considered while caring for ED patients. For each diagnosis, the symptoms, signs, workup, and comments and treatment considerations are addressed.

Although we must consider acute disease processes that a particular complaint might represent, serious diagnoses frequently can be effectively ruled out with reasonable certainty on the basis of historical information and physical examination. Frequently this can be accomplished with minimal ancillary testing. It is important to remember that most tests are far from perfect. Before ordering tests, we must first understand from the literature the test characteristics (sensitivity and specificity) and then consider what the result will mean given the pretest probability of disease. For example, although ESR is a "good test for temporal arteritis (TA)," a 20-year-old patient with a headache and a high ESR is unlikely to have TA. Conversely, a low ESR in an 80-year-old patient with a headache and temporal tenderness would not be adequate evidence for us to abandon our concern for TA.

The authors have used the medical literature to provide a range for the frequency with which symptoms, signs, recognized patterns of disease, and diagnostic tests are present (or positive) in the presence of disease (sensitivity). We have concentrated on sensitivity to limit the number of critical diagnoses missed. The following system has been used:

+	(< 5%)
++	(6% to 30%)
+++	(31% to 69%)
++++	(70% to 94%)
+++++	(95% to 100%)

Specificity (the frequency of negative results in those without disease) is also indicated when possible. If a test is highly sensitive, it is likely to be positive if the disease is present. However, as sensitivity rises, specificity generally falls, which increases the likelihood of false-positive results.

To limit the size of this text, the great majority of references used in its preparation are listed on the supporting World Wide Web site, *www.signsandsymptoms.com.* This site also provides a medical formula calculator and links to other World Wide Web sites and intelligent search agents of medical interest (see Appendix A).

In addition to a critical review of the literature, optimal medical decision-making requires consideration of the value of each possible outcome that may occur, given treatment alternatives. For example, we may recommend hospital admission to patients with a low risk of myocardial infarction based on our decision that information available indicates they are at low risk for MI. In this decision, we generally do not consider the value (utility) patients or society at large place on other disposition alternatives, nor do we consider their risk-taking strategies. Unfortunately, there is no validated framework currently available for routinely measuring patient utilities or other outcome measures and integrating them formally into medical decisions.

Given the uncertainties of the medical literature and in the values of possible outcomes, how are ED patient care decisions made? We elicit a careful history and perform a directed physical examination. We always consider the possible threats to life and limb and are able to rule them out in many patients without a great deal of ancillary testing. In the minority of patients for whom a serious diagnosis remains a possibility, thoughtful use of appropriate tests or observation helps to "rule in" or "rule out" the entities of concern. At such time as we, and our patients, decide that the level of risk for an emergent condition is sufficiently low to warrant making a presumptive diagnosis of a nonemergent problem, we treat and discharge the patient with outpatient follow-up.

Although as emergency physicians we will establish a diagnosis in most patients at risk for significant complications, at times we will miss a critical diagnosis in those with emergent conditions. We can protect our patients (and ourselves) by providing discharge instructions that specifically inform patients of events that should lead to their re-presentation to the emergency department. We should arrange for the patient to be reexamined in an appropriate time frame and prescribe a follow-up physician visit to ensure adequacy of our intervention and for further evaluation as indicated. Patients should be instructed to seek further medical attention if their symptoms worsen or persist for longer than a specified time interval. It is perhaps most important that we be honest with our patients and ourselves. We can limit risk to patients through an informed evaluation, but risk can never be completely eliminated.

Mark A. Davis, MD, MS

Great efforts have been made to check the accuracy of the information contained in the book; however, practitioners should use only those treatments, drugs, and drug dosages with which they have experience and for which they have cross-referenced dosages from other sources.

Acknowledgements

Occasionally in our pursuits we meet someone whose intellect, insight, and strength of character change us and the world in which we live. On behalf of the legions of students, colleagues, patients, and friends who have benefited from his tireless efforts, I want to thank Jerry Hoffman.

This text is the product of tremendous effort on the part of many friends and colleagues who served as authors and editors. I appreciate their dedication to the project. Special thanks to Kathy Falk at Mosby, for her insight and support in keeping this project on track. Thanks to Baxter Larmon for his work on the Code Blue "Unstable"/"Stable" reference card, to Kenneth Lawrence for reviewing the drug treatment recommendations, and to Jonathan Edlow for reviewing the manuscript. And, Mandy Folan's work at Beth Israel Deaconess Medical Center was, as always, outstanding.

Contents

Appendixes

CHAPTER 1

Abdominal Pain

ELIZABETH CHAR and JOHN WONG

Abdominal pain is a common complaint of ED patients. Although in most cases the cause of the pain is benign, great care must be taken not to miss emergent conditions requiring treatment. Elderly patients and those with comorbid conditions are especially at high risk for having a serious abdominal condition. Medical and surgical emergencies arising from pathologic conditions outside of the abdomen must also be considered.

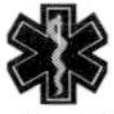

ABDOMINAL AORTIC ANEURYSM

An abdominal aortic aneurysm (AAA) is caused by dilation of the aorta secondary to weakening of all layers of the aortic wall. A leaking AAA generally causes intense pain that can be confused with the pain of a renal stone.

Symptoms

- Severe abdominal pain ++++
- Flank or back pain with radiation to the groin or legs
- Syncope

Signs

- Pulsatile abdominal mass ++++
- Diffuse abdominal tenderness
- Abdominal bruit ++
- Hypotension (late finding) +++
- Hematuria ++
- Flank ecchymosis (late sign)
- Evidence of peripheral embolization +
- Ischemic lower extremities

- High output cardiac failure (rare)
- GI bleed (rare)

Workup

- A CT scan should be obtained for the hemodynamically stable patient because it is highly sensitive and specific and also can demonstrate retroperitoneal hemorrhage, rupture, leakage, and other potential diagnoses.
- An ED ultrasound can be used in the hemodynamically unstable patient as arrangements are being made for transfer to the operating room. Ultrasound confirms an enlarged aortic diameter, but it is unreliable in detecting rupture, leakage, or retroperitoneal hemorrhage.

Comments and Treatment Considerations

Femoral pulses usually are normal even after rupture. If the patient is unstable, immediately consult surgery and do not send the patient for a CT scan. AAAs are often asymptomatic until they rapidly expand, leak, or rupture.

REFERENCES[www]

Ernst C: Abdominal aortic aneurysm, *N Engl J Med* 328:1167, 1993.

Johansen K, Kohler TR, Nicholls SC, et al: Ruptured abdominal aortic aneurysm: the Harborview experience, *J Vasc Surg* 13:240, 1991.

Marston WA, Ahlquist R, Johnson G Jr, Meyer AA: Misdiagnosis of ruptured abdominal aortic aneurysms, *J Vasc Surg* 16:17, 1992.

Siegel C, Cohan R: CT of abdominal aortic aneurysm, *Am J Roentgenol* 163:17, 1994.

[www]Additional references are available on the following web site: www.signsandsymptoms.com.

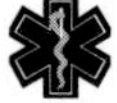

MESENTERIC ISCHEMIA

Ischemic disease of the intestines (small bowel is most common) can be hyperacute, chronic recurrent, or acute on chronic. The classic symptoms and signs attributed to ischemia are actually those of infarction. Diagnosis after infarction is associated with high mortality. Mesenteric ischemia should be considered for patients at risk, such as elderly patients with vascular disease or atrial fibrillation and those who have severe abdominal pain that cannot be adequately explained.

Symptoms

Symptoms vary depending on location.

- Superior mesenteric artery embolism (50%): acute onset of severe, poorly localized, unrelenting abdominal pain followed by nausea, vomiting, and diarrhea. Patients usually have a history of cardiovascular disease (myocardial infarct, dysrhythmia, or valvular disease), a previous embolism ++, or evidence of embolism elsewhere ++.
- Superior mesenteric artery thrombosis (25%): gradual onset of abdominal pain. Patients may have a history of intestinal angina (postprandial abdominal pain relieved by vomiting), weight loss, and diarrhea or a history of vasculitis, prothrombic disorder, or atherosclerosis.
- Nonocclusive mesenteric ischemia (20%): history of low flow state (sepsis, congestive heart failure, hypotension, or previous treatment with vasopressors, digoxin, or beta-blockers). Abdominal pain is typically of gradual onset.
- Mesenteric vein thrombosis (5%): progressive onset of abdominal pain, nausea, and vomiting and history of venous thrombosis +++.

Signs

- Pain is classically out of proportion to physical findings.
- Abdominal examination varies depending on the stage of ischemia. Often, physical findings arise late in the disease and range from mild localized or generalized tenderness to peritoneal signs. Occult blood may precede other signs, but its absence does not rule out the diagnosis.
- Usually afebrile with stable vital signs until becoming hypovolemic or septic

Workup

- Angiography is the test of choice for exploring arterial causes.
- Laboratory abnormalities, such as acidosis and leukocytosis, occur relatively late in the ischemic process.

- CT with triple contrast may show dilated fluid-filled loops of thick-walled bowel, luminal dilatation, pneumatosis intestinalis (intramural gas), or mesenteric or portal venous gas as the disease progresses. CT is the test of choice for demonstrating mesenteric venous thrombosis.
- Plain abdominal radiographs are rarely helpful but may show thumbprinting (smooth indentations on the colon), dilated, thickened bowel loops, gasless abdomen or ileus, or gas in the bowel wall or portal vein (late signs).

Comments and Treatment Considerations

Early diagnosis is critical and is based primarily on the history and physical examination. Early angiographic or surgical intervention is necessary to prevent death.

REFERENCES[www]

Bradbury A, McBride B, Ruckley C: Mesenteric ischemia: a multidisciplinary approach, *Br J Surg* 82:1446, 1995.

Kurland B, Brandt LJ, Delany HM: Diagnostic tests for intestinal ischemia, *Surg Clin North Am* 72:85, 1992.

Lange H, Jackel R: Usefulness of plasma lactate concentration in the diagnosis of acute abdominal disease, *Eur J Surg* 160:381, 1994.

Schneider TA, Longo WE, Ure T, Vernava AM III: Mesenteric ischemia: acute arterial syndromes, *Dis Colon Rectum* 37:1163, 1994.

Stoney R, Cunningham C: Acute mesenteric ischemia, *Surgery* 114:489, 993.

[www]Additional references are available on the following web site: www.signsandsymptoms.com.

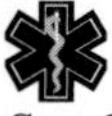

ACUTE MYOCARDIAL INFARCTION

See Chapter 7, Chest Pain.

Comments and Treatment Considerations

Elderly patients may have atypical symptoms of acute myocardial infarction (MI) (i.e., absence of chest pain or tightness). Many of these patients complain of dyspnea +++, but a significant number have gastrointestinal complaints alone, usually consisting of abdominal pain or discomfort ++ or nausea and vomiting. Patients also may have silent or asymptomatic MIs. The percentage of patients with atypical presentations of acute MI increases with age.

REFERENCES[www]

Arnow WS: Prevalence of presenting symptoms of recognized acute myocardial infarction and unrecognized healed myocardial infarction in elderly patients, *Am J Cardiol* 60:1182, 1987.

Lusiani L, Perrone A, Pesavento R, et al: Prevalence, clinical features, and acute course of atypical myocardial infarction, *Angiology* 45:49, 1994.

Wroblewski M, Mikulowski P, Steen B: Symptoms of myocardial infarction in old age: clinical case, retrospective and prospective studies, *Age Aging* 15:99, 1986.

[www]Additional references are available on the following web site: www.signsandsymptoms.com.

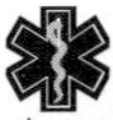

PERFORATED ULCER

A perforated ulcer is commonly caused by nonsteroidal anti-inflammatory drug use or by *H. pylori* disease (up to one third may have no such history). Perforation with spillage of gastric or duodenal contents into the abdomen can lead to severe peritonitis.

Symptoms

- Severe abdominal pain of sudden onset ++++; may cause back pain in posterior penetrating ulcer
- Nausea
- Vomiting
- Older patients may have only minimal pain +++.

Signs

- Diffuse abdominal pain with diminished bowel sounds
- Acute peritonitis
- Rigid abdomen +++
- Hypovolemia

- Hypotension
- Tachycardia
- Fever

Workup

- Abdominal series to look for free air ++++. Plain films can detect 1 to 2 ml of free air, but the patient must be in a left lateral decubitus position for 10 to 20 minutes and then upright for 10 minutes. This is impractical for most patients with a perforated viscus, so the sensitivity may be limited. Many studies report that 5 to 30 ml of free air is required before routine plain films can identify perforation.
- CT scans identify free air in the abdomen and can rule out other diagnoses that may mimic the presentation of a perforated viscus.
- WBC is insensitive +++, as are amylase and alkaline phosphatase.

Comments and Treatment Considerations

The duration of perforation is an independent risk factor for death, so patients who have an acute abdominal condition should have hollow viscus injury expeditiously diagnosed. Most of these injuries are related to peptic ulcer disease, but perforation can occur in the small or large intestine, usually as a result of malignancy, trauma, or diverticular disease. Intestinal perforations may present more insidiously than perforations of the stomach or duodenum.

REFERENCES[www]

Gunshefski L, Flancbaum L, Brolin RE, et al: Changing patterns in perforated peptic ulcer disease, *Am J Surg* 56:270, 1990.

Miller TA: Emergencies in acid-peptic disease, *Gastroenterol Clin North Am* 17:303, 1988.

Stapakis JC, Thickman D: Diagnosis of pneumoperitoneum: abdominal CT versus upright chest film, *J Comput Assist Tomogr* 16:713, 1992.

[www]Additional references are available on the following web site: www.signsandsymptoms.com.

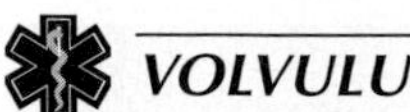

VOLVULUS

See also Malrotation and Volvulus in Chapter 18, The Irritable Child and Vomiting.

Symptoms

Adults (sigmoid colon, 60%; cecal, 40%; small bowel, very rare):

- Severe, colicky abdominal pain
- Abdominal distention
- Recurrent episodes +++
- Constipation
- Nausea
- Vomiting

Signs

Adults:

- Diffuse abdominal tenderness
- Markedly tympanitic and distended abdomen
- Peritoneal signs, fever, and shock if ischemic

Workup

Adults:

- Abdominal plain films identify the dilated loop of bowel in 80% of the sigmoid volvulus and 50% of cecal (Fig. 1-1).
- Barium enema (BE)
- Sigmoidoscopy

Comments and Treatment Considerations

If the neonate is ill-appearing with bilious vomiting, obtain an immediate surgical consultation and provide intravenous hydration. Surgical consultation is also required for adults with volvulus.

REFERENCES

Frizelle F, Wolff B: Colonic volvulus, *Adv Surg* 29:131, 1996.

Kealey WD, McCallion WA, Brown S, et al: Midgut volvulus in children, *Br J Surg* 83:105, 1996.

Mason J: The evaluation of acute abdominal pain in children, *Emerg Med Clin North Am* 14:629, 1996.

Pelucio M, Haywood Y: Midgut volvulus: an unusual case of adolescent abdominal pain, *Am J Emerg Med* 12:167, 1994.

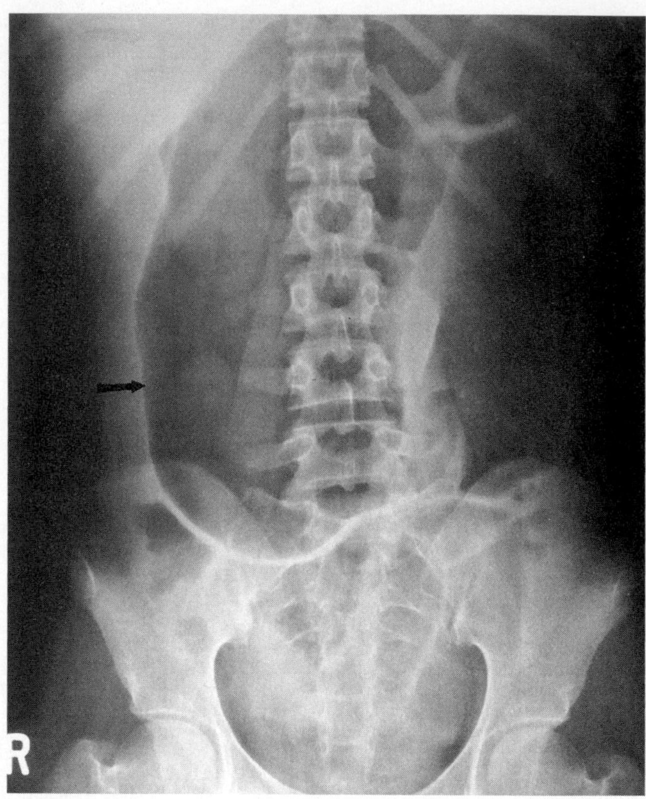

Fig. 1-1 Sigmoid volvulus. Anteroposterior supine view of abdomen reveals markedly distended sigmoid colon *(arrow)*.

INTUSSUSCEPTION

Intussusception—a "telescoping" of intestine usually occurring at the junction of the terminal ileum and ileocecal valve—occurs most commonly in children under 2 years. Approximately 5% of cases occur in adults. Less than 50% of patients have the classic clinical triad of abdominal pain, currant jelly stools, and a palpable abdominal mass. Lethargy may be a predominant finding in some patients.

Symptoms

- Episodic colicky abdominal pain ++++ in an otherwise healthy child (90% to 95% of cases) or in an adult (5% to 10% of cases)
- Nausea and vomiting ++++
- Bloody stool +++
- Diarrhea ++
- Poor oral feeding by a child and episodes of crying and drawing up the legs

Signs

- Palpable abdominal mass +++ classically described as sausage shaped
- Abdominal tenderness +++
- Dehydration and lethargy between episodes of pain may be the only signs of intussusception in young children.
- Occult blood in stool +++
- Currant jelly (bloody, mucoid) stool ++

Workup

- Abdominal series, which may be normal ++ or may show evidence of a bowel obstruction +++, mass effect +++, or the classic target sign (bull's eye) (Fig. 1-2).
- Barium enema has long been the gold standard for diagnosing and sometimes treating and reducing ++++ intussusception. Use of air or gas enemas (GE) has increased (may improve reduction rate). Neither BE nor GE should be done in adults, since both the high likelihood of a pathologic condition (lead points and malignancy) and the higher risk of perforation with an enema under pressure are indications for operation.
- Routine laboratory tests are not helpful in the diagnosis of intussusception.
- Ultrasound also has been useful in the diagnosis of intussusception (sensitivity up to +++++, specificity 88%).
- CT may demonstrate an intraluminal mass or may be helpful in ruling out other causes of acute abdominal conditions,

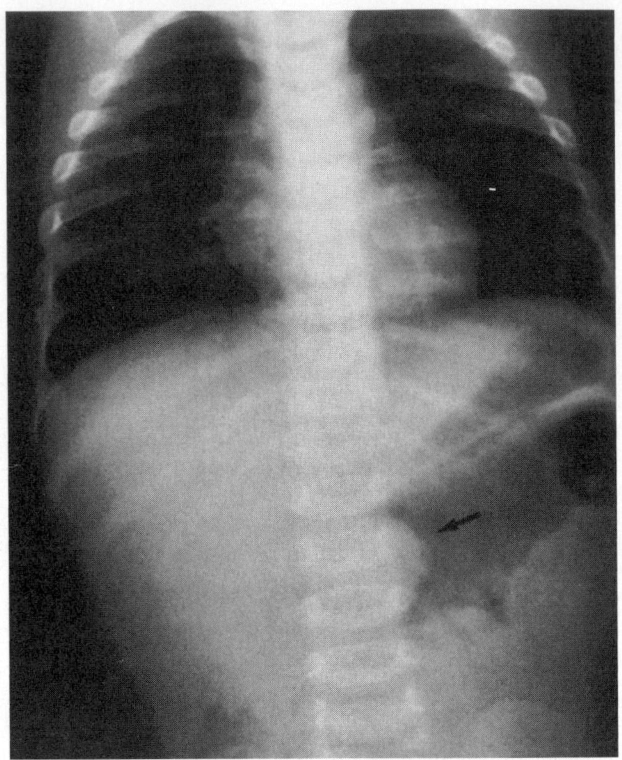

Fig. 1-2. Intussusception. Anteroposterior supine view of abdomen demonstrates soft tissue density *(arrow)* in distended small bowel. (From Rosen P: *Diagnostic radiology in emergency medicine,* St Louis, 1992, Mosby.)

especially in adults, in whom 70% to 90% of intussusceptions are caused by a tumor.

Comments and Treatment Considerations

Consider intussusception whenever evaluating a young child with a possible abdominal process or an altered mental status. The recurrence rate is 6% to 12%.

REFERENCES[www]

Daneman A, Alton DJ: Intussusception: issues and controversies related to diagnosis and reduction, *Radiol Clin North Am* 34:743, 1996.

Luks FI, Yazbeck S, Perrault G, et al: Changes in the presentation of intussusception, *Am J Emerg Med* 10:574, 1992.

Prater JM, Olshenki FC: Adult intussusception, *Am Fam Physician* 47:447, 1993.

[www]Additional references are available on the following web site: www.signsandsymptoms.com.

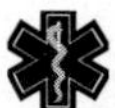

OVARIAN TORSION

Ovarian torsion is a twisting of an ovary that compromises ovarian blood supply, leading to ovarian infarction if not rapidly diagnosed and treated.

Symptoms

- Abrupt onset of severe unilateral or nonlocalized lower abdominal or pelvic pain
- Nausea
- Vomiting
- Recurrent episodes
- Mild fever
- Urinary symptoms

Signs

- Unilateral lower abdominal or pelvic tenderness, tender adnexal mass +++
- Progression to peritoneal signs

Workup

- Pregnancy test
- Transvaginal ultrasound without delay is the imaging study of choice. Addition of color Doppler may increase specificity.
- Laparoscopy can be used for diagnosis and treatment.

Comments and Treatment Considerations

In infants and small children, the reproductive organs are higher in the abdomen.

REFERENCES

Gordon JD, Hopkins KL, Jeffrey RB, Giudice LC: Adnexal torsion: color Doppler diagnosis and laparoscopic treatment, *Fertil Steril* 61:383, 1994.

Meyer JS, Harmon CM, Harty MP, et al: Ovarian torsion: clinical and imaging presentation in children, *J Pediatr Surg* 30:1433, 1995.

Shust N, Hendricksen D: Ovarian torsion: an unusual cause of abdominal pain in a young girl, *Am J Emerg Med* 13:307, 1995.

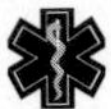

TESTICULAR TORSION

See Chapter 26, Scrotal Pain.

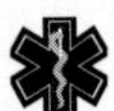

ECTOPIC PREGNANCY

See Chapter 34, Vaginal Bleeding. Always consider ectopic pregnancy in women of childbearing age who have lower abdominal pain.

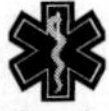

BOWEL OBSTRUCTION

In developed countries, approximately 50% of all small bowel obstructions are caused by adhesions, 15% by incarcerated or strangulated hernias, and 15% by neoplasms.

Symptoms

- Abdominal pain +++++
- Nausea ++++
- Vomiting ++++
- No flatus or stool passage
- Bloating ++++
- Inguinal pain or a bulge or mass in the scrotum if an incarcerated hernia is the cause of the obstruction

Signs

- Abdominal distention ++++

- Abdominal tenderness ++++
- Fever ++
- Tender palpable mass if hernia is present
- Peritonitis if hernia is strangulated

Workup

- Abdominal series ++++, but may be negative early
- WBC not particularly helpful +++
- CPK, LDH, alkaline phosphatase, and amylase have not shown any consistent correlation to the diagnosis of small bowel obstruction.

Comments and Treatment Considerations

Treatment of small bowel obstruction comprises insertion of a nasogastric tube, intravenous fluids with the patient NPO, surgical consultation, and hospital admission.

REFERENCES[www]

Holder WD Jr: Intestinal obstruction, *Gastroenterol Clin North Am* 17:317, 1988.

Sarr MG, Bulkley GB, Zuideman GD: Preoperative recognition of intestinal strangulation obstruction, *Am J Surg* 145:176, 1983.

Simpson A, Sandeman D, Nixon SJ, et al: The value of an erect abdominal radiograph in the diagnosis of intestinal obstruction, *Clin Radiol* 36:41, 1985.

[www]Additional references are available on the following web site: www.signsandsymptoms.com.

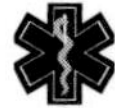

CHOLECYSTITIS, CHOLANGITIS, AND COMMON BILE DUCT OBSTRUCTION

Gallbladder disease generally presents as biliary colic, a "benign" condition in which gallstones cause colicky right upper quadrant pain that is easily treated with mild analgesics. Cholelithiasis is most common in obese women in their fourth decade.

However, it is important not to miss patients who have cholecystitis (inflammation of the gallbladder), common bile duct obstruction, or cholangitis (inflammation of the biliary duct system), for which hospital admission and specific treatments are required. Approximately 10% of cholecystitis occurs in the absence of documented gallstones.

Symptoms

- Acute onset of colicky severe right upper quadrant or epigastric pain
- Nausea and vomiting +++
- Fever is variably present with cholecystitis and cholangitis.

Signs

- Right upper quadrant tenderness ++++
- Localized peritonitis
- Murphy's sign (arrest of respiration with palpation of the right upper quadrant)
- Low grade fever and tachycardia are variably present in cholecystitis.

Workup

- Ultrasound is sensitive in identifying stones and can confirm clinical suspicion of cholecystitis ++++. It may indicate cholelithiasis, dilated gallbladder, thickened wall, pericholecystic fluid, or sonographic Murphy's sign. It has limited sensitivity for acute ductal dilatation +++ associated with obstruction.
- Radionuclide cholescintigraphy has similar sensitivity to ultrasound for cholecystitis ++++ but is more specific (93% vs 64%). It is more sensitive for detecting obstruction.
- Hepatic aminotransferases, alkaline phosphatase, bilirubin, and amylase may be elevated.

Comments and Treatment Considerations

Radionuclide cholescintigraphy is the most sensitive and specific test to rule out cholecystitis and common bile duct obstruction. Ultrasound is quicker and noninvasive, is generally more readily available, can be done at the bedside, and offers more anatomic detail of the hepatic ducts and pancreas. Radionuclide cholescintigraphy should be performed when clinical evaluation suggests cholecystitis or obstruction and ultrasound studies are negative.

REFERENCES[www]

Babb R: Acute acalculous cholecystitis, *J Clin Gastroenterol* 15:238, 1992.

Davis L, McCarroll K: Correlative imaging of the liver and hepatobiliary system, *Semin Nucl Med* 3:208, 1994.

Samuels BI, Freitas JE, Bree RL, et al: A comparison of radionuclide hepatobiliary imaging and real-time ultrasound for the detection of acute cholecystitis, *Radiology* 147:207, 1983.

[www]Additional references are available on the following web site: www.signsandsymptoms.com.

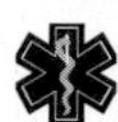

ACUTE APPENDICITIS

The most important factors in diagnosing appendicitis are the history and physical examination. Because patients come to the ED at various times within the course of the disease and may have atypical symptoms, a period of observation and reexamination may be necessary.

Symptoms

- Abdominal pain that begins periumbilically or diffusely and localizes to the right lower quadrant over the next 12 to 48 hours ++++
- Anorexia ++++
- Nausea and vomiting +++
- Diarrhea ++

Signs

- Abdominal tenderness ++++
- Fever +++
- Rebound tenderness +++
- Rovsing sign (peritoneal irritation producing right lower quadrant pain with palpation of the left lower quadrant)
- Psoas sign (pain with active flexion against resistance or passive extension of the right hip) ++
- Obturator sign (pain with passive internal rotation of the flexed right hip) ++
- Voluntary or involuntary guarding
- Cervical motion tenderness ++

Workup

- Appendicitis is a clinical diagnosis.
- The value of a white blood cell (WBC) count is limited ++++; specificity, 40% to 75%.
- C-reactive protein, ESR, WBC differential, abdominal x-rays have unproven value.
- CT scan with rectal contrast ++++; specificity, 90% to 97%
- Abdominal ultrasound; accuracy varies widely according to experience.
- CT and ultrasound may be helpful in diagnosing other causes of abdominal pain when the diagnosis of acute appendicitis is in doubt.

Comments and Treatment Considerations

Elderly patients and children are more likely to have atypical presentations and are more likely to have appendiceal perforation at the time of presentation to the ED.

REFERENCES[www]

Izbicki JR, Knoefel WT, Wilker DK, et al: Accurate diagnosis of acute appendicitis: a retrospective analysis of 686 patients, *Eur J Surg* 158:227, 1992.

Lyons D, Waldron R, Ryan T, et al: An evaluation of the clinical value of the leukocyte count and sequential counts in suspected appendicitis, *Br J Clin Prac*tice 41:794, 1987.

Reynolds SL: Missed appendicitis in a pediatric emergency department, *Pediatr Emerg Care* 9:1, 1993.

[www]Additional references are available on the following web site: www.signsandsymptoms.com.

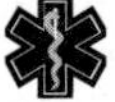

COLONIC DIVERTICULITIS

Diverticulitis is generally a disease of older adults and typically presents with left lower quadrant pain and tenderness, similar to the right-sided pain and tenderness of appendicitis.

Symptoms

- Abdominal pain, usually in the left lower quadrant ++++
- Nausea and vomiting

- Constipation
- Diarrhea

Signs

- Left lower quadrant tenderness, guarding, rebound
- Fever
- General peritonitis with tachycardia, high fever, and sepsis if colonic perforation occurs

Workup

- Diverticulitis is primarily a clinical diagnosis.
- A CT scan with intravenous and oral contrast (with rectal contrast if needed) demonstrates pericolic inflammation, abscess (both at the site of perforation and at distant sites in the abdomen), and involvement of other organs.
- WBC is of limited value +++.
- Abdominal x-rays may be useful for ruling out free air or bowel obstruction but otherwise provide little diagnostic information.

Comments and Treatment Considerations

By the age of 85, a majority of the population will have diverticular disease. Between 10% and 35% of these individuals will have an episode of acute diverticulitis.

REFERENCES[www]

Hulnick DH, Megibow AJ, Balthazar EJ, et al: Computed tomography in the evaluation of diverticulitis, *Radiology* 152:491, 1984.

Morris J, Steallato TA, Haaga JR, et al: The utility of computed tomography in colonic diverticulitis, *Ann Surg* 204:128, 1986.

Pohlman T: Diverticulitis, *Gastroenterol Clin North Am* 17:357, 1988.

[www]Additional references are available on the following web site: www.signsandsymptoms.com.

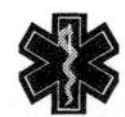

ACUTE PANCREATITIS

Pancreatitis can be acute or chronic. Diagnosis is generally clinical and can be confirmed by ancillary testing.

Symptoms

- Epigastric or left upper quadrant pain ++++
- Back pain ++

Signs

- Abdominal tenderness ++++
- Vomiting ++++
- Abdominal distention
- Guarding
- Dehydration (as a result of third spacing and possible hemorrhage)

Workup

- Amylase ++++; specificity, 70% to 95%
- Lipase ++++; specificity, 87% to 99%
- CT scan (contrast enhanced) ++++; specificity, near 100%; CT is generally not required in the ED.
- Ultrasound is useful for viewing the biliary tract but is unable to visualize the pancreas due to overlying bowel gas in 25% to 40%.
- Plain x-ray films (abdominal series) may be useful to check for free air (perforated viscus) if the diagnosis is in doubt.

Comments and Treatment Considerations

Severe pancreatitis is life threatening (5%) and can lead to many complications, including hemorrhage, hypocalcemia, coagulation abnormalities, hypoxia, ARDS, cardiovascular decompensation, and renal failure. The most common causes of acute pancreatitis are biliary obstruction and toxins (alcohol and medications), which account for 70% of all cases. About 10% to 20% of cases are idiopathic. Generally, patients with acute pancreatitis must be admitted for observation and analgesia. Typically patients do not require NGT or antibiotics.

REFERENCES[www]

Calleja GA, Barkin JS: Acute pancreatitis, *Med Clin North Am* 77:1037, 1993.

Clavien PA, Robert J, Meyer P, et al: Acute pancreatitis and normoamylasemia: not an uncommon combination, *Ann Surg* 210:614, 1989.

Gumaste V, Dave P, Sereny G: Serum lipase: a better test to diagnose acute alcoholic pancreatitis, *Am J Med* 92:239, 1992.

---

wwwAdditional references are available on the following web site: www.signsandsymptoms.com.

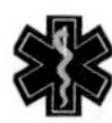

PELVIC INFLAMMATORY DISEASE AND TUBOOVARIAN ABSCESS

Pelvic inflammatory disease (PID) and tuboovarian abscess (TOA) are associated with a history of new or multiple sexual partners, frequent intercourse, recent insertion of an intrauterine device, lower socioeconomic status, younger age, history of smoking, and previous PID or sexually transmitted diseases.

Symptoms

- Lower abdominal or pelvic pain that is dull, constant, and poorly localized +++++
- Vaginal discharge ++++
- Abnormal vaginal bleeding ++
- Urinary symptoms ++
- Dyspareunia

Signs

- Lower abdominal tenderness ++++
- Adnexal mass or tenderness ++++
- Cervical motion tenderness
- Mucopurulent endocervical discharge
- Endocervix that is erythematous, edematous, or friable in association with temperature of >38° C +++

Workup

- Pregnancy test
- Cervical cultures for gonorrhea
- Cervical swab or urine sample for *Chlamydia* testing
- Wet mount for clue cells (bacterial vaginosis) and *Trichomonas*

- Pelvic ultrasound to rule out tuboovarian abscess in select cases
- Consider syphilis and HIV testing

Comments and Treatment Considerations

Ectopic pregnancy and PID have considerable overlap of symptoms. Appendicitis or other gastrointestinal pathologic conditions should also be considered.

Because of the potential complications of untreated PID, the empiric use of antibiotics is common after a presumptive diagnosis is made on clinical examination. Several treatment options can be followed for early PID, including ceftriaxone 250 mg IM (gonorrhea) and doxycycline 100 mg po bid × 14 days (chlamydia). Do not use doxycycline in pregnant women. Consider admission for IV antibiotics, especially in advanced cases. For treatment of bacterial vaginosis, administer metronidazole 500 mg bid × 7 days (avoid in pregnancy). For trichomoniasis, use metronidazole 2 g as a single dose (avoid in pregnancy).

REFERENCES

Gilbert DN, Moellering RC, Sande MA: Guide to antimicrobial therapy, Antimicrobial Therapy, Inc. 1998.

Newkirk G: Pelvic inflammatory disease: a contemporary approach, *Am Fam Physician* 53:112, 1996.

Soper D: Pelvic inflammatory disease, *Infect Dis Clin North Am* 8:821, 1994.

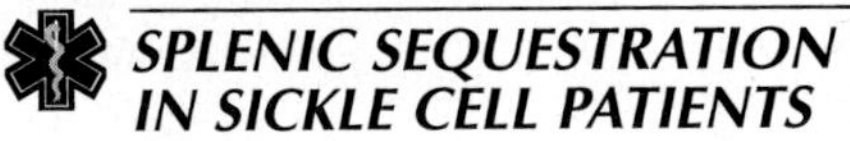

SPLENIC SEQUESTRATION IN SICKLE CELL PATIENTS

Symptoms

- Abdominal pain
- Acute weakness
- Syncope
- Thirst

Signs

- Abdominal fullness or tenderness

- Large spleen
- Pallor
- Tachycardia

Workup

- Hemoglobin: rapid fall of >2 g/dl despite an elevated reticulocyte count
- Platelets: mild to moderate thrombocytopenia

Comments and Treatment Considerations

Sequestration crisis most commonly occurs in patients between 6 months to 3 years of age for those with hemoglobin SS, and older children or adults with hemoglobin SC and S/B-thalassemia disease. Hospital admission is required.

REFERENCES

Baumgartner F, Klein S: The presentation and management of the acute abdomen in the patients with sickle-cell anemia, *Am Surg* 55:660, 1989.

Galloway S, Harwood-Nuss A: Sickle cell anemia: a review, *J Emerg Med* 6:213, 1988.

Pollack C: Emergencies in sickle cell disease, *Emerg Med Clin North Am* 11:365, 1993.

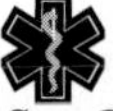

DIABETIC KETOACIDOSIS

See Chapter 22, Mental Status Change and Coma.
Abdominal pain can be a symptom of an underlying cause of diabetic ketoacidosis or a symptom of the disease itself. Abdominal processes should be evaluated thoroughly.

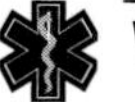

VIRAL HEPATITIS

See Chapter 19, Jaundice.

BLACK WIDOW (LATRODECTUS) SPIDER BITE

Muscle pain and fasciculations caused by binding of the toxin (venom) to membrane receptors can result in excessive stimulation of the motor end plates. Muscle spasms may involve the abdomen and can lead to the erroneous diagnosis of an acute surgical condition.

Symptoms

- Severe muscle pain and muscle spasms of the involved area, which may progress to the abdomen, back, and other areas
- Pain usually begins within 30 minutes to 2 hours at the site of the bite and is followed by painful muscle cramping in 3 to 4 hours.

Signs

- Muscle fasciculations

Workup

- A history of likely exposure (working in a cool, dark place or on a construction site or in a wood pile)
- The physical examination may uncover the spider bite.
- No specific laboratory tests are useful.

Comments and Treatment Considerations

Treatment consists of benzodiazepines and analgesia. Administration of 10% calcium gluconate (adults, 10 to 20 ml; children, 0.2 to 0.3 ml/kg) may provide transient relief and can be repeated as necessary.

REFERENCES

Olson KR et al, editors: *Poisoning and drug overdose,* Norwalk, Conn, 1994, Appleton & Lange.

Pearigen PD: Unusual causes of abdominal pain, *Emerg Clin North Am* 14:593, 1996.

CHAPTER 2

Agitation and Psychosis

ERIC LEGOME

Agitated or violent behavior can be caused by a medical disorder ("organic"), a psychiatric disorder ("functional"), or both. Although the distinction between organic and functional is somewhat artificial, it provides a useful model for evaluating an agitated patient. The differential diagnosis of each includes emergent conditions that may require different treatment strategies. Many medical illnesses have the capability to alter CNS functioning and produce delusions, dementia, delirium, and other disordered thinking. Psychosis is a disorder characterized by a gross distortion or disorganization of a person's mental capacity, affective response, and capacity to recognize reality, communicate, and relate to others in a way that meets the demands of everyday life. Many new "psychiatric" patients initially have an unrecognized medical illness that caused or exacerbated their psychiatric symptoms. Furthermore, patients with psychiatric diseases manifesting as psychosis have a higher incidence of medical illness and die of medical diseases at a rate higher than that of the general population.

The goal in the ED is to conduct a brief but thorough examination to exclude the most common and dangerous physical disorders mimicking psychiatric illness and to control dangerous behaviors.

While by no means definite, certain physical and historical factors may favor an organic rather than a functional etiology. Aspects that suggest an organic etiology include autonomic disturbances, including severe hypertension or hypotension, hyperthermia, tachypnea, and tachycardia. Other findings may include abnormal vital signs, diaphoresis, pupillary abnormalities, gait disturbances or focal neurologic deficits, weight loss, systemic signs and symptoms, and incontinence. A patient with a fluctuating level of consciousness or a disturbance of attention, orientation, and recent memory is also more likely to have an organic etiology. Nonauditory hallucinations and delusions (e.g., visual, olfactory, tactile) are specific but insensitive for organic disease. Auditory hallucinations that are ego-syntonic (patient is concerned about the content of the voices, but not that they are occurring) are classically described for schizophrenia and other psychiatric disorders.

A careful history for previous diseases including HIV, SLE or other inflammatory conditions, endocrinologic disorders, and cancer is essential to the evaluation. A history of drug dependence, intravenous drug abuse, or detoxification is inversely correlated with a functional cause of agitation or psychosis. However, drug abuse is common among those with functional psychosis, and it is often not possible to establish a firm diagnosis for chronic abusers. A full accounting of any medications must be sought.

Other crucial information to obtain during the evaluation is the patient's age, family history, and premorbid function. Patients who are younger than 40 years of age, have no previous psychiatric history, a productive premorbid function, and an acute onset of symptoms most likely have an organic cause of their illness. Conversely, a slowly progressive decline in a younger patient or a patient with a family history of schizophrenia is more likely to have a functional cause.

Treatment for agitated psychosis usually includes a neuroleptic, benzodiazepine, or both. The treatment goal is to provide for the patient's and the staff's safety while alleviating the patient's distress and agitation to allow for an appropriate evaluation. Droperidol (adults: 2.5 to 5.0 mg IV/IM, may repeat) and lorazepam (adults: 1 to 2 mg IV/IM, may repeat; watch for respiratory depression) are among the many medical treatment alternatives. When using neuroleptics without benzodiazepines, consider concomitant use of benztropine or diphenhydramine to reduce the risk of acute dystonia and akathisia. Haloperidol is an acceptable alternative to droperidol.

LEGAL ISSUES

Although laws differ between states, some general principles govern treatment of psychotic patients and their ability to participate in or refuse medical care. In general, for medical therapy to be delivered against their will, psychotic patients must have a profound lack of insight and understanding of their illness, be considered a danger to themselves or others, or be gravely disabled.

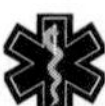

SELECTED ORGANIC CAUSES

This chapter addresses common psychiatric causes of psychoses. Medical conditions are addressed in other chapters. The box on pp. 25 and 26 lists selected organic causes to consider when evaluating psychotic patients.

REFERENCES

Anderson WH, Kuehnle JC: Diagnoses and early management of acute psychosis, *N Engl J Med* 305:1128, 1981.

Dubin WR, Weese KJ, Zeezardia JA: Organic brain syndrome, the quiet impostor, *JAMA* 249:60, 1983.

Frame DS, Kercher E: Acute psychosis: functional versus organic, *Emerg Med Clin North Am* 9:123, 1992.

Hall RCW, Gardner ER, Popkin MK, et al: Unrecognized physical illness prompting psychiatric admission: a prospective study, *Am J Psychiatry* 138:629, 1981.

Lipowski ZL: Delirium (acute confusional state), *JAMA* 258:1789, 1997.

Pine DS, Douglas CJ, Charles E, et al: Patients with multiple sclerosis presenting to psychiatric hospitals, *J Clin Psychiatry* 56:297, 1995.

Resnick, Burton BT: Droperidol vs. haloperidol in the initial management of acutely agitated patients, *J Clin Psychiatry* 45:298, 1984.

Richards RR, Derlet RW, Duncan DR: Chemical restraint for the agitated patient in the emergency department: lorazepam versus droperidol, *J Emerg Med* 16:567, 1998.

Rosenthal RN, Miner CR: Differential diagnosis of substance-induced psychosis and schizophrenia in patients with substance abuse disorders, *Schizophr Bull* 23:187, 1997.

SELECTED ORGANIC CAUSES OF PSYCHOSES

Drug Intoxications
Opiates
Designer drugs
Alcohol
Cocaine
LSD
PCP

Drug Withdrawal
Alcohol
Benzodiazepines
Tricyclic antidepressants

Medications (Increased in Elderly)
Serotonin reuptake inhibitors (serotonin syndrome)
Neuroleptics (neuroleptic malignant syndrome)
Isoniazid
Anticholinergics
Antibiotics
Sympathomimetics
Cimetidine
Steroids
Insulin and hypoglycemics
Antiarrhymics
Antiparkinsonians

Infections
Sepsis
Meningitis
Encephalitis
HIV
Neurosyphilis

Seizures
Temporal lobe
Postictal states

SELECTED ORGANIC CAUSES OF PSYCHOSES—cont'd

Neoplasm
Hemispheric
Temporal lobe
Posterior fossa

Cerebrovascular Disease
Stroke
Intracranial hemorrhage
Multiple sclerosis
CNS vasculitis
SLE
TTP

CNS (Other)
Dementia
Pick's disease
Jakob-Creutzfeldt disease
Parkinson's disease
Wilson's disease
Pseudobulbar palsy

Endocrine
Hyperthyroidism, hypothyroidism
Carcinoid
Pheochromocytoma
Cushing's disease
Addison's disease
Hyperparathyroidism

Other
Nutritional disorders
Acute intermittent porphyria

Entries in *italics* are the most common causes.

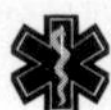

PSYCHIATRIC CAUSES

As listed below, psychiatric diagnoses in general are defined by criteria published in DSM-IV, the manual of psychiatric disorders. These diagnoses are based on consensus among leaders in the field. Limited information is available in the medical and psychiatric literature suggesting the prevalence of particular signs and symptoms of the diagnoses.

SCHIZOPHRENIA

Schizophrenia is a common and heterogeneous disorder that currently has no known cure. There is often a combination of positive symptoms, which are the production of abnormal actions and thoughts, and negative symptoms, which are the absence of usual occurring interests, thoughts, gestures, and actions. According to the DSM-IV, six major criteria must be present to establish the diagnosis, including the provision that symptoms must be present for at least 6 months. The prevalence of schizophrenia in the general population has been fairly constant at ~0.5 %.

Schizophrenia has five subtypes—paranoid, disorganized, catatonic, undifferentiated, and residual—that are defined by the prominent symptomatology and signs at the time of evaluation. Prodromal symptoms of depression, perplexity, and fear are often present before onset. As the diagnosis is partially dependent on a time course of symptoms, it is not unusual (>70%) to fail to achieve a definitive diagnosis on initial presentation.

To establish the diagnosis, the patient must fit six DSM-IV diagnostic criteria. (DSM criteria are noted below in italics, *A-F*.)

Symptoms

Characteristic, or type *A*, symptoms define the illness. Two or more of the following need be present for 1 month (or less if treated):

- Delusions
- Hallucinations
- Disorganized speech
- Grossly disorganized or catatonic behavior
- Negative symptoms: (e.g., anhedonia, avolition)

One or more major areas of functioning including work, relationships, or self-care are significantly diminished *(B),* with continuity for at least 6 months of this worsening *(C).*

Other mood or schizoaffective disorders are not concurrently diagnosed *(D),* and a substance abuse or medical condition is not the direct cause *(E).*

If the patient has an underlying developmental disorder, there must be a development of prominent hallucinations or delusions *(F).*

Signs

- Positive signs: disorganized speech, disorganized or catatonic behavior, excessive motor activity that is apparently purposeless, echolalia or echopraxia
- Negative signs: flat affect, motor immobility, mutism, and maintenance of a rigid posture

Workup

- History is the most important clue toward establishing the diagnosis.
- Detailed neurologic examination
- Serum glucose, if indicated
- Oxygen saturation, if indicated
- Evaluation for possible medical etiologies as indicated
- CT, if evidence of focal neurologic process, advanced age, or other suggestion of organic cause
- Lumbar puncture, if fever or evidence of meningeal irritation
- ESR, if concern of collagen vascular or rheumatologic disorder
- EEG, if consideration of underlying ongoing seizure or prolonged postictal state
- MRI, if consideration of demyelinating disease

Comments and Treatment Considerations

Acute psychosis secondary to schizophrenia requires ED psychiatric consultation and generally hospital admission.

REFERENCES

American Psychiatric Association: *Diagnostic and statistical manual of mental disorders,* ed 4 (DSM-IV), Washington, DC, 1994, The Association.

Battaglia J, Moss S, Rush J, et al: Haloperidol, lorazepam, or both for psychotic agitation? A multicenter, prospective, double-blind, emergency department study, *Am J Emerg Med* 15:335, 1997.

Ellison JM, Jacobs D: Emergency psychopharmacology: a review and update, *Ann Emerg Med* 15:962, 1986.

SCHIZOPHRENIFORM DISORDER

Schizophreniform disorder is diagnosed using similar criteria for schizophrenia, where the episode lasts between 1 and 6 months.

SCHIZOAFFECTIVE DISORDER

Schizoaffective disorder is defined by DSM-IV as an uninterrupted period of illness during which a major depressive episode, a manic episode, or mixed manic-depressive episode co-exists with type A symptoms of schizophrenia.

BRIEF PSYCHOTIC DISORDER

A brief psychotic disorder is a time-limited disorder that may occur in response to a significant life stressor (e.g., death in family), may be seen postpartum, or may occur without a stressor. The duration is at least 1 day with a maximum duration of 1 month. The patient eventually returns to his or her previous level of functioning.

SHARED PSYCHOTIC DISORDER

Shared psychotic disorder is a delusional development that exists in a patient with a close relationship to another individual with similar symptoms. Symptoms and signs are similar to those of schizophrenia.

PSYCHOTIC DISORDER—NOT OTHERWISE SPECIFIED

Due to the nature of emergency medicine, the time course of the patient's illness often cannot be followed. This category takes into account the lack of available information to make a specific diagnosis. The diagnosis applies to psychotic patients whose problems cannot be clearly defined as organic or functional. A definitive diagnosis of psychiatric disease is not made until medical conditions have been fully considered.

MAJOR DEPRESSION WITH PSYCHOTIC SYMPTOMS

The patient must meet criteria for a major depressive episode and have the following diagnostic symptoms:

- *Mood-congruent psychotic features*—delusions or hallucinations that are consistent with the depressive's ideation (e.g., death, deserved punishment, nihilism)
- *Mood-incongruent psychotic features*—delusions or hallucinations whose themes may not involve typical depressive ideation, including such themes as persecution and thought broadcasting

ANXIETY DISORDER

Patients with anxiety disorder manifest excessive anxiety and worry about a number of events and activities for at least 6 months. They find it difficult to control, and the anxiety is associated with at least three symptoms (see symptoms below). The diagnosis may be modified if combined with specific concerns (e.g., social phobias, separation anxiety, somatization disorder).

Acutely, patients may have panic attacks notable for somatic complaints and signs of adrenergic hyperactivity.

Symptoms

- Restlessness
- Fatigability
- Difficulty with concentration
- Irritability
- Muscle tension
- Sleep disturbance
- Somatic medical complaints

Signs

- Tachycardia
- Hypertension
- Diaphoresis (It is imperative to rule out concomitant medical illness that can also cause autonomic changes.)

Comments and Treatment Considerations

Patients with an anxiety disorder or panic attack may have acute chest pain or other somatic complaints that are difficult to distinguish from organic disease in the ED. In general, an organic cause is presumed with appropriate evaluation for possible psychiatric etiology. Treatment of anxiety may be indicated whether the symptom is caused by a medical or psychiatric condition.

REFERENCES

American Psychiatric Association: *Diagnostic and statistical manual of mental disorders,* ed 4 (DSM-IV), Washington, DC, 1994, The Association.

CHAPTER 3

The Alcoholic Patient

DAN GROSSMAN

Alcohol-intoxicated patients frequently receive treatment in the ED. Although they generally need only a period of observation until reaching clinical sobriety, they are at risk for occult trauma, infection, co-ingestion, or other pathologic conditions that may be mistakenly attributed to alcohol. Unfortunately, the history and physical examination often yield limited information in alcoholic patients, so a high index of suspicion with appropriate diagnostic testing is necessary. Determination of alcohol level is generally unnecessary unless co-ingestion is a possibility or if needed to verify significant ethanol ingestion. Administration of thiamine (100 mg IV) and a blood sugar check (or administration) should be considered for all patients with alteration in mental status (see Chapter 22, Mental Status Change and Coma).

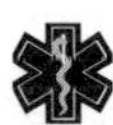 *INTRACRANIAL HEMORRHAGE*

Head trauma and coagulopathy are common among alcoholic patients. Between 8% and 18% of alcohol-intoxicated ED patients with minor head injury have positive CT scans, and up to 5% need a craniotomy. Alcohol plays a role in many head injuries and often contributes to unfavorable outcomes. Some patients who appear to have alcohol withdrawal seizures actually have structural lesions demonstrated on CT scans.

Management generally consists of serial neurologic examinations with a determination that the mental status of the patient is improving. A neurologic examination must be normal before patients can be discharged. CT scanning of the head is indicated in the following situations: the patient has a focal neurologic examination or evidence of head trauma, alcohol does not explain initial findings, or the patient's mental status does not improve during ED observation.

See Chapter 15, Headache.

REFERENCES[www]

Brickley MR, Shepherd, JP: The relationship between alcohol intoxication, injury severity, and Glasgow coma score in assault patients, *Injury* 26:311, 1995.

Cook LS, Levitt MA, Simon B, Williams VL: Identification of ethanol-intoxicated patients with minor head trauma requiring computed tomography scans, *Acad Emerg Med* 1:227, 1994.

Feussner JR, Linfors EW, Blessing CL, Starmer CF: Computed tomography brain scanning in alcohol withdrawal seizures: value of neurologic examination, *Ann Intern Med* 94:519, 1981.

[www]Additional references are available on the following web site: www.signsandsymptoms.com.

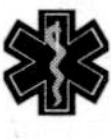

CO-INTOXICATION WITH ETHYLENE GLYCOL, METHANOL, AND ISOPROPYL ALCOHOL

Diagnosing a co-ingestion of nonethanol alcohols without a reliable history can be difficult. The patient may appear intoxicated but not have an odor of ethanol on the breath. Classically, patients ingesting methanol or ethylene glycol appear ill, have an anion gap, metabolic acidosis, and an osmolal gap. Isopropyl alcohol can cause hypoglycemia and ketosis without acidosis.

See Chapter 32, Toxic Ingestion, Approach to.

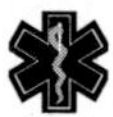

INFECTION

Alcoholics can have fevers for reasons unrelated to an acute infection (e.g., from delirium tremens, seizures, or intracranial bleeds). However, when fever is present, a source of infection must be sought, and admitting the patient should be strongly considered whether or not one is found. In one study, 58% of alcoholics had an infectious cause of fever. Alcoholics are prone to pneumonia, tuberculosis, spontaneous bacterial peritonitis (if cirrhosis and ascites), spontaneous bacteremia, endocarditis, and salmonellosis.

REFERENCES[www]

Adams HG, Jordan C: Infections in the alcoholic, *Med Clin North Am* 68:179, 1984.

Wrenn KD, Larson S: The febrile alcoholic in the emergency department, *Am J Emerg Med* 9:57, 1991.

[www]Additional references are available on the following web site: www.signsandsymptoms.com.

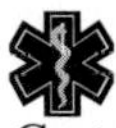

GASTROINTESTINAL BLEEDING

Gastrointestinal bleeding (GIB) can be occult or acutely life threatening. Coagulopathy is common among chronic alcoholics as a result of thrombocytopenia and decreased production of clotting factors by the liver. Furthermore, if the liver is cirrhotic, then esophageal and gastric varices are often present and are prone to rupture.

See Chapter 6, Bleeding.

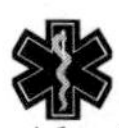

ALCOHOLIC KETOACIDOSIS

Alcoholic ketoacidosis (AKA) principally occurs after the cessation of a drinking binge by a malnourished chronic alcoholic. Increased hepatic ketone formation, active lipolysis, and inadequate peripheral ketone utilization all contribute to the accumulation of ketoacids and the resulting elevated anion gap acidosis that physiologically defines AKA. The diagnosis of AKA is established by the findings of an elevated anion gap acidosis with concurrent ketosis in the absence of a history of diabetes mellitus or a markedly elevated glucose. Co-morbidities such as alcoholic pancreatitis, liver disease, or gastritis that share symptoms and signs with AKA also should be considered.

Symptoms

- Anorexia
- Nausea
- Vomiting
- Abdominal pain
- Orthostatic dizziness

Signs

- Odor of ketones on the breath
- Tachycardia
- Orthostatic hypotension
- Tachypnea, particularly with Kussmaul respirations
- Diaphoresis
- The abdomen usually reveals only mild to moderate diffuse tenderness. Marked distention, the absence of bowel sounds, or the presence of peritoneal signs should raise the concern for other concomitant intraabdominal pathologic conditions.
- Abnormalities in orientation or level of consciousness ++ (may also indicate other pathologic conditions)

Workup

- Glucose (may be normal, low, or mildly elevated +)
- Electrolytes, magnesium, BUN, creatinine
- Serum ketones
- ABG: generally not necessary. Mixed acid-base disorders are very common, as are electrolyte disorders including hypokalemia, hypomagnesemia, hyponatremia, and hypocalcemia.

Comments and Treatment Considerations

Volume repletion with glucose administration (after thiamine 100 mg IV) and electrolyte repletion (K, Mg) are generally curative. Bicarbonate administration is unnecessary. Co-morbidities must be treated. If diagnosed and treated appropriately, AKA has low mortality.

REFERENCES[www]

Braden GL, Strayhorn CH, Germain MJ, et al: Increased osmolal gap in alcoholic acidosis, *Arch Intern Med* 153:2377, 1993.

Miller PD, Heinig RE, Waterhouse C: Treatment of alcoholic acidosis: the role of dextrose and phosphorus, *Arch Intern Med* 138:67, 1978.

Palmer JP: Alcoholic ketoacidosis: clinical and laboratory presentation, pathophysiology, and treatment, *J Clin Endocrinol Metab* 12:381, 1983.

Wrenn KD, Slovis CM, Minion GE, Rutowski R: The syndrome of alcoholic ketoacidosis, *Am J Med* 91:119, 1991.

[www]Additional references are available on the following web site: www.signsandsymptoms.com.

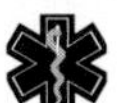

HYPOTHERMIA

Hypothermia, defined as a core temperature of less than 35° C, may occur in healthy patients after acute cold exposure or in patients with medical or social conditions that limit adaptive mechanisms or temperature perception. Alcohol blunts temperature sensation in intoxicated patients and increases heat loss through vasodilation, thereby increasing the risk of severe hypothermia. Resuscitative measures, including establishment of airway control, in addition to rapid rewarming, are necessary for severe hypothermia. Arrhythmia treatment may be ineffective until core temperature is >32° C. Attempts to resuscitate patients in cardiac arrest should be continued until their core temperature is at least 35° C. Evaluation and treatment for possible infection or other conditions leading to hypothermia are required.

Symptoms

Vary with degree of hypothermia and underlying medical condition

- Nausea
- Dizziness
- Chills
- Pruritus
- Dyspnea
- Confusion

Signs

Vary with degree of hypothermia and underlying medical condition

- Patient cool to touch
- Dysrhythmia
- Shivering
- Paradoxic undressing in early stages
- Hypotension
- Altered mental status
- Respiratory depression
- Decreased bowel sounds
- Apathy
- Abdominal rigidity
- Decreased level of consciousness
- Dysarthria
- Muscular rigidity
- Frostbite

Workup

- Core temperature evaluation with a rectal probe, since many oral and rectal thermometers do not read below 35° C.
- Rapid blood glucose determination
- Thorough physical examination to exclude a primary medical or surgical condition
- Chest x-rays, urinalysis, blood and urine cultures (41% of hypothermic patients in one study were infected)
- Serum electrolytes
- Hematocrit
- CT scanning: consider in particular head CT if altered mental status
- DIC panel
- Serum CPK to rule out rhabdomyolysis
- Blood alcohol level and directed toxicologic screen
- ECG may show Osborne (J) waves
- Thyroid function tests (for later confirmation of myxedema)

Comments and Treatment Considerations

Passive rewarming with blankets in a warm room is indicated for patients with mild hypothermia. After securing the airway and initiating ACLS procedures, the treatment for severe hypothermia (cardiovascular instability, T <32.2° C, failure to rewarm using other methods, endocrinologic dysfunction, peripheral dilation caused by trauma or toxic materials, impaired thermoregulation) is active rewarming. Controversy surrounds the effectiveness of active external rewarming methods (e.g., heat lamps, warm baths, or warmed blankets). Severe hypothermia should be treated with active core rewarming methods that may include warmed humidified inhalation gases; warmed intravenous fluids; peritoneal, NGT, or Foley warm fluid lavage; or cardiopulmonary bypass. Patients should receive intravenous fluids and cardiac resuscitation (including CPR, drug, and electrical therapy) as needed. Resuscitation is rarely successful until a temperature of 28° to 30° C is achieved.

REFERENCES[www]

Danzl DF, Pozos RS, Auerbach PS, et al: Multicenter hypothermia study, *Ann Emerg Med* 16:1042, 1987.

Lewin S, Brettman LR, Holzman RS, et al: Infections in hypothermic patients, *Arch Intern Med* 141:920, 1981.

Reuler JAB: Hypothermia: pathophysiology, clinical setting, and management, *Ann Intern Med* 89: 519, 1978.

Weyman AE, Greenbaum DM, Grace WJ: Accidental hypothermia in an alcoholic population, *Am J Med* 56:13, 1974.

White JD: Hypothermia: the Bellevue experience, *Ann Emerg Med* 11:417, 1982.

[www]Additional references are available on the following web site: www.signsandsymptoms.com.

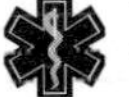

DELIRIUM TREMENS

See Chapter 22, Mental Status Change and Coma.

CHAPTER 4

Back Pain, Lower

MICHAEL WEITZ

Lower back pain is the most common complaint in the ambulatory setting, second only to the common cold in resultant missed workdays. The emergency physician must distinguish emergent conditions presenting as back pain (see the box on p. 41) from self-limited, musculoskeletal problems.

The majority of patients with lower back pain have an identifiable cause and do not have "red flags" that lead to an evaluation beyond the usual history and physical examination. Ancillary testing is of limited value in these cases. In one large study, 1/2500 x-ray studies demonstrated a clinically unsuspected finding. A lumbar spine series delivers a gonadal dose equivalent to a daily chest x-ray for 6 years. Obliques and coned laterals add little information and add radiation exposure.

Although the lifetime incidence of sciatica is 40%, only a minority of patients with acute back pain have signs and symptoms clearly caused by nerve root compression. Back pain is typically self-limited, with significant resolution, regardless of therapy, in 50% of patients by week 1, 80% by week 2, and 90% by 2 months. Sciatica resolves by 6 weeks in more than 50% of patients. The natural history of disk herniation with radiculopathy is that 90% to 95% improve without surgery. A stable neurologic deficit, due to nerve root compression from a herniated disc, is generally *not* an indication for early surgery. An evolving motor neurologic deficit or bowel or bladder dysfunction requires urgent surgical evaluation and treatment.

Back or flank pain also may be the chief complaint of patients with pyelonephritis.

"RED FLAGS" FOR POTENTIALLY SERIOUS DISEASE

Tumor or Infection

Age over 50 or under 20

History of cancer

Constitutional symptoms such as fever, chills, or weight loss; risk factors for spinal infection (recent urinary tract infection or pyelonephritis, intravenous drug abuse, immune suppression); pain that worsens when supine or severe nighttime pain

Cauda Equina Syndrome

Recent onset of bladder dysfunction (e.g., urinary retention, increased frequency, or overflow incontinence). Similar bowel dysfunction may occur but usually is seen later, if at all.

Saddle anesthesia

Severe or progressive neurologic deficit in lower extremity not clearly due to pain only.

Fracture

Major trauma; minor trauma in older or osteoporotic patients

Abdominal Aortic Aneurysm

Abdominal pain

Pulsatile abdominal mass

Atherosclerotic disease

REFERENCES

Agency for Health Care Policy and Research: Practice guideline: *Acute low back problems in adults—assessment and treatment,* pub no 95-0643, Dec 1994.

Hadler NM: Regional back pain, *N Engl J Med* 315:1090, 1986.

Kelsey JL, White AA: Epidemiology and impact of low back pain, *Spine* 5:133,1980.

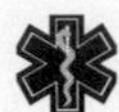

ABDOMINAL AORTIC ANEURYSM

See Chapter 1, Abdominal Pain.

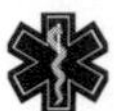

CAUDA EQUINA SYNDROME

Cauda equina syndrome is caused by compression of the cauda equina, the thecal sac that contains the group of nerve roots remaining after termination of the spinal cord at approximately the L1-L2 level. Symptoms of cauda equina syndrome are dominated by bladder (and possibly bowel) complaints, as well as motor and sensory deficits. In a patient with back or leg pain or caudal anesthesia with incontinence or urinary retention, the possibility of cauda equina syndrome must be evaluated immediately because it represents a surgical emergency regardless of etiology. Cauda equina compression is most typically the result of massive central disc herniation, but also can be caused by an epidural abscess, hemorrhage, or tumor.

Symptoms

- Low back pain ++++
- Urinary retention or incontinence ++++
- Sciatica may be bilateral
- Lower extremity weakness
- Fecal retention or incontinence
- Saddle anesthesia

Signs

- Urinary retention ++++
- Decreased rectal tone or perianal sensation (anal wink)
- Motor deficit
- Sensory deficit

Workup

- Urinary catheter to check for residual urine after patient attempts to completely empty bladder
- Emergent MRI to rule out the diagnosis
- CT myelogram may be substituted if MRI not available

Comments and Treatment Considerations

Emergent assessment and treatment are necessary, as outcome is time dependent; neurosurgical or orthopedic consultation must be arranged immediately.

REFERENCES

DePalma AF, Rothman RH: *The intervertebral disc,* Philadelphia, 1970, WB Saunders.

Kostiuk JP: *J Bone Joint Surg* 68A:381, 1986.

Scott PJ: Bladder paralysis in cauda equina lesions from disc prolapse, *J Bone Joint Surg* 47B:224, 1965.

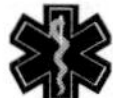

TUMOR

A spinal tumor or spinal cord compression should be considered as possible causes of lower back pain in older patients and in those who have a history of cancer.

Symptoms

- Back pain without a significant identifiable precipitant
- Constitutional symptoms
- Sensory or motor deficits that involve the spinal cord or cauda equina

Signs

- Spinous process tenderness
- Sensory or motor deficit if the spinal cord or cauda equina is involved

Workup

- Lumbosacral spine films have limited sensitivity.
- ESR sensitivity ++++, but poor specificity
- Bone scan sensitivity ++++, but nonspecific
- MRI +++++
- CT scan if MRI not available
- CBC is neither sensitive nor specific.

Comments and Treatment Considerations

If tumor is diagnosed, prompt x-ray therapy is generally required. Emergent neurosurgical or orthopedic consultation is appropriate.

REFERENCES

Deyo RA, Diehl AK: Cancer as a cause of back pain, *J Gen Intern Med* 3:230, 1988.

Fernbach JC, Langer F, Gross AE: The significance of low back pain in older adults, *Can Med Assoc J* 115:898, 1976.

Liang M: Roentgenograms in primary care patients with acute low back pain: a cost-effective analysis, *Arch Intern Med* 142:1108, 1982.

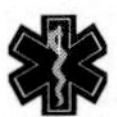

SPINAL INFECTIONS

Infections involving the spine include osteomyelitis, epidural abscess, and discitis. The first two conditions can coexist, since vertebral osteomyelitis is a major risk factor for the development of an epidural abscess. These conditions are more common in diabetics, alcoholics, intravenous drug addicts, immunosuppressed patients, patients with prior spinal column abnormality or trauma or invasive procedure, and patients with prior urinary tract and pelvic infections. About 20% of patients with an epidural abscess may have no systemic or local predisposing factor. Osteomyelitis often is not diagnosed until 8 to 10 weeks after initial presentation, which consequently leads to significant morbidity. Discitis or disc space infection is typically diagnosed 6 months after the onset of symptoms but may be more acute following disc excision.

Symptoms

- Unrelenting back pain +++++
- Fever +++ (50% of patients with vertebral osteomyelitis are *afebrile* at presentation)
- Patients with epidural abscess also may have radicular pain, leg weakness, sensory deficit, neck pain or stiffness, bladder dysfunction.

Signs

- Midline bony and percussion tenderness +++
- Discitis manifests as well-localized midline pain featuring limited motion and exquisite discomfort produced by any jarring movement. Most patients have referred pain of femoral or sciatic distribution.

Workup

- MRI is the gold standard +++++ and also differentiates acute transverse myelopathy from spinal cord ischemia.
- ESR is sensitive in advanced disease, but is nonspecific.
- Bone scan ++++, but low specificity
- CT scan +++, but misses 50% of epidural abscesses
- CT myelogram can be performed if MRI is not available, contraindicated, or nondiagnostic.
- Lumbosacral spine films are neither sensitive nor specific for infection. Discitis may be demonstrated radiographically by disc space narrowing, sclerosis of subchondral bone, and irregularity of the bony endplates.
- Blood cultures may help to direct antibiotic therapy ++.
- CBC has little value +++.

Comments and Treatment Considerations

An epidural abscess is an orthopedic and neurosurgical emergency requiring rapid evaluation and treatment. Treatment for epidural abscess consists of decompressive laminectomy with abscess drainage and prolonged course of antibiotics. Osteomyelitis is generally treated with an extended administration of intravenous antibiotics. *Staphylococcus aureus* is the most common causative organism in both osteomyelitis and epidural abscess, although other organisms such as *Escherichia coli, Pseudomonas aeruginosa,* or tuberculosis may be causative. An antibiotic course is begun in the ED after cultures are obtained and may include a penicillinase-resistant penicillin in combination with either a third-generation cephalosporin or an aminoglycoside.

Treatment of discitis ranges from conservative therapy with antibiotics and spinal immobilization to surgical debridement and decompression of the disc space.

REFERENCES

DeSouza LJ: Disc space infection in children, late adolescents, and adults, *Minn Med,* May 1980.

Hlavin ML, Kaminski HJ, Ross JS, Ganz E: Spinal epidural abscess: a ten-year perspective, *Neurosurgery* 27:177, 1990.

Kemp HBS, Jackson JW, Jeremiah JD, Hall AJ: Pyogenic infections occurring primarily in intervertebral discs, *Joint Bone Joint Surg* 55B:698, 1973.

Ross PM, Fleming JL: Vertebral body osteomyelitis: spectrum and natural history, *Clin Orthop* 118:190, 1976.

Smith AS, Blaser SI: Infectious and inflammatory processes of the spine, *Radiol Clin North Am* 29:809, 1991.

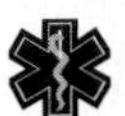

PYELONEPHRITIS

Urinary tract infection (UTI), including both cystitis and pyelonephritis, may present with back pain. Cystitis typically causes a low lumbar or sacral aching pain, whereas the pain of pyelonephritis typically localizes to the costovertebral angle on the side of the infected kidney. Patients with cystitis usually have dysuria and the other classic symptoms of UTI.

Pyelonephritis can present without urinary symptoms, and back pain is occasionally the chief complaint. Although many risk factors for pyelonephritis are the same as those for cystitis (urinary retention, instrumentation or indwelling catheter, pregnancy, immunosuppression), additional risk factors for pyelonephritis include anatomic abnormalities of the kidney (bifid ureter, ureteral valves, renal scarring from prior infections, and renal calculi). Pyelonephritis is more common in women than men, although men are more likely to have predisposing anatomic abnormalities. Chronic prostatitis also predisposes men to UTI.

Symptoms

- Fever and chills, occasionally rigors
- Nausea or vomiting
- Flank pain
- Dysuria, frequency, and urgency may be present whenever cystitis coexists with pyelonephritis.

Signs

- Unilateral costovertebral angle tenderness usually present
- Fever
- Malaise
- Unlike musculoskeletal back pain, the back pain of pyelonephritis does not radiate, nor is it exacerbated by movement
- Flank tenderness to percussion should be elicited.

Workup

- In men, examination of the genitalia and prostate is warranted if UTI is a diagnostic concern.
- Urinalysis: pyuria, bacteruria, and occasionally hematuria
- CBC: leukocytosis with a neutrophil predominance
- Blood urea nitrogen (BUN) and creatinine are useful if renal insufficiency is suspected.
- Urine cultures are indicated when urinalysis is abnormal and the clinical scenario suggests pyelonephritis.
- Blood cultures are rarely useful.

Comments and Treatment Considerations

Gram-negative organisms, particularly *E. coli* (90%), are the predominant causative organisms. Many patients, especially otherwise healthy young women, can be treated with oral antibiotics on an outpatient basis. A fluoroquinolone (ciprofloxacin 500 mg po bid, norfloxacin 400 po bid, and others) is appropriate except in pregnancy and children, in which case a cephalosporin is often used. Trimethoprim-sulfamethoxazole is no longer first-line therapy in many parts of the United States because resistance continues to emerge. Patients who appear toxic, are immunocompromised, are elderly or otherwise debilitated, are unable to take oral fluids or medications, or have failed oral antibiotics require hospitalization. Men with pyelonephritis should be strongly considered for hospitalization for parenteral antibiotic therapy. Pyelonephritis requires 14 days of antibiotic therapy.

REFERENCES

Childs S: Current diagnosis and treatment of urinary tract infections, *Urology* 40:295, 1992.

Faro S: New considerations in treatment of urinary infections in adults, *Urology* 390:1, 1992.
Stramm W, Hooton TM: Management of urinary tract infection in adults, *N Engl J Med* 329:1328, 1993.
Wilrhe MT, et al: Diagnosis and management of urinary tract infection in adults, *Br Med J* 305:1137, 1992.

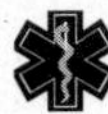

VERTEBRAL COMPRESSION FRACTURES

See Chapter 5, Back Pain, Upper.

CHAPTER 5

Back Pain, Upper

GERIANNE DUDLEY

In comparison to lower back pain, upper or thoracic back pain is an uncommon presenting complaint. In the absence of trauma, musculoligamentous strain or degenerative vertebral disease is usually responsible for producing this symptom. However, upper back pain is the chief complaint in several clinically important conditions, and failure to consider these disease entities can lead to missing a critical diagnosis. Because the heart, lungs, esophagus, great vessels, and abdominal organs are innervated by visceral afferents, the location and radiation of pain overlap considerably. Therefore pathologic conditions of the chest and abdomen must be considered in the evaluation of patients with upper back pain.

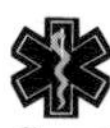 *AORTIC DISSECTION*

See Chapter 7, Chest Pain.

Aortic dissection is characterized by entrance of blood into the aortic media and is associated with a mortality rate of 1% per hour in the first 48 hours if untreated. Back pain occurs in some patients (++) with proximal dissections and in many (+++) with distal dissections.

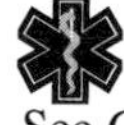 *ACUTE MYOCARDIAL INFARCTION*

See Chapter 7, Chest Pain.

Although acute myocardial infarction typically presents with chest pain, radiation to other anatomic sites is common. Some patients (++) who have angina report pain radiating to the interscapular region. A few patients (+) have thoracic back pain only. In patients with signs and symptoms highly suggestive of an acute myocardial infarction in combination with significant interscapular back pain, consideration should be given to an acute aortic dissection with coronary artery involvement, especially when thrombolytic therapy is being considered.

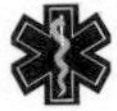

PULMONARY EMBOLISM, PNEUMOTHORAX, AND PNEUMONIA

See Chapter 7, Chest Pain.

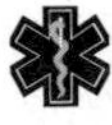

PERFORATED ULCER, ABDOMINAL AORTIC ANEURYSM, GALLBLADDER DISEASE, AND PANCREATITIS

See Chapter 1, Abdominal Pain.

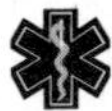

SPINAL OSTEOMYELITIS, EPIDURAL ABSCESS, AND TUMOR

See Chapter 4, Back Pain, Lower.

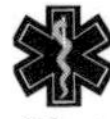

VERTEBRAL COMPRESSION FRACTURE

Vertebral compression fracture, defined as a 15% to 20% reduction of anterior, posterior, or central vertebral body height, occurs in 25% of women over age 50, often after trivial injury (bending, lifting, cough, or sneeze). Risk factors include prolonged postmenopausal state, glucocorticoid use, smoking, alcohol abuse, and medical diseases known to affect calcium or bone metabolism (e.g., renal failure). In patients less than age 60 prevalence is higher in men and is generally the result of trauma.

Symptoms

- Acute, severe pain at the fracture site is typical; however, minor fractures in elderly or postmenopausal patients may be asymptomatic.
- Pain may radiate anteriorly to the flank or abdomen and increase with movement or Valsalva.
- Radicular pain or symptoms of spinal cord compression (bilateral leg pain, paresthesias, incontinence) are very rare.
- Nausea and vomiting may be encountered due to an ileus.

Signs

- Spinal tenderness over fracture site
- Paravertebral muscle spasm
- Ileus (abdominal distention and decreased bowel sounds)
- Kyphosis and loss of height
- Weakness, sensory deficits, incontinence, or diminished deep tendon reflexes (spinal cord compression) +

Workup

- Anteroposterior and lateral spine films. If available, previous x-rays are helpful to determine age of fracture.
- MRI, if evidence of neurologic deficits

Comments and Treatment Considerations

Treatment is based on the stability of the fracture. More than 90% of compression fractures are stable. If compression is greater than 25% to 50%, angulation is greater than 20 degrees, or if there is a fracture at more than one level, the fracture may be considered unstable. Patients with stable fractures and with no evidence of ileus or spinal cord compression can be discharged home with narcotic medication, bed rest, and early medical follow-up; otherwise, they should be admitted and receive medical and orthopedic or neurosurgical consultation.

REFERENCES[www]

Lukert BP: Vertebral compression fractures: how to manage pain, avoid disability, *Geriatrics* 49:22, 1994.

Ryan PJ, Fogelman I: Osteoporotic vertebral fractures: diagnosis with radiography and bone scintigraphy, *Radiology* 190:669, 1994.

Santavirta S, Konttinen YT, Heliovaara M, et al: Determinants of osteoporotic thoracic vertebral fracture: screening of 57,000 Finnish women and men, *Acta Orthop Scand* 63:198, 1992.

[www]Additional references are available on the following web site: www.signsandsymptoms.com.

CHAPTER 6

Bleeding

LYNNE MCCULLOUGH and CAROLYN SACHS

Bleeding is a common presentation in the emergency department. In most cases, the cause of the bleeding is readily identifiable (e.g., as a result of trauma or originating from the gastrointestinal tract). Evaluation and treatment is directed at the specific cause.

Rarely, bleeding is caused or exacerbated by an underlying blood element defect including platelet abnormalities (either in number or function), problems with coagulation factors, and vascular disorders. Systemic bleeding disorders should be suspected when patients have unusually severe bleeding, spontaneous hemorrhage without trauma, or bleeding from multiple sites.

In general, patients with abnormalities of platelet number (thrombocytopenia) or function (thrombocytopathia) and those with vascular disorders (e.g., capillary fragility) have gingival bleeding, petechiae or easy bruising, gastrointestinal bleeding, excessive menses, hematuria, or prolonged bleeding after dental work. Once controlled, bleeding does not ordinarily recur. Coagulation factor deficiencies typically lead to delayed or recurrent bleeding, since, although initial hemostasis is normal, an inadequate fibrin clot forms. This process leads to the formation of deep muscular hematomas, hemarthroses, and rarely, retroperitoneal bleeding.

See Chapter 33, Trauma, Approach to.

REFERENCES

Bick RL: Coagulation abnormalities in malignancy: a review, *Semin Thromb Hemost* 18:353, 1992.

Walker IR: The bleeding disorders: current concepts and management, *Can Fam Physician* 34:2539, 1988.

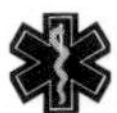

GASTROINTESTINAL BLEEDING

The goal when evaluating gastrointestinal bleeding in the ED is to resuscitate and stabilize patients with an acute GI bleed. In addition, attempts are made to determine the nature and extent of the bleed, whether it is acute or chronic, and to identify the 10% to 20% of patients who may rebleed. Upper gastrointestinal bleeding (UGIB) is bleeding occurring proximal to the ligament of Treitz; lower gastrointestinal bleeding (LGIB), the less frequent of the two, is distal and usually is due to colonic bleeding.

The five most common causes of nonvariceal UGIB are duodenal and gastric ulcers (50%), gastric erosions (30%), Mallory-Weiss syndrome (10%), and esophagitis. Duodenal ulcers are more common than gastric ulcers. Gastric ulcers are more often associated with the use of nonsteroidal antiinflammatory drugs and aspirin. Esophageal varices account for a significant minority of UGIB admissions. Many patients with known esophageal varices have GI bleeding originating from other locations.

Perirectal disease, diverticulosis, and angiodysplasia account for the majority of significant LGIB. In patients with a history of AAA grafts or occlusive aortoiliac disease, aortoenteric fistulas, a condition with high mortality, should be considered. A decreased hematocrit can lead to cardiac ischemia, particularly in elderly patients with coronary artery disease.

Symptoms

- Red or coffee-ground hematemesis with or without melena indicates UGIB.
- Bright red rectal bleeding usually occurs with LGIB but can be seen with a vigorous UGIB.
- Hematochezia can be associated with either UGIB or LGIB.

- Patients with UGIB may have no symptoms other than hematemesis or melena +++.
- The volume of hematemesis is a poor guide for estimating volume loss.
- For Mallory-Weiss tears, patients have a history of hematemesis and alcohol consumption ++++; repetitive vomiting +++; and aspirin use, coughing, heavy lifting, and pregnancy +.
- Patients with simultaneous UGIB and acute myocardial infarction may report only dizziness, syncope, or acute confusion +++ and not chest pain.

Signs

- Hematemesis
- Gross or occult blood in stool
- Hypotension occurs late (typically with about 1500 ml blood loss).
- Tachycardia may appear earlier in hypovolemia.
- Cool, clammy extremities and altered mental status occur late (after significant volume loss).
- Hepatomegaly, ascites, palmar erythema, and spider nevi are suggestive of variceal disease.

Workup

- Two large-bore intravenous lines, type and crossmatch blood
- Nasogastric aspirate is sensitive ++++ but has low specificity, since many foods and medications can give false-positive results on hemoccult testing. Duodenal bleeds and an acidic stomach can cause false-negative results.
- CBC: immediate hematocrit values may not reflect blood loss. Serial values after rehydration are required.
- Endoscopy: use for diagnosis and treatment of UGIB with active bleeding is controversial, but is a standard practice in many institutions. In some patients with a low clinical risk of rebleed, endoscopy may allow for discharge and outpatient follow-up.
- Sigmoidoscopy can be used in patients with stable LGIB.
- Arteriography or radionuclide scanning may be considered if

endoscopy or sigmoidoscopy fails to locate the source despite ongoing bleeding.
- Abdominal films have very low sensitivity and are of little value, except when perforation is suspected (see Chapter 1, Abdominal Pain).
- An elevated BUN:creatinine ratio (>25:1) is often thought to suggest a UGI source; in rapid bleeds, the BUN can be very high (40 mg/dl).
- ECG in patients with likely coronary artery disease

Comments and Treatment Considerations

Nasogastric tubes are generally indicated for diagnosis of possible UGIB but not for treatment. Iced lavage is not beneficial and can cause hypothermia and arrhythmias, as well as prolong bleeding time; it should not be done. Most clinicians do room temperature lavage to remove clots and determine cessation of bleeding, although even this has not been shown to improve the outcome. Endoscopy and medical therapies are frequently used for unstable patients, although the evidence of their efficacy in these circumstances is limited.

Endoscopy may allow for cautery or injection sclerosis in ongoing bleeds. Octreotide, a longer-acting somatostatin analog, appears to control active peptic ulcer bleeding in some patients. The majority of Mallory-Weiss tears stop bleeding spontaneously.

Variceal bleeding should be ruled out in patients with known or suspected liver disease. Sclerotherapy has an immediate effect in many patients; octreotide may be as effective. Pharmacologic control of variceal bleeding can also be achieved in many patients with the use of vasopressin, terlipressin (a vasopressin derivative), and somatostatin. Infusion of somatostatin before endoscopy for variceal bleeding reduces bleeding and facilitates sclerotherapy.

For UGIB, H2-receptor antagonists can be used for gastric erosions but are not beneficial for bleeding peptic ulcers or for preventing rebleeding. Omeprazole, a proton pump inhibitor, appears more effective than H2 blockers in preventing rebleeding. Antacid therapy has no role in treating acute bleeds. Sengstaken-Blakemore tube tamponade controls 85% of acute variceal bleeds but is rarely used.

High-risk patients who may be considered for admission to the ICU include those with any of the following: ongoing bleeding, hypotension, prolonged prothrombin time, altered mental status, >8% drop in hematocrit, age >75, or unstable comorbid disease. Independent predictors of an adverse outcome include an initial hematocrit <30%, initial systolic blood pressure <100 mm Hg, red blood in nasogastric lavage, history of cirrhosis or ascites on examination, or history of vomiting red blood. Surgical consultation should be obtained because surgery may be necessary if medical management is ineffective.

Less acutely ill patients at risk for rebleed may be admitted to a non-ICU setting. Some low-risk patients with GIB can be safely evaluated as outpatients. However, patients with significant UGIB should not be discharged from the ED without first having an endoscopic evaluation. All discharged patients should be referred for timely follow-up. In particular, most patients with a presumptive diagnosis of bleeding due to hemorrhoids or anal fissure require outpatient sigmoidoscopy to rule out other pathologic conditions.

REFERENCES[www]

Avgerinos A, Nevens F, Raptis S, et al: Early administration of somatostatin and efficacy of sclerotherapy in acute oesophageal variceal bleeds: the European Acute Bleeding Oesophageal Variceal Episodes (ABOVE) randomized trial, *Lancet* 350:1495, 1997.

Berstad A: Antacids, pepsin inhibitors, and gastric cooling in the management of massive upper gastrointestinal haemorrhage, *Scand J Gastroenterol* 22 (suppl):33, 1987.

Collins R, Langman M: Treatment with histamine H2 antagonists in acute upper gastrointestinal hemorrhage: implications of randomized trials, *N Engl J Med* 313:660, 1985.

Imperiale TF, Teran JC, McCullough AJ: A meta-analysis of somatostatin versus vasopressin in the management of acute esophageal variceal hemorrhage, *Gastroenterology* 109:1289, 1995.

Kollef MH, O'Brien JD, Zuckerman GR, Shannon W: BLEED: a classification tool to predict outcomes in patients with acute upper and lower gastrointestinal hemorrhage, *Crit Care Med* 25:1125, 1997.

[www]Additional references are available on the following web site: www.signsandsymptoms.com.

Lin HJ, Tseng GY, Lo WC, et al: Predictive factors for rebleeding in patients with peptic ulcer bleeding after multipolar electrocoagulation: a retrospective analysis, *J Clin Gastroenterol* 26:113, 1998.

Lin HJ, Perng CL, Wang K, et al: Octreotide for arrest of peptic ulcer hemorrhage: a prospective, randomized controlled trial, *Hepatogastroenterology* 42:856, 1995.

Longstreth GF: Epidemiology of hospitalization for acute upper gastrointestinal hemorrhage: a population-based study, *Am J Gastroenterol* 90:206, 1995.

Longstreth GF, Feitelberg SP: Outpatient care of selected patients with acute non-variceal upper gastrointestinal haemorrhage, *Lancet* 345:108, 1995.

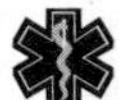

THROMBOCYTOPENIA

A low platelet count can result from decreased production, increased utilization, or destruction, as well as from splenic sequestration. Thrombocytopenia should be considered, especially in patients with mucous membrane bleeding or petechial hemorrhages.

Causes of failed platelet production include aplastic and megaloblastic anemia, infection (including HIV), alcohol-induced bone marrow suppression, and bone marrow infiltration with leukemia or with myelodysplastic cells.

Causes of increased platelet destruction or utilization include idiopathic thrombocytopenic purpura, thrombotic thrombocytopenic purpura, and hemolytic-uremic syndrome; drugs, including heparin, quinidine, gold salts, rifampin, sulfa, oral diabetic agents, and ticlopidine; and states of intravascular coagulation (sepsis, metastatic cancer, traumatic brain damage, and obstetric complications such as HELLP and ARDS).

Causes of splenic sequestration should also be considered, including cirrhosis and mononucleosis with secondary splenomegaly, Gaucher's disease, and myelofibrosis with myeloid dysplasia.

Symptoms

- Gingival bleeding

- Prolonged bleeding after dental work
- Epistaxis
- Easy bruising
- Excessive menses
- Hematuria
- GI bleeding

Signs

- Multiple scattered petechiae, purpura, or ecchymosis
- Epistaxis
- Other bleeding

Workup

- CBC with platelets
- Evaluation of a peripheral blood smear
- Urinalysis (hematuria)
- LFTs and rheumatologic tests, as clinically indicated
- Platelet function studies and bone marrow analysis, although important in the evaluation of otherwise unexplained thrombocytopenia, are not indicated in the emergency setting.

Comments and Treatment Considerations

No treatment is indicated for the majority of cases of thrombocytopenia. Patients with a platelet count below 10,000/mm^3 are thought to be at risk for spontaneous intracranial hemorrhage, and thus replacement is generally recommended at that level. Platelet transfusion may be considered even with a level as high as 50,000/mm^3 in the presence of severe ongoing bleeding. One unit of platelets usually raises the platelet count by 10,000/mm^3. The same precautions taken to prevent allergic reactions when transfusing other blood products should be followed when transfusing platelets (i.e., pretreatment with acetaminophen and diphenhydramine). For patients who have ongoing heavy bleeding, single donor platelet units can be transfused to minimize antigenic exposure with multiple transfusions. If TTP or DIC has not been ruled out, platelets should not be transfused, since this can aggravate the thrombotic process.

REFERENCES

Coller BS: Disorders of platelets. In Ratnoff OD, Forbes CD, editors: *Disorders of hemostasis*, Orlando, Fla, 1984, Grune & Stratton.

Glatt AE, Anand A: Thrombocytopenia in patients infected with human immunodeficiency virus: treatment update, *Clin Infect Dis* 21:415, 1995.

Goebel RA: Thrombocytopenia, *Emerg Med Clin North Am* 11:445, 1993.

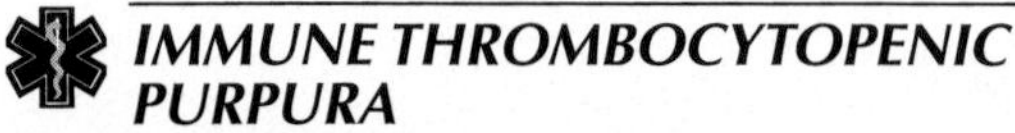

IMMUNE THROMBOCYTOPENIC PURPURA

Immune thrombocytopenic purpura (ITP) can be either an acute or chronic condition. The acute form is caused by immune complexes binding to or cross-reacting with platelets, often as the result of a viral infection. Acute ITP occurs predominantly in children, usually younger than 6 years of age, and is self-limited. Chronic ITP has an insidious onset, occurs three times more commonly in females than in males, and is seen most commonly between the ages of 20 and 40.

Symptoms

- Acute: see Thrombocytopenia
- Chronic: see Thrombocytopenia
- Menometrorrhagia may occur

Signs

- See Thrombocytopenia

Workup

- The physical examination and laboratory evaluation should focus on the elimination of other causes of thrombocytopenia.
- See Thrombocytopenia
- Bone marrow biopsy is routinely performed on an outpatient basis to rule out an atypical presentation of aplastic anemia, acute leukemia, or a metastatic tumor.

Comments and Treatment Considerations

Expectant management is often all that is indicated. With the acute childhood form, intravenous immunoglobulin or corticosteroids can be used for symptomatic patients with platelet counts in the 10,000 to 20,000/mm^3 range.

Platelet transfusion is of transient benefit and is considered a heroic measure reserved for life-threatening hemorrhage despite conventional treatment. Consultation with a hematologist and follow-up are required.

REFERENCES[www]

Bussel JB, Goldman, A, Imbach P, et al: Treatment of acute idiopathic thrombocytopenia of childhood with intravenous infusions of gamma globulin, *J Pediatr* 106:886, 1985.

George JN, Woolf SH, Raskob GE, et al: Idiopathic thrombocytopenic purpura: a practicc guideline developed by explicit methods for the American Society of Hematology, *Blood* 88:3, 1996.

Imbach P: Immune thrombocytopenic purpura and intravenous immunoglobulin, *Cancer* 68(suppl):1422, 1991.

Lightsey AL, McMillan R, Koenig, HM: Childhood idiopathic thrombocytopenic purpura: aggressive management of life-threatening complications, *JAMA* 232:734, 1975.

[www]Additional references are available on the following web site: www.signsandsymptoms.com

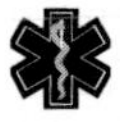

THROMBOTIC THROMBOCYTOPENIC PURPURA

Classically, thrombotic thrombocytopenic purpura (TTP) is diagnosed when at least four of the following five elements are present, in the absence of another explanation: microangiopathic hemolytic anemia (MAHA), thrombocytopenia, decreased renal function, fever, and neurologic abnormalities. The cause of this disease process is uncertain, but it is characterized by microthrombi (deposits composed of platelets and fibrin) within the lumina of capillaries and arterioles in various locations, creating a variable clinical presentation.

Symptoms

- Neurologic abnormalities are seen most commonly (headache, confusion, cranial nerve palsies, hemiparesis, or coma).
- Other symptoms (dependent on organ system involved)
- See Thrombocytopenia

Signs

- See Thrombocytopenia

Work-up

- CBC with platelets
- Urinalysis (may suggest a hemolytic anemia or proteinuria)
- Peripheral blood smear (schistocytes, reticulocytosis)
- Bilirubin (indirect)
- LDH
- Electrolytes (elevated BUN, creatinine)

Comments and Treatment Considerations

Once recognized, this disease process constitutes an emergency and should prompt emergency consultation with a hematologist. The primary treatment is plasma exchange transfusion. While waiting for this to be arranged, the emergency physician may consider glucocorticoids and antiplatelet therapy (dipyridamole or aspirin) in patients with acute life-threatening presentations. Platelets should not be transfused unless the patient has an uncontrollable, life-threatening hemorrhage, since this can exacerbate the thrombotic process.

REFERENCES[www]

Bell WR, Braine HG, Ness PM, Kickler TS: Improved survival in thrombotic thrombocytopenic purpura-hemolytic uremic syndrome, *N Engl J Med* 32:398, 1991.

Bukowski RM: Thrombotic thrombocytopenic purpura: a review, *Prog Hemost Thromb* 6:287, 1982.

Harkness DR, Byrnes JJ, Lian ECY, et al: Hazard of platelet transfusion in thrombotic thrombocytopenic purpura, *JAMA* 246:1931, 1981.

[www]Additional references are available on the following web site: www.signsandsymptoms.com.

Shephard KV, Bukowski RM: The treatment of thrombotic thrombocytopenic purpura with exchange transfusion, plasma infusion, and plasma exchange, *Semin Hematol* 24:178, 1987.

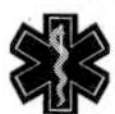

RENAL DISEASE AND UREMIA

Patients dependent on hemodialysis often report bleeding, which reflects the multifactorial nature of hemostatic abnormalities in renal failure. Their bleeding tendency results from a qualitative and a mild quantitative platelet problem, as well as from frequent coagulation factor deficiencies acquired as a result of a nephrotic state (the anticoagulant properties of retained uremic toxins), chronic anemia, and the fact that they receive anticoagulation with dialysis.

Workup

- CBC with platelets
- Bleeding time is not generally performed in the ED, although it is the hemostatic test most consistently abnormal with uremia.

Comments and Treatment Considerations

It is important to establish the adequacy and timing of recent dialysis, as dialysis may transiently improve platelet function. Correcting the anemia associated with renal failure (by transfusion of packed red blood cells to an optimum hematocrit of 26% to 30%) also improves platelet function. Platelet replacement has minimal efficacy because the transfused platelets rapidly acquire the uremic deficiency. Nonetheless, in life-threatening hemorrhage, both platelet and cryoprecipitate transfusions are indicated. Desmopressin (DDAVP), a synthetic analogue of vasopressin, increases platelet adhesion through stimulation of the release of von Willebrand factor and factor VIII, resulting in a shortening of the bleeding time in many uremic patients. The drawbacks associated with the use of DDAVP include tachyphylaxis after three or four doses and the side effects of headache, flushing, nausea, and abdominal cramps. Conjugated estrogens are also effective in reducing bleeding, although the mechanism is unclear.

REFERENCES

Eberst ME, Berkowitz LR: Hemostasis in renal disease: pathophysiology and management, *Am J Med* 96:168, 1994.

Hodde LA, Sandroni S: Emergency department evaluation and management of dialysis patient complications, *Am J Emerg Med* 10:317, 1992.

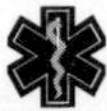

HEMOLYTIC UREMIC SYNDROME

Hemolytic uremic syndrome (HUS) is a serious multisystem disease usually affecting young children, with a peak incidence between 6 months and 4 years of age. It usually follows a prodromal infectious illness (well described following diarrhea caused by *Escherichia coli* serotype 0157:H7). HUS is both clinically and pathologically similar to TTP, with a predominance of renal symptomatology. Important abnormalities include hemolytic anemia, azotemia, thrombocytopenia, and frequently, encephalopathy.

Symptoms

- Similar to TTP, although neurologic manifestations less common
- Abdominal pain (may be severe)
- Rectal bleeding
- Symptoms of circulatory fluid overload including fatigue and generalized weakness, shortness of breath, and swelling

Signs

- Pale, weak, ill appearing
- Petechiae or purpura
- Neurologic abnormalities (irritable, obtunded, or focal defects possible), somnolent, and varying respiratory difficulty as a result of congestive heart failure
- Abdominal tenderness, possibly as a result of hepatic and splenic enlargement or a surgical condition
- Hypertension

Workup

- CBC with platelets (anemia and thrombocytopenia secondary to destruction or consumption)

- Urinalysis—red and white blood cells, cellular casts, and a significant amount of protein
- Electrolytes, calcium, phosphate—acute renal failure pattern (elevated BUN and creatinine, hyperkalemia, hyponatremia, hyperphosphatemia, hyperuricemia, hypocalcemia)
- Liver function tests
- PT and PTT

Comments and Treatment Considerations

Treatment is generally supportive and focuses on renal failure and its complications. This is an area of active investigation.

REFERENCES

Musgrave JE, Talwakar YB, Puri HC, et al: The hemolytic-uremic syndrome: a clinical review, *Clin Pediatr* 17:218, 1978.

Musgrave JE, Talwakar YB, Puri HC, et al: Hemolytic uremic syndrome in adults, *Arch Intern Med* 140:353, 1980.

Seigler RL: Management of hemolytic-uremic syndrome, *J Pediatr* 112:1014, 1988.

Stewart CL, Tina LU: Hemolytic uremic syndrome, *Pediatr Rev* 14:218, 1993.

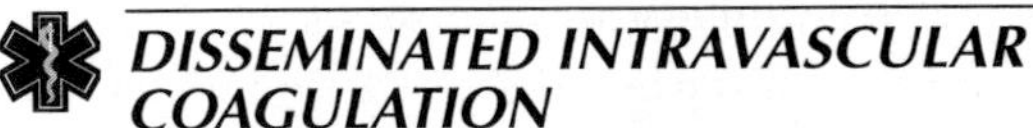

DISSEMINATED INTRAVASCULAR COAGULATION

Disseminated intravascular coagulation (DIC) is a severe blood clotting abnormality that affects multiple organ systems and occurs in patients with a serious preexisting medical or surgical problem. Many conditions have been associated with the development of DIC including infection, acid-base disturbances, malignancies, burns, traumatic injuries, vascular disorders, transfusion reactions, massive transfusions, and obstetric complications. The emergency physician must initiate the treatment for DIC, as well as diagnose and treat the underlying condition.

DIC is characterized by an imbalance in the system of coagulation and fibrinolysis. It is thought to occur as a result of the release of tissue factor that triggers the coagulation cascade. Small fibrin clots are formed and deposited at the same time fibrinolysis is stimulated, and the process results in the consumption of both coagulation factors and platelets.

Symptoms

- Bleeding and/or thrombosis
- Bleeding from multiple sites, including areas of venipuncture, into the urine, from the gastrointestinal tract, and most commonly, from the skin and mucous membranes

Signs

- See Thrombocytopenia
- Bleeding
- Purpura
- Signs of microthrombi formation and subsequent tissue ischemia (e.g., gangrene, purpura fulminans, renal cortical necrosis, ARDS) can be seen in any organ system.
- CNS findings stemming from an intracerebral hemorrhage

Workup

- CBC with platelets (thrombocytopenia)
- PT and PTT (may be prolonged)
- Fibrinogen level (decreased)
- Fibrin degradation products and D-dimers (elevated)
- Blood smear (fragmented RBCs)

Comments and Treatment Considerations

Initially, management should be focused on establishing hemodynamic stability while assessing and treating the underlying condition. Further management then focuses on the replacement of depleted coagulation factors. Usually, fibrinogen is deficient, and this can be replaced with cryoprecipitate. The PT is the best indicator of factor depletion; when two to three times greater than normal, fresh frozen plasma should be given. Each unit of FFP contains 200 to 250 units of each factor and is usually given 2 units at a time. It is also prudent to administer folate and vitamin K (use phytonadione, since it has a more rapid onset of action; maximum IV rate is 1 mg/minute).

Heparin is a highly controversial treatment for thromboses and is rarely used in the ED. It does not reliably reverse abnormal coagulation and can exacerbate a bleeding diathesis. Likewise, antifibrinolytic agents are also used only with extreme caution. Platelet replacement is effective only transiently and should be given according to the guidelines for general thrombocytopenia, outlined above.

REFERENCES[www]

Bick RL: Disseminated intravascular coagulation: objective criteria for diagnosis and management, *Med Clin North Am* 78:511,1994.

Contreras M, Ala FA, Greaves M, et al: Guidelines for the use of fresh frozen plasma. British Committee for Standards in Haematology, Working Party of the Blood Transfusion Task Force, *Transfus Med* 2:57, 1992.

Fruchtman S, Aledort LM: Disseminated intravascular coagulation, *J Am Coll Cardiol* 8:159, 1986.

[www]Additional references are available on the following web site: www.signsandsymptoms.com.

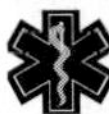

LIVER DISEASE AND HEPATIC FAILURE

The pathophysiologic abnormalities associated with liver disease result in hemostatic problems that range from subclinical coagulopathy, unmasked by the performance of a procedure, to brisk, active hemorrhage that can be life threatening. If the patient has liver disease as a result of alcoholism, thrombocytopenia results not only from splenic sequestration, but also from decreased production.

Symptoms

- Fatigue
- Anorexia
- Pruritus
- Gastrointestinal bleeding
- Increasing abdominal girth

Signs

- Jaundice
- Hematemesis
- Melena or bright red blood from rectum
- Ascites
- Spider nevi

- Asterixis
- Altered mental status

See Hepatic Encephalopathy in Chapter 22, Mental Status Change and Coma.

Workup

- CBC with platelets
- PT and PTT
- Liver function tests
- Tests to rule out infections when indicated (aspiration of ascites, chest x-ray, urinalysis, blood and urine cultures)

Comments and Treatment Considerations

Intervention is indicated for active bleeding or when preparing for an invasive procedure. Packed red blood cells should be replaced as needed to maintain hemodynamic stability. Fresh frozen plasma (generally begin with two units) immediately supplies missing coagulation factors. The effects of vitamin K are delayed. If vitamin K is administered in the ED, the subcutaneous and intramuscular routes should be avoided because they can cause significant bleeding or hematoma. Platelets are transfused only when bleeding is severe because the transfused platelets rapidly acquire a qualitative defect. DDAVP also can be helpful in reducing the bleeding time in patients with liver disease, as it does with renal failure, and should be considered in the treatment of the bleeding patient with significant liver disease. Infections such as spontaneous bacterial peritonitis and pneumonia are common in patients with hepatic failure.

REFERENCES

Levine RF, Spivak JL, Meagher RC: Effect of ethanol on thrombopoiesis, *Br J Haematol* 62:345, 1986.

Mammen EF: Coagulopathies of liver disease, *Clin Lab Med* 14:769, 1994.

Paramo JA, Rocha E: Hemostasis in advanced liver disease, *Semin Thromb Hemost* 19:184, 1993.

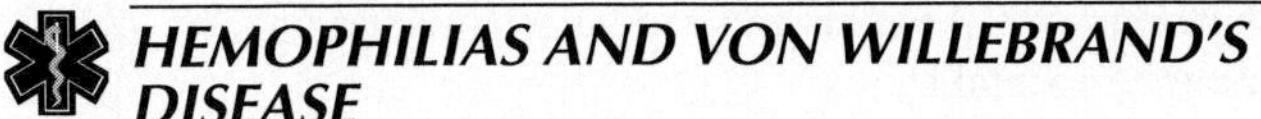

HEMOPHILIAS AND VON WILLEBRAND'S DISEASE

Hemophilia A (factor VIII) and B (factor IX) are both X-linked recessive, coagulation factor disorders. In both hemophilia A and B a normal level of factor is present, but its coagulant activity is diminished. Hemophilia A is far more common. The clinical presentation varies according to the degree of coagulant activity present. In addition to coagulant activity, factor VIII stimulates platelet adhesion. When this function is diminished, von Willebrand's disease results.

Symptoms and Signs

Hemophilia

- Hemarthrosis or muscle hematoma is most common. Chronic joint destruction can occur because of repetitive hemarthrosis often caused by minimal trauma.
- Bleeding also can occur elsewhere, including the CNS, and may indicate more severe factor dysfunction. In severe cases (when factor activity is less than 1%), spontaneous hemorrhage is more common.

von Willebrand's disease

- Generally less symptomatic than hemophilia
- Epistaxis, excessive bruising, or prolonged bleeding after minor surgery (e.g., dental extractions) Hemarthroses or soft tissue bleeding, as seen with hemophilia, is less common.

Workup

- Platelet count (to exclude a quantitative platelet disorder)
- PT and PTT

Hemophilias

Coagulation screening tests typically show a normal PT and a prolonged PTT, demonstrating a defect in the intrinsic pathway. All screening tests can be normal in hemophilia, however, if the factor activity is greater than 30%. The type of factor deficiency (VIII versus IX) can be established only by specific assay.

von Willebrand's disease

Factor activity can be assessed by performing a ristocetin cofactor assay. (This is not routinely performed in the ED.) The bleeding time typically is prolonged.

Comments and Treatment Considerations

Patients with hemophilia should not receive intramuscular injections, have arterial blood gases drawn, nor have central venous access attempted without prior and continued factor replacement, since life-threatening hemorrhage may occur.

Prompt hemostasis is the goal of therapy. Specific treatment varies with the site and severity of hemorrhage.

Mild to moderate hemophilia may respond to treatment with desmopressin (DDAVP), and it is helpful to know if the patient has responded to this treatment in the past. When efficacious, DDAVP can produce a threefold increase in factor VIII activity. The usual dose is 0.3 μg/kg IV over 15 to 30 minutes. A response is typically seen within 1 hour. Tachyphylaxis often occurs after three or four doses.

Severe hemophilia or any severity with serious bleeding (determined either by location or amount) requires treatment with specific factor concentrates. Dosing of factor concentrates varies according to the site and degree of hemorrhage. In general, a patient factor activity level of $<1\%$ should be assumed, and treatment should ensure 50% activity after treatment for most bleeds and 100% activity after treatment for life-threatening bleeding.

Hemophilia A: Doses range from 15 to 30 U/kg as an initial dose for minor hemorrhage (epistaxis, after dental extraction, into joints or muscles) to 50 U/kg for life-threatening bleeding (CNS, retropharynx/pharynx, retroperitoneum, or for patients who need emergent surgery).

Hemophilia B: Initial doses range from 30 U/kg for minor bleeding to 50 U/kg for major hemorrhage.

Circulating antibodies may be formed to infused factor precipitates; this occurs in approximately 15% of patients with severe hemophilia A and 10% of patients with hemophilia B. If a patient is unresponsive to usual therapy, antibodies may be present and can be assayed by the Bethesda inhibitor assay (BIA). The level present can be used as a guide for choosing the most efficacious type of factor replacement therapy.

If the bleeding is life threatening and factor concentrates are not readily available, cryoprecipitate (one bag contains approximately 100 U of factor VIII) or FFP (1 unit of FFP raises factor IX activity by 3%) can be used.

REFERENCES[www]

Brettler DB, Levine PH: Factor concentrates for treatment of hemophilia: which one to choose? *Blood* 73:2067, 1989.

Hoyer LW: Hemophilia A, *N Engl J Med* 330:38, 1994.

Logan LJ: Treatment of von Willebrand's disease, *Hematol Oncol Clin North Am* 6:1079, 1992.

Manucci PM, Cattaneo M: Desmopressin: a nontransfusional treatment of hemophilia and von Willebrand disease, *Haemostasis* 22:276, 1992.

[www]Additional references are available on the following web site: www.signsandsymptoms.com.

CHAPTER 7

Chest Pain

MARK LOUDEN

Chest pain is one of the most frequent presenting complaints in the ED. The patient's history is the single most important source of information for distinguishing between emergent, urgent, and benign conditions. Timely ECG and chest x-rays are often invaluable, whereas blood tests are rarely helpful in the initial evaluation.

PNEUMOTHORAX, TENSION PNEUMOTHORAX, AND PNEUMOMEDIASTINUM

A pneumothorax may occur in patients with trauma, or it may be iatrogenic (e.g., central line insertion or aspiration of pleural effusion) or spontaneous. Spontaneous pneumothoraces are most likely to occur in patients who are tall and thin and smoke cigarettes. Spontaneous pneumothoraces also are associated with Marfan's syndrome, smoking crack cocaine, and *Pneumocystis carinii* pneumonia. Other severe injuries or conditions can mask all symptoms.

Pneumomediastinum may present in the same way as pneumothorax (spontaneous or traumatic), but it is sometimes accompanied by throat pain or dysphagia.

Tension pneumothorax is caused by the buildup of pressure outside of the lung, compressing the mediastinum and limiting venous return and cardiac output. Tension pneumothorax should be suspected in trauma patients who are hypoxic or hypotensive, patients who have a known pneumothorax (or if having a procedure that may cause one), and those receiving mechanical ventilation who deteriorate clinically.

Symptoms

- Acute onset of chest pain or discomfort (often pleuritic) ++++
- Dyspnea +++
- Both chest pain and dyspnea +++

Signs

Pneumothorax

- A healthy patient with a small pneumothorax (usually less than 15% to 20% volume) may have no physical signs.
- Tachypnea
- Tachycardia
- Decreased breath sounds
- Hyperresonance to percussion (may be masked by hemothorax)
- Subcutaneous emphysema
- Patients with preexisting cardiopulmonary disease or other associated injuries may be cyanotic or in shock.

Tension pneumothorax

- Hypotension
- Tracheal deviation (later finding)
- Distended neck veins (later finding)

Pneumomediastinum

- Hamman's sign (crepitance heard over the heart during systole) +++
- Subcutaneous emphysema +++

Workup

- Needle thoracostomy followed by tube thoracostomy before chest x-ray for patients with a pneumothorax who are in shock or without a pulse
- Chest x-rays (Figs. 7-1 and 7-2): Moderate (15% to 60% volume) or large (>60%) pneumothoraces usually are evident. If pneumothorax is suspected, an additional film taken during maximal expiration may increase sensitivity.
- ECG is used primarily to evaluate for other potential causes of chest pain, as well as in the pulseless patient to determine the presence of cardiac rhythm.

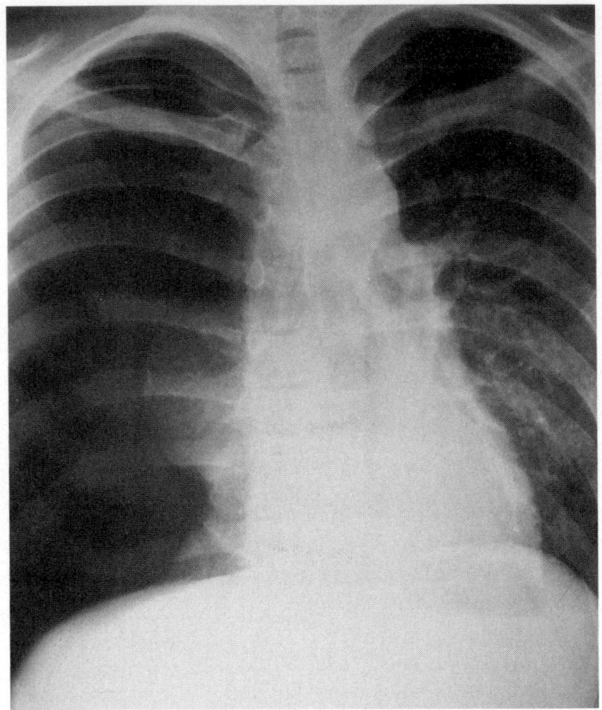

Fig. 7-1 Tension pneumothorax. Anteroposterior chest radiograph demonstrates shift of the mediastinal structures to the left, indicating tension. (Courtesy Michael Zucker, MD, Los Angeles.)

- CT scans are more sensitive than chest x-rays, but since small pneumothoraces are of little clinical significance, CT is not warranted.
- Contrast-enhanced esophagography is indicated in patients with pneumomediastinum, especially if a spontaneous rupture is suspected (Boerhaave's syndrome) or if trauma has caused penetration of the esophagus (see Esophageal Rupture).

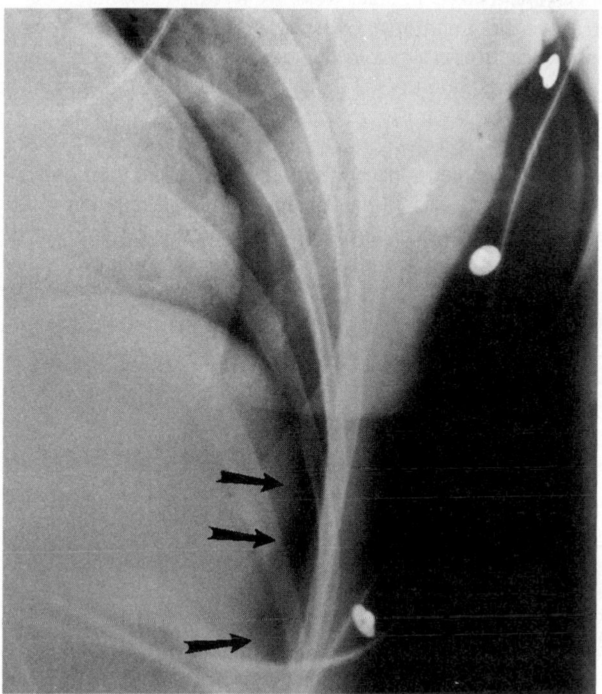

Fig. 7-2 Nontension pneumothorax. Anteroposterior supine chest radiograph shows left deep sulcus sign *(arrows)*. (Courtesy Michael Zucker, MD, Los Angeles.)

Comments and Treatment Considerations

Patients with a very small spontaneous pneumothorax (<15%) frequently can be given 100% O_2 in the ED and be observed, since spontaneous reabsorption is expected at a rate of 1% of the hemithorax per day. Simple pneumothoraces (<25%) can be aspirated through a small catheter (with 45% to 87% success rate) and observed for 4 to 6 hours (for recurrence or for reexpansion pulmonary edema).

For some patients, placement of a small diameter catheter attached to a one-way valve may allow for ED discharge with daily follow-up.

Larger pneumothoraces and those associated with underlying lung disease, empyema, hemothorax, or trauma or in patients with severe cardiopulmonary disease and those who are to be transported by air should have a tube thoracostomy.

Management of pneumomediastinum is conservative if the esophagus or bronchi have not been injured.

REFERENCES[www]

Aitchison F, Bleetman A, Munro P, et al: Detection of pneumothorax by accident and emergency officers and radiologists on single chest films, *Arch Emerg Med* 10:343, 1993.

Delius RE, Obeid FN, Horst HM, et al: Catheter aspiration for simple pneumothorax: experience with 114 patients, *Arch Surg* 124:833, 1989.

Light RW: Management of spontaneous pneumothorax, *Am Rev Respir Dis* 148:245, 1993.

Markos J, McGonigle P, Phillips MJ: Pneumothorax: treatment by small-lumen catheter aspiration, *Aust N Z J Med* 20:775, 1990.

Panacek EA, Singer AJ, Sherman BW, et al: Spontaneous pneumomediastinum: clinical and natural history, *Ann Emerg Med* 21:1222, 1992.

Seow A, Kazerooni EA, Pernicano PG, Neary M: Comparison of upright inspiratory and expiratory chest radiographs for detecting pneumothoraces, *Am J Roentgenol* 166:313,1996.

[www]Additional references are available on the following web site: www.signsandsymptoms.com.

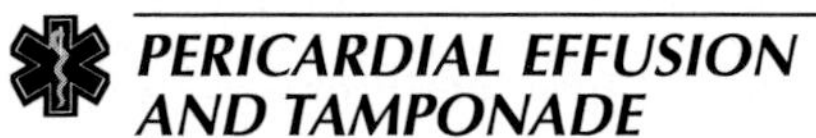

PERICARDIAL EFFUSION AND TAMPONADE

Pericardial tamponade is caused by elevated pressure in the pericardial space, resulting in equilibration of pericardial, left ventricular, and right ventricular diastolic pressures, which leads to a decrease in preload and cardiac output. An effusion usually is present in pericarditis, but it does not result in tamponade in most cases. The rate at which an effusion develops may determine whether tamponade results. Rapid accumulation of fluid is most likely to develop from penetrating injuries, such as stab or missile wounds, complications of central line insertion, or rupture of myocardium after myocardial infarction. It also may follow retrograde aortic dissection. Tamponade from medical causes of pericarditis is more likely when the underlying cause is a malignancy and when a patient with an existing effusion becomes acutely, severely dehydrated (see also Pericarditis).

Symptoms

- Chest pain and tightness
- Shortness of breath
- Peripheral edema
- Dyspnea on exertion
- Altered mental status

Signs

- Tachycardia
- Narrow pulse pressure
- Pulsus paradoxus
- Kussmaul's sign (distention of neck veins with inspiration)
- Pericardial friction rub
- Beck's triad—hypotension, muffled heart sounds, and neck vein distention—is a very late event.

Workup

- Echocardiography is the study of choice.
- Central venous pressure or Swan-Ganz pressure monitoring may be useful but should not delay echocardiography.
- If the etiology is traumatic or from aortic dissection, a thoracic surgeon should be consulted. Preparations should be made for pericardiocentesis, pericardial window, or thoracotomy.
- Pericardiocentesis should be performed immediately for patients in shock.
- Patients with penetrating trauma resulting in tamponade, with loss of vital signs in or en route to the ED, are among the few who may benefit from thoracotomy in the ED.

REFERENCES [www]

Markiewicz W, Borovik R, Ecker S: Cardiac tamponade in medical patients: treatment and prognosis in the echocardiographic era, *Am Heart J* 111:1138, 1986.

McGregor M: Pulsus paradoxus, *N Engl J Med* 301:480, 1979.

Whye D, Barish R, Almquist T, et al: Echocardiographic diagnosis of acute pericardial effusion in penetrating chest trauma, *Am J Emerg Med* 6:21, 1988.

[www]Additional references are available on the following web site: www.signsandsymptoms.com.

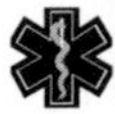

ACUTE MYOCARDIAL INFARCTION AND ISCHEMIA

Acute myocardial infarction (MI) accounts for 650,000 hospital admissions each year and is one of the leading causes of death in the United States. A missed diagnosis of MI can have fatal or debilitating consequences. Furthermore, a missed diagnosis of MI is the most common and most costly cause of malpractice litigation. Reasons for a missed diagnosis of MI include failure to consider the diagnosis in an atypical presentation, misinterpreting or not ordering appropriate tests (such as an ECG), or inappropriately relying on a single, normal ECG or serum marker for MI to rule out infarction.

Epidemiologic risk factors for coronary artery disease include history of hypertension, diabetes, smoking, elevated serum cholesterol, male sex, age over 40, and family history of premature coronary artery disease. However, these do not effectively predict acute ischemia in the ED. The most important diagnostic factors in the ED are (1) symptoms consistent with MI, (2) past history of ischemic heart disease, and (3) an abnormal ECG (see below). Up to one half of patients have unstable angina before MI. Cocaine abuse can induce ischemia in younger individuals who have no other risk factors.

Symptoms

- Chest pain ++++ in acute MI or ischemia is typically heavy, squeezing, tight, or pressure-like in quality, but may be sharp

++, burning, or indigestion-like ++, pleuritic +, or even absent.

- Painless MI is more common in the elderly and in patients with diabetes. The frequency of chest pain decreases steadily after age 65 to 70 and is present in only 50% at age 80, after which dyspnea is the most common symptom. Pain typically localizes to the retrosternal area or, less often, the left chest. It may localize to the epigastrium or back. It may radiate to, or even primarily localize to, the arm, shoulder(s), jaw, or neck +++. The pain usually is not positional +. The upper limit of constant pain duration is difficult to define but is usually measured in hours, not days.
- Dyspnea
- Diaphoresis +++
- Nausea +++
- Dizziness
- Palpitations
- Apprehension
- Syncope
- Sudden death

Signs

- Tachycardia (+++ anterior MIs)
- Bradycardia (+++ inferior MIs)
- Diaphoresis ++
- Premature beats
- Hypertension or hypotension
- Vomiting
- Murmurs; a new murmur with pathologic qualities may indicate papillary muscle dysfunction or rupture (producing mitral regurgitation) or perforation of the interventricular septum.
- Gallops
- Rales
- Altered mental status
- Evidence of peripheral vascular disease (e.g., diminished pedal pulses, femoral bruits, or claudication) also increases the likelihood of coronary artery disease.
- Signs of cerebral ischemia may coexist in 10% of elderly patients.

Workup

- 12-Lead ECG may be normal ++ or reveal nondiagnostic or nonspecific ST segment or T wave changes ++. An abnormal ECG places the patient at high risk for MI and other complications.
- ST segment elevation of more than 1 mm in two contiguous leads along with chest pain suggests acute infarction +++.
- ST depression (also of more than 1 mm) may indicate ischemia or a non-Q wave MI (a non-Q wave MI will evolve in one third of patients with chest pain and ST depression).
- New bundle-branch block in the clinical setting of MI also should be regarded as evidence of ischemia. Ischemia is difficult to identify in the presence of preexisting left bundle-branch block (LBBB) or paced ventricular rhythm, both of which produce ST elevations. Criteria that, if present with LBBB, aid in the detection of ischemia or infarction but, if absent, do not rule these out, include (1) ST segment elevation of more that 1 mm concordant with the QRS complex (sensitivity ++, specificity 92% to 94%), (2) ST segment depression of more than 1 mm in leads V1, V2, or V3 (sensitivity ++, specificity 82% to 96%), and (3) ST segment elevation of more than 5 mm discordant with the QRS complex (sensitivity +++, specificity 88% to 92%).
- No standard has been established for how often ECGs should be repeated in the ED, but additional tracings should be considered after therapeutic interventions, as well as after changes in clinical condition.
- Right-sided chest leads are useful in identifying acute ischemia in the right ventricle and are particularly warranted in patients with inferior MI or hypotension.
- ST-segment trend monitoring is a new technology with potential for detecting changes without repetition of the 12-lead ECG.
- Chest x-rays are useful, especially for identifying CHF or other potential causes of chest pain such as pneumonia, pneumothorax, and aortic dissection.

- Serum markers of myocardial infarction, such as creatine kinase, myocardial bound (CKMB), and troponins I and T are useful for prognosis but are not adequately sensitive when measured on a single occasion +++ to rule out MI.
- Radionuclide scans (such as technetium sestamibi, which irreversibly binds ischemic tissue) may be useful in evaluating low-risk patients in the ED ++++.
- Echocardiography may provide evidence of ischemia in patients who show no other diagnostic evidence.
- Early stress testing may expedite risk stratification and enable early discharge for some low-risk patients.

Comments and Treatment Considerations

Cautions:

1. Pain relieved after a "GI cocktail" may still be ischemic pain; never use nitroglycerine as a diagnostic test.
2. Patients with panic disorder, histrionic traits, or psychosis may also have MIs.
3. Overall, many presentations of MI are atypical, especially in diabetic or elderly patients.
4. Beware of the patient who minimizes significant symptoms.
5. Chest wall tenderness, or partial or full reproducibility of chest pain (with pressure applied to the chest), may be present in patients with acute MI ++.

Barring contraindications, all patients with suspected AMI should receive aspirin (25% to 50% reduction in mortality; dose 81 to 325 mg), beta-blockers (15% reduction in mortality; e.g., metoprolol 5 mg every 5 min for total of 15 mg if heart rate and blood pressure tolerate), low flow oxygen, and nitrates (sublingual nitroglycerine, nitroglycerine paste to skin, or intravenous nitroglycerin; see Appendix B for doses).

Immediate thrombolysis or percutaneous transluminal coronary angioplasty (PTCA) should be considered for the following: (1) chest pain that lasts more than 30 minutes and less than 12 hours and (2) ST elevation greater than 1 mm in two contiguous limb leads, ST elevation greater than 2 mm in two contiguous precordial leads, or new bundle-branch block. Choice of revascularization method depends on availability and experience at the institution and on the presence or absence of contraindications to individual methods. Patients with unstable angina (USA) should receive the same initial care as those with MI, with the exception of immediate revascularization.

A diagnosis of MI can be ruled out in 5% to 10% of patients who meet the criteria for thrombolysis. The majority of these have USA +++ or other diagnoses, including pericarditis, pancreatitis, esophagitis, and aortic dissection.

REFERENCES[www]

Bayer AJ, Chadha JS, Farag RR, Pathy MS: Changing presentation of myocardial infarction with increasing old age, *J Am Geriatr Soc* 34:263, 1986.

Bode C, Smalling R, Berg G: Randomized comparison of coronary thrombolysis achieved with double-bolus retaplase (recombinant plasminogen activator) and front-loaded, accelerated alteplase (recombinant tissue plasminogen activator) in patients with acute myocardial infarct, *Circulation* 94:891, 1996.

Brady WJ, Aufderheide TP: Left bundle-branch block pattern complicating the electrocardiographic evaluation of acute myocardial infarction, *Acad Emerg Med* 4:56, 1997.

Every N, Parsons LS, Hlatky M, et al: A comparison of thrombolytic therapy with primary coronary angioplasty for acute myocardial infarction, *N Engl J Med* 335:1253,1996.

Gitter MJ, Goldsmith SR, Dunbar DN, Sharkey SW: Cocaine and chest pain: clinical features and outcome of patients hospitalized to rule out myocardial infarction, *Ann Intern Med* 115:277, 1991.

GUSTO Angiographic Investigators: The effects of tissue plasminogen activator, streptokinase, or both on coronary artery patency, ventricular function, and survival after acute myocardial infarction, *N Engl J Med* 329:1615, 1993.

ISIS-2: Randomized trial of intravenous atenolol among 16,027 cases of suspected acute myocardial infarction, *Lancet* 2:57, 1986.

Ohman EM, Armstrong PW, Christenson RH, et al: Cardiac troponin T levels for risk stratification in acute myocardial ischemia, *N Engl J Med* 335:1333,1996.

Ryan TJ, Anderson JL, Antman EM, et al: ACC/AHA guidelines for the management of patients with acute myocardial infarction, *J Am Coll Cardiol* 28:1328,1996.

[www]Additional references are available on the following web site: www.signsandsymptoms.com.

Sgarbossa EB, Pinski SL, Barbagelata A, et al: Electrocardiographic diagnosis of evolving acute myocardial infarction in the presence of left bundle-branch block, *N Engl J Med* 334:481, 1996.

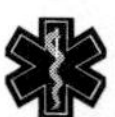

PULMONARY EMBOLUS

Pulmonary embolus (PE) is caused by an obstruction of flow in the pulmonary arteries due to arterial occlusion. This occurs most commonly from the embolization of blood clots from the deep veins of the legs (the subject for the following discussion). Fat (after long bone fractures), air, amniotic fluid, blood clots from other locations, and other substances are rare causes of PE. At least one of the following risk factors is present in 90% of patients with PE: immobility, heart disease, cancer, estrogen therapy, previous deep venous thrombosis (DVT) or PE, hypercoagulability, or abnormal thrombolysis. Not all patients with cancer or hypercoagulability are known at the time of presentation.

Symptoms

- Chest pain ++++ (two thirds of patients with chest pain describe pleuritic pain)
- Dyspnea ++++
- Cough +++
- Hemoptysis ++
- The classic triad of dyspnea, pleuritic chest pain, and hemoptysis is seldom present ++.
- Syncope ++

Signs

- Tachypnea >16/min ++++
- Rales +++
- P2 >A2 +++
- Tachycardia +++
- Fever (low grade) +++
- Diaphoresis +++
- Hypotension (in massive PE)
- Hypoxia (by pulse oximetry)
- Pleural friction rub

- Evidence of DVT (calf swelling—one calf with circumference 2 cm greater than opposite calf) ++

Workup

- Ventilation-perfusion (V/Q) scans should be interpreted in Bayesian fashion. To rule out PE, patients with anything other than a "normal" or "low-probability" V/Q scan in the setting of a low pretest probability should generally be sent for angiography. (A low-probability scan without consideration of pretest probability is falsely negative in 10% to 15% of patients.) Similarly, a "low-probability" or "intermediate-probability" scan does not rule out PE in a patient with a moderate or high pretest probability. These patients should also generally be sent for angiography.
- ECG pattern of S1-Q3-T3 is present in a small minority of patients. Most ECGs are abnormal in PE, but nearly half reveal only nonspecific ST-T wave changes. However, ECG may be helpful in diagnosing other pathologic conditions such as MI or pericarditis.
- Chest x-ray findings are abnormal in most patients with PE but are nonspecific. X-rays may show atelectasis +++, pleural effusion +++, pleural-based opacities ++, elevated hemidiaphragm, decreased vascularity, ++ and prominent central artery ++.
- ABG (and by extrapolation, a normal pulse oximetry reading) does not exclude the possibility of PE. Although ABGs may reveal hypoxia Pao_2 <60 (++) or an increased A-aDo_2, some patients with PE have a Pao_2 >80 (++) and may have a normal A-a gradient (++).
- Doppler flow or duplex scans are currently the standard tests for establishing DVT, although venography is the gold standard. In patients with symptoms or signs of DVT, the results of these tests may indicate the need for anticoagulation, thus obviating the need for pulmonary scans or angiography.
- Plasma D-dimer levels tests show promise, but currently no standardized, rapid assay has consistently proved to be of clinical use.
- Spiral CT angiography has compared well with V/Q scintigraphy but does not reliably demonstrate thromboemboli in

subsegmental arteries. If CT is used as an alternative to V/Q, patients with negative CT scans but with moderate or high clinical suspicion should be considered for pulmonary angiography.

- Pulmonary angiography is the gold standard for diagnosis of PE, although it is time- and labor-intensive, is not without risk (up to 0.5% mortality, 6% complications), and is inconclusive in up to 3%.

Comments and Treatment Considerations

Standard therapy for PE includes early anticoagulation (consider before diagnosis is confirmed if suspicion is high and likelihood of complications low) with intravenous heparin. Ideally, heparin should be dosed by weight-based protocol and is followed by oral anticoagulation. This regimen may soon be replaced by low-molecular-weight heparin, which is as safe and effective as heparin but is easier to administer (no intravenous line required) and monitor (no PT or PTT necessary). Low-molecular-weight heparin may allow for outpatient therapy in some cases.

Thrombolytics or surgical embolectomy is reserved for severe PE (cardiogenic shock, pulmonary hypertension, and right ventricular strain) because of high complication rates. Thrombolytics should be administered either before heparin or after heparin is discontinued and PTT is < 80. Surgical consultation for vena cava filters may be considered when medical treatment is contraindicated.

REFERENCES[www]

Allescia G et al: Invasive and noninvasive diagnosis of pulmonary embolus. Preliminary results of the Prospective Investigative Study of Acute Pulmonary Embolism Diagnosis (PISA-PED), *Chest* 107(suppl):33, 1995.

Goodman LR, Curtin JJ, Mewissen MW, et al: Detection of pulmonary embolism in patients with unresolved clinical and scintigraphic diagnosis: helical CT versus angiography, *Am J Roentgenol* 164:1369, 1995.

[www]Additional references are available on the following web site: www.signsandsymptoms.com.

Perrier A, Desmarais S, Goehring C, et al: D-dimer testing for suspected pulmonary embolism in outpatients, *Am J Respir Crit Care Med* 156:492, 1997.

PIOPED Investigators: Value of the ventilation perfusion scan in the diagnosis of pulmonary embolism, *JAMA* 263:2753, 1990.

Stein PD, Goldhaber SZ, Henry JW, Miller AC: Arterial blood gas analysis in the assessment of suspected acute pulmonary embolism, *Chest* 109:78, 1996.

Stein PD, Hull RD, Saltzman HA, Pineo G: Strategy for diagnosis of patients with suspected acute pulmonary embolism, *Chest* 103:1553, 1993.

Stein PD, Saltzman HA, Weg JG: Clinical characteristics of patients with acute pulmonary embolism, *Am J Cardiol* 68:1723, 1991.

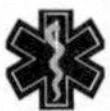

TRAUMATIC AORTIC RUPTURE

Aortic rupture is usually caused by a sudden impact or deceleration (e.g., high-speed motor vehicle collision, a fall from a height, or a pedestrian struck by an automobile). Most of the victims of aortic rupture die before arrival in the ED. The majority of those who reach the ED may survive if they are diagnosed and treated promptly. Many patients are unconscious or have other serious injuries that may mask symptoms of great vessel injury. If the EMS reports that passengers were not wearing seat belts, that the car was not equipped with airbags, or that the steering wheel or dashboard was damaged, then vessel injury should be seriously considered.

Symptoms

- Chest pain +++
- Dyspnea ++
- Back pain ++
- Hoarseness
- Dysphagia
- Painful extremity

Signs

- Abrasions
- Ecchymosis

- Tenderness of the chest wall
- Pseudo-coarctation—elevated blood pressure in the upper extremities with absent femoral pulses ++
- Harsh precordial or interscapular murmur ++

Workup

- Supine chest x-ray—wide mediastinum (>8 cm at the level of the aortic knob +++, nonspecific)
- Supine chest x-ray—blurred, indistinct, or wide aortic arch ++++, nonspecific
- Supine chest x-ray—absent aortopulmonary window, wide right paratracheal stripe (>5 mm), abnormal or absent left paratracheal stripe, tracheal deviation to the right, nasogastric tube deviation to the right, apical pleural cap, or downward displacement of the left mainstem bronchus
- Fractures of the first two ribs may be a sign of trauma to the upper chest; however, this finding alone does not establish aortic trauma.
- None of these signs, or any combination, is 100% sensitive or specific. If any are present in the proper clinical setting, further imaging is necessary, although a completely normal upright chest x-ray suggests that an aortic rupture is unlikely.
- Available methods for determining the presence or absence of aortic disruption include helical thoracic CT, transesophageal echocardiography (TEE), and aortography (the gold standard).
- In stable patients, helical CT may be preferred, since it reduces the need for aortography by more than 50%.
- Aortography may be necessary for those with indeterminate CT scans and possibly for definition of the anatomy of lesions identified on positive CT scans.
- TEE may be useful (where available and feasible) in unstable patients, especially those requiring immediate operative intervention for other injuries.

Comments and Treatment Considerations

Treatment for traumatic aortic rupture is surgical repair without delay.

REFERENCES[www]

Gavant ML, Flick P, Menke P, Gold RE: CT aortography of thoracic aortic rupture, *Am J Roentgenol* 166:955, 1996.

Smith MD, Cassidy M, Souther S, et al: Transesophageal echocardiography in the diagnosis of traumatic rupture of the aorta, *N Engl J Med* 332:356, 1995.

Sturm JT, Hankins DG, Young G: Thoracic aortography following blunt chest trauma, *Am J Emerg Med* 8:92, 1990.

Warren RL, Akins CW, Conn AK, et al: Acute traumatic disruption of the thoracic aorta: emergency department management, *Ann Emerg Med* 21:391, 1992.

Woodring JH, Loh FK, Kryscio RJ: Mediastinal hemorrhage: an evaluation of radiographic manifestations, *Radiology* 151:15, 1984.

[www]Additional references are available on the following web site: www.signsandsymptoms.com.

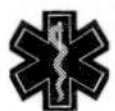

ACUTE AORTIC DISSECTION

Acute aortic dissection is dissection of the media of the aortic wall by a column of blood. It occurs most commonly in the thoracic aorta, and the age of onset is usually at least 50 years. A history of hypertension is usually (80%) present. Aortic dissection is rare in those younger than 40 years of age unless other predisposing conditions are present, such as Marfan's syndrome, Ehlers-Danlos syndrome, congenital heart disease, iatrogenic trauma (e.g., cardiac catheterization), bicuspid aortic valve, or pregnancy. AAD should also be considered when acute dysfunction of more than one organ system is observed.

Symptoms

- Chest pain is the most common symptom ++++ and is classically sudden in onset and ripping or tearing in quality.
- Anterior chest pain is more common in ascending aortic dissection ++++; back pain is more common in descending aortic dissection ++++. Coexisting anterior chest pain and back pain is seen less frequently.
- Pain may migrate as the dissection progresses and may also

involve the limbs, particularly if the dissection obstructs the origin of a limb vessel.
- Neurologic deficits ++
- Syncope +
- Nausea
- Diaphoresis
- Light-headedness

Signs

- Hypertension (early)
- Hypotension (late)
- Tachycardia
- Pulse deficits in extremities +++
- Aortic insufficiency (+++ in patients with ascending aorta involvement)
- Murmur over the thoracic inlet
- Tamponade
- Acute stroke + - ++
- Hemoptysis, hematemesis, Horner's syndrome, and SVC syndrome (rare)

Workup

- Laboratory tests are of little value except for a type and crossmatch and a baseline hematocrit.
- Chest x-rays are abnormal in most patients, but findings may be subtle. Mediastinal widening +++ and an indistinct aortic knob +++ are the two features most useful for predicting dissection. Tracheal or esophageal deviation, irregular aortic contour +++, change in aortic diameter compared to previous films, and left pleural effusion ++ have been reported. The calcium sign, or displacement of calcified intima (calcium ring > 6 mm from outer border of the aorta), is infrequent +.
- The best choice for establishing a definitive diagnosis is controversial. Since mortality is high and occurs quickly (50% within 48 hours of onset), the choice may be dictated by what is (most rapidly) available (Table 7-1). The preference of the surgeon who would provide definitive care for proximal dissections is also important.

Table 7-1 Diagnostic Tests for Aortic Dissection

Test	Comments
Spiral chest CT +++++	Generally rapidly available
Transesophageal echocardiography +++++	Can be done at bedside Accuracy operator dependent
Aortography +++++	Gold standard Also evaluates valves and branches 95% accurate Invasive, time consuming; may miss thrombosed false channel
MRI +++++	May be preferable for stable patients Sensitivity, 90% to 100%; specificity 94% to 99% Visualizes origins of branches Time consuming; difficult to monitor; availability varies, frequent delays

Comments and Treatment Considerations

Treatment should begin before confirmation of the diagnosis and should include infusions for control of pulse rate, blood pressure, and cardiac contractility (to minimize further progression of the dissection), such as a combination of sodium nitroprusside and a beta-blocker (e.g., esmolol drip). Early consultation with a cardiothoracic surgeon is essential. Proximal dissection is generally managed surgically, distal dissection medically. Caution: anticoagulation or thrombolysis following a misdiagnosis as MI or PE can lead to death.

REFERENCES[www]

Nienaber CA, Kodolitsch YV, Nicolas V, et al: The diagnosis of thoracic aortic dissection by noninvasive imaging procedures, *N Engl J Med* 328:1, 1993.

[www]Additional references are available on the following web site: www.signsandsymptoms.com.

Sarasin FP, Louis-Simonet M, Gaspoz JM, Junod AF: Detecting acute thoracic aortic dissection in the emergency department: time constraints and choice of the optimal diagnostic test, *Ann Emerg Med* 28:278, 1996.

Sommer T, Fehske W, Holzknecht N, et al: Aortic dissection: a comparative study of diagnosis with spiral CT, multiplanar transesophageal echocardiography, and MR imaging, *Radiology* 199:347, 1996.

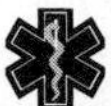

ESOPHAGEAL RUPTURE

Esophageal rupture is a dangerous condition. Early symptoms can be nonspecific, so less than half are correctly diagnosed within the first 12 hours, after which time mortality is 25%. Mortality exceeds 60% after 24 hours.

Spontaneous esophageal rupture, or Boerhaave's syndrome, occurs when esophageal pressure is significantly increased (e.g., vomiting against a closed glottis). This usually creates a small, vertical tear of the lower esophagus (90%), on the left side (90%). Other phenomena reported to induce an esophageal tear include hiccups, childbirth, weight lifting, forceful swallowing, and blunt trauma. The causes of esophageal rupture include Boerhaave's syndrome (15%), trauma (20%), foreign bodies (15%), and iatrogenic causes (50%).

Symptoms may mimic and are often misdiagnosed as perforated ulcer, acute MI, dissecting aortic aneurysm, pulmonary embolism, acute pancreatitis, spontaneous pneumothorax, lung abscess, biliary colic, mesenteric vascular occlusion, incarcerated diaphragmatic hernia, and other entities. Although esophageal rupture is most common after age 50 and is rare in children, it can occur at any age.

Symptoms

- Chest pain +++++, commonly severe, acute, and pleuritic that is generally left sided and preceded by vomiting
- Abdominal or back pain
- Dyspnea
- Dysphagia
- Nausea

Signs

- Vital signs may be normal early in the course of this disease but progress to shock.
- Tachypnea
- Fever
- Hamman's sign ++
- Chest examination provides evidence of pleural effusion.
- Subcutaneous emphysema +++
- Meckler's triad of vomiting, lower chest pain, and subcutaneous emphysema may be present.

Workup

- Chest x-ray ++++. The most common findings are effusion or infiltrate. Although effusion is more common in this entity, a patient with chest pain, dyspnea, and an effusion is more likely to have a PE (based on the prevalence of the two diseases). "V sign of Naclerio," a V-shaped hypodense area outlining fascial planes behind the heart, may be an early radiographic sign ++. Mediastinal emphysema (pneumomediastinum) may be present +++.
- Esophagography may be diagnostic ++++. If it is negative and concern for the diagnosis persists, proceed to a second study.
- Esophagoscopy
- CT (with or without oral contrast)
- ECG is helpful only to screen for myocardial ischemia as an alternative diagnosis.
- Pleurocentesis may yield the diagnosis when performed. For pleural fluid studies, a pH of <6.0 is an indicator of esophageal rupture; when esophagography findings are negative, methylene blue given orally may be detected in pleural drainage.
- Routine laboratory tests are of no value in making this diagnosis.

Comments and Treatment Considerations

Treatment of esophageal rupture requires aggressive supportive care, including drainage of gastric and pleural contents and intravenous antibiotics. Early thoracotomy with primary surgical closure of the esophageal defect is usually necessary in spontaneous or traumatic esophageal rupture. Conservative therapy is employed in some cases associated with iatrogenic or foreign-body causes and in very late presentations of spontaneous rupture, in which operative mortality approaches that of supportive care.

REFERENCES[www]

Bradley SL, Paroleiro PC, Payne WS, Gracey DR: Spontaneous rupture of the esophagus, *Arch Surg* 116:755, 1981.

DelCastillo J, Boyar C, Hess F, Miller J: Atraumatic panmural rupture of the esophagus: Boerhaave syndrome, *Ann Emerg Med* 12:385, 1983.

Walker WS, Cameron EWJ, Walbaum PR: Diagnosis and management of spontaneous transmural rupture of the oesophagus (Boerhaave's syndrome), *Br J Surg* 72:204, 1985.

[www]Additional references are available on the following web site: www.signsandsymptoms.com.

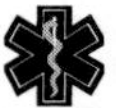

PNEUMONIA

Pneumonia is common and, depending on the etiology and general health of the patient, can be treated with outpatient antibiotics or require admission to the ICU. Patients with asthma, COPD, diabetes, CHF, renal failure, asplenic state (splenectomy or sickle cell patients), chronic liver disease, predilection for aspiration, malnutrition, recent hospitalization (<1 year), and age >65 are at particular risk. In winter, influenza pneumonia (potentially severe and complicated by staphylococcal infection) and respiratory syncytial virus should be considered in adults and children, respectively. A history of occupational exposure to animals may suggest unusual but potentially severe forms of pneumonia, such as hantavirus (rodent droppings), plague (rodents), tularemia (rabbits), Q fever, or psittacosis (pet birds). Foreign body aspiration is particularly prevalent in patients under age 3 and involves food in 61%. Tuberculosis (and respiratory isolation) should be considered in patients at risk for this disease.

Symptoms

- Cough
- Sputum production
- Pleuritic chest pain
- Fever
- Dyspnea/shortness of breath (less frequent in the elderly)
- Altered mental status

Signs

- Fever
- Tachypnea
- Tachycardia
- Diaphoresis
- Crackles
- Egophony
- Dullness to percussion
- Pleural friction rub
- Wasting
- Cyanosis
- Altered mental status
- Hypotension
- Decreased urine output
- Abdominal signs in elderly and the very young

Workup

- Chest x-ray: Standard posteroanterior and lateral (if possible) chest films should be obtained in patients whose symptoms and signs suggest the possibility of pneumonia. When only an anteroposterior film can be obtained, special attention should be paid to the heart shadow, behind which an infiltrate may hide. Plain films of children with a history of foreign body aspiration are normal in 33%; abnormal x-rays findings reveal obstructive emphysema (66%), mediastinal shift (55%), pneumonia (26%), atelectasis (18%), or radiopaque objects (only 3%).
- Arterial blood gases are not useful for diagnosis but may aid in assessing ventilatory status.
- Complete blood count is not generally useful unless risk of neutropenia (neutrophil count <1000/ml).
- Creatinine is indicated for sick patients in whom antibiotics may cause renal toxicity or require renal clearance.
- Blood cultures have low yield in patients who are likely to be treated as outpatients. Cultures are usually negative and seldom alter therapy for admitted patients. Higher yields are

seen in severely ill patients, although this infrequently influences management.

- Skin tests for tuberculosis should be obtained in patients at risk (homeless, alcoholic, immigrant, HIV-infected) who have not been vaccinated with BCG. Patients with symptoms and x-ray findings consistent with active tuberculosis should be isolated while awaiting skin test and microbiologic results.
- Sputum cultures are seldom useful because of the difficulty in obtaining an adequate (uncontaminated) specimen and the high incidence of false positives. Sputum induction for AFB or PCP should be done in a negative pressure room approved for such procedures.
- Thoracentesis should be considered when effusion accompanies pneumonia so that the need for drainage can be determined. The most important test to obtain on the pleural fluid is the pH (pH < 7.0 suggests need for chest tube drainage). Also important are cell count with differential, LDH, protein, glucose, gram stain, culture, and AFB and fungal stains and cultures.

Comments and Treatment Considerations

Findings that suggest the need for admission include a pulse >100 to 125 (in adults), respiratory rate (RR) of > 20 to 30 (in adults), temperature $>38.3^\circ$ C, hypotension, evidence of extrapulmonary involvement, or acutely altered mental status. Severe pneumonia, suggesting the need for ICU admission, is indicated by a respiratory rate (in adults) of >30, shock, and urine output less than 20 ml/hr. Radiographic features that predict increased mortality include multilobar involvement, cavitation, rapid spreading if $>50\%$ increase in 48 hours, and effusion.

Apical infiltrates suggest consideration of reactivation tuberculosis; cavitation suggests anaerobic abscess, staphylococcus, or *Pseudomonas* infection. Lymphadenopathy on chest x-rays suggests tuberculosis, fungal disease, or neoplasm. Tuberculosis may have an atypical appearance in HIV patients. Although possibly suggestive, the pattern of infiltrate does not reliably distinguish between etiologies for pneumonia.

Choice of therapy should be directed toward pathogens suspected after initial workup but should not be delayed in a seriously ill patient. The increasing prevalence of resistant strains of pneumococcus (and others) makes penicillin and amoxicillin obsolete. A macrolide antibiotic is generally adequate for outpatient therapy in an otherwise healthy patient. If the pathogen is presumably bacterial (patient with purulent sputum or COPD), second- or third-generation cephalosporins (e.g., cefuroxime, ceftriaxone, cefotaxime) are reasonable choices.

For hospitalized, nonimmunosuppressed patients, initial therapy with erythromycin (minimum is 15 to 20 mg/kg/day IV in divided doses q6h) and a second- or third-generation cephalosporin is usually adequate. ICU patients should be administered third-generation cephalosporins, erythromycin (1.0 g IV q6h), and vancomycin.

Patients with known or suspected *Pneumocystis* and a Pao_2 <70 should be treated with corticosteroids (prednisone 40 mg po, then bid, then taper) 15 to 30 minutes before specific antimicrobial therapy (e.g., TMP/SMX, 15 mg of TMP component/kg/day IV divided q 6 to 8 hr).

REFERENCES[www]

American Thoracic Society: Guidelines for the initial management of adults with community-acquired pneumonia: diagnosis, assessment of severity, and initial antimicrobial therapy, *Am Rev Respir Dis* 148:1418, 1993.

Bartlett JG, Mundy LM: Community-acquired pneumonia, *N Engl J Med* 333:1618, 1995.

Burton EM, Brick WG, Hall JD, et al: Tracheobronchial foreign body aspiration in children, *South Med J* 89:195, 1996.

Chalasani NP, Valdecanas MA, Gopal AK, et al: Clinical utility of blood cultures in adult patients with community-acquired pneumonia without defined underlying risks, *Chest* 108:932, 1995.

[www]Additional references are available on the following web site: www.signsandsymptoms.com.

Fine MJ, Auble TE, Yealy DM, et al: A prediction rule to identify low-risk patients with community acquired pneumonia, *N Engl J Med* 336:243, 1997.

Gilbert DN, Moellering RC, Sande MA: Guide to antimicrobial therapy, 1988, Antimicrobial Therapy, Inc.

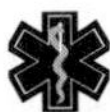

ACUTE CHEST SYNDROME AND SICKLE CELL DISEASE

Acute chest syndrome is a clinical syndrome found in sickle cell patients that may lead to death.

Symptoms

- Severe chest pain ++++
- Fever ++++
- Shortness of breath +++
- Bone pain +++

Signs

- Tachypnea
- Rhonchi +++
- Hypoxia
- Elevated temperature

Workup

- Chest x-ray may show pulmonary infiltrates +++.
- ABG, if needed, to assess ventilatory status (Pao_2 <80 +++)
- Hematocrit shows anemia; reticulocyte count should be elevated.

Comments and Treatment Considerations

The cause of acute chest syndrome is uncertain; it may represent pulmonary infarction, but cultures of blood and sputum are positive in a small percentage of patients. Treatment may include intravenous hydration, oxygen, broad-spectrum antibiotics covering *Staphylococcus aureus, Mycoplasma, Streptococcus pneumonia, and Haemophilus influenzae* (particularly if questionable vaccination history), heparin, and transfusion. Since the effect of treatment on outcome is not clear, patients may need to be admitted to the ICU.

REFERENCES

Charache S, Scott JC, Charache P: Acute chest syndrome in adults with sickle cell disease, *Arch Intern Med* 139:67, 1979.

Poncz M, Kane E, Gill FM: Acute chest syndrome in sickle cell disease: etiology and clinica correlates, *J Pediatr* 107:861, 1985.

van Agtmael MA, Cheng JD, Nossent HC: Acute chest syndrome in adult Afro-Caribbean patients with sickle cell disease, *Arch Intern Med* 154:557, 1994.

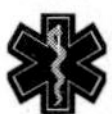

PERICARDITIS

Symptoms

- Chest pain is the most common presenting symptom +++. The pain is usually pleuritic but sometimes is dull; it may radiate to the left trapezius, is aggravated by supine posture, and is often alleviated by sitting up. The pain may last hours or days and is usually constant, but may be intermittent.
- Dyspnea ++
- Fever
- Fatigue
- Malaise
- Abdominal pain
- Syncope

Signs

- Pericardial friction rub +++, classically of three components, is best heard over the left sternal border and is usually accentuated by sitting up and leaning forward. Only one or two components may be present, and it may be audible only intermittently or over a limited area. When only a single component is present, it can be confused with a murmur.

Workup

- ECG may be abnormal ++++. Changes may evolve in four stages (Table 7-2).
- Ratio of the ST segment elevation to T wave amplitude (ST/T) of 0.25 or greater suggests pericarditis.
- Echocardiography is useful for demonstrating pericardial fluid (effusion, blood) and for determining whether tamponade is present or imminent (see Pericardial Effusion and Tamponade).
- Erythrocyte sedimentation rate (Westergren) may be elevated (over 50 mm/hr) +++ but is nonspecific.
- Chest x-rays are normal unless there is an effusion of 250 ml or other conditions coexist.

Comments and Treatment Considerations

The majority of cases are idiopathic (40% to 60%) or viral (20%). Other causes include lupus and other collagen-vascular diseases, malignancy (especially lymphoma, melanoma, and breast and lung carcinomas), uremia, bacterial infection or tuberculosis, rheumatic fever, trauma, myocardial infarction (Dressler's syndrome), cardiac surgery, radiation therapy, and certain medications.

Pericarditis usually follows viral symptoms by 2 to 4 weeks but may be concurrent. Pericardial hemorrhage leading to tamponade and death, although rare, has been reported after thrombolysis when pericarditis was misdiagnosed as myocardial infarction.

Table 7-2 ECG Evolution of Acute Pericarditis (Leads I, II, aVL, aVF, V3-6)

Stage	PR Segment	ST Segment	T Waves
I	Depressed or baseline	Elevated	Upright
II	Baseline or depressed	Baseline	Upright
III	Baseline	Baseline	Inverted
IV	Baseline	Baseline	Upright or inverted

REFERENCES[www]

Ginzton LE, Laks MM: The differential diagnosis of acute pericarditis from the normal variant: new electrocardiographic criteria, *Circulation* 65:1004, 1982.

Ilan Y, Oren R, Ben-Chetrit E: Acute pericarditis: etiology, treatment and prognosis: a study of 115 patients, *Jpn Heart J* 315, 1991.

Spodick DH: ECG in acute pericarditis; distributions of morphologic and axial changes by stages, *Am J Cardiol* 33:470, 1974.

Spodick DH: Pericardial rubs: prospective, multiple observer investigation of pericardial friction in 100 patients, *Am J Cardiol* 35:357, 1975.

Sternbach GL: Pericarditis, *Ann Emerg Med* 17:214, 1988.

[www]Additional references are available on the following web site: www.signsandsymptoms.com.

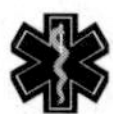

ESOPHAGEAL FOREIGN BODIES

Esophageal foreign bodies take many forms: they may be smooth or blunt, food or nonorganic objects, and ingestion may be intentional or accidental. History may be absent, and symptoms vary; the diagnosis and management largely depend on a high index of suspicion, the nature of the object ingested, and the symptoms and signs present. Although less than 1% of foreign body ingestions result in perforation or other serious complications, they account for 15% of esophageal perforations. Once past the esophagus, most foreign bodies pass through the GI tract without complication.

Symptoms

- Suspected ingestion in small children +++, but more than half of children with an esophageal foreign body have no such history; up to 18% are asymptomatic.
- Choking, gagging, or coughing that has resolved on arrival to the ED is a common presentation.
- Poor feeding
- Drooling

- Vomiting
- Difficulty swallowing
- Older children and adults usually report chest, throat or neck pain, dysphagia, or foreign body sensation.

Signs

- Physical signs are absent in most of childhood ingestions +++.
- Drooling
- For delayed cases, see Esophageal Rupture

Workup

- Oropharyngeal examination or indirect laryngoscopy may reveal a foreign object lodged high in the aerodigestive tract.
- Soft tissue neck x-rays may identify a foreign body, soft tissue swelling (especially in delayed cases, suggesting infection), or retropharyngeal air (suggesting perforation).
- X-rays of the chest and abdomen are useful for localizing and identifying some objects, such as coins, button batteries, and other highly radiopaque objects. Coins in the esophagus generally are oriented parallel to the esophagus, as opposed to tracheal coins, which are generally transverse. Diagnostic yield for ingested organic objects, such as fish or chicken bones (representing 60% of adult presentations), is low (false negative in up to 71%). Plastic and aluminum are also not generally visualized.
- Esophagoscopy is the ideal procedure when an object is obstructive, is sharp or irregular, or has a high risk of causing perforation. It can be both diagnostic and therapeutic. Negative findings, or presence only of abrasions or esophagitis, are common.
- CT scan, with or without contrast, may be useful in the diagnosis of perforation (see Esophageal Rupture).
- Esophagography may be useful for identifying obstructive objects or demonstrating perforation, but it carries the risk of vomiting and aspiration and may delay definitive diagnosis and therapy.

Comments and Treatment Considerations

Ingestions of button batteries pose particular problems. They may contain high concentrations of caustic potassium hydroxide or various potentially toxic metals (e.g., mercury). If lodged in the esophagus, they should be *immediately* removed (endoscopically if available). Once past the esophagus, observation while awaiting spontaneous passage may be employed.

Spasmolytic drugs such as glucagon (0.5 to 2.0 mg IM or slow IVP) are reported to aid in the passage of lower esophageal foreign bodies (usually food), but the success rate may not differ from that for placebo. Carbonated beverages might also assist passage. Smooth objects, such as coins, lodged in the distal esophagus will pass spontaneously in 60% and may be observed.

Esophageal foreign bodies present for prolonged periods (from 12 to 24 hours) and those in the proximal and middle thirds of the esophagus should be removed. The standard method for removal is endoscopy, but Foley catheter retrograde removal and bougienage (using a dilator to advance the object into the stomach) have been described. Any object, smooth or not, that is present for a prolonged period may cause perforation of the esophagus. Refer adults for further evaluation to rule out obstructing esophageal lesions.

REFERENCES[www]

Brady PG: Esophageal foreign bodies, *Gastroenterol Clin North Am* 20:691, 1991.

Conners GP: A literature-based comparison of three methods of pediatric esophageal coin removal, *Pediatr Emerg Care* 13:154, 1997.

Harned RK II, Strain JD, Hay TC, Douglas MR: Esophageal foreign bodies: safety and efficacy of Foley catheter extraction of coins, *Am J Roentgenol* 168:443, 1997.

Rimell FL, Thome A Jr, Stool S, et al: Characteristics of objects that cause choking in children, *JAMA* 274:1763, 1995.

Tibbling L, Bjorkhoel A, Jansson E, Stenkvist M: Effect of spasmolytic drugs on esophageal foreign bodies, *Dysphagia* 10:126, 1995.

[www]Additional references are available on the following web site: www.signsandsymptoms.com.

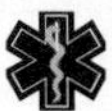 *PANIC DISORDER*

Panic disorder (PD) occurs in up to 25% of ED patients with chest pain. The quality of pain is often indistinguishable from ischemic pain. Since patients with PD often have coexistent CAD, a diagnosis of panic disorder is infrequently made in the ED. Many patients with panic disorder have coexisting symptoms of depression, including suicidal ideation (10%).

Symptoms

- Chest pain
- Dyspnea
- Palpitations
- Dizziness
- Sweating
- Trembling
- Fear of losing control
- Fear of dying
- Acral paresthesias
- Prior history of similar events
- Fear of additional attacks

Signs

- Tachycardia
- Tachypnea
- Normal examination

Workup

- ECG
- Chest x-rays are useful for ruling out other diagnoses.

Comments and Treatment Considerations

ED physicians must be careful not to miss possible myocardial infarction in patients with panic disorder who are at risk, as well as not to overlook the potential for suicide in patients with chest pain and other psychiatric symptoms.

REFERENCES[www]

Carter SC, Servan-Schreiber D, Perlstein WM: Anxiety disorders and the syndrome of chest pain with normal coronary arteries: prevalence and pathophysiology, *J Clin Psychiatry* 58(suppl 3):70, 1997.

[www]Additional references are available on the following web site: www.signsandsymptoms.com.

Fleet RP, Dupuis G, Kaczorowski J, et al: Suicidal ideation in emergency department chest pain patients: panic disorder a risk factor, *Am J Emerg Med* 15:345, 1997.

Fleet RP, Dupuis G, Marchand A, et al: Panic disorder in emergency department chest pain patients: prevalence, co-morbidity, suicidal ideation, and physician recognition, *Am J Med* 101:371, 1996.

Yingling KW, Wulsin LR, Arnold LM, Rouan GW: Estimated prevalence of panic disorder and depression among consecutive patients seen in an emergency department with acute chest pain, *J Gen Intern Med* 8:231, 1993.

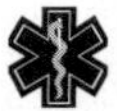

CHEST PAIN IN CHILDREN

Chest pain is a common presenting complaint in children, accounting for an estimated 650,000 ED visits annually and 0.6% of all visits. Most are due to non-life-threatening conditions, and only 2% require hospital admission. Causes include chest wall pains (24% to 41%), idiopathic (12% to 21%), pulmonary disease (cough, pneumonia, asthma combine for 21%), minor trauma (5%), and psychogenic (5% to 9%). Cardiac causes (including SVT and bradycardia, among others) constitute less than 5%. The vast majority of cases require only a history and physical for diagnosis. Family history of MI is actually associated with decreased likelihood of an organic cause of pain.

Symptoms

- Chest pain of acute onset and pain awakening a child from sleep are associated with organic disease (3 and 3.6-fold increased likelihood, respectively).
- Features or past medical history suggestive of one of the entities discussed in the previous sections (especially pneumonia, pneumothorax, pericarditis or pericardial tamponade, traumatic aortic rupture, or esophageal foreign body—the others being very uncommon in children) should also elicit further clinical investigation.
- Kawasaki's disease is a rare cause of pain and one of the few causes of ischemic cardiac disease in children.

Signs

- Fever (12-fold increased likelihood of organic disease), tachycardia, and other abnormal physical findings may warrant additional testing in the ED.

Workup

- Laboratory tests are rarely useful.
- Chest x-rays in children selected on the basis of history and physical are positive in 11% of children with chest pain. If pneumonia is excluded, positive findings are present in only 2%.
- ECGs are positive in 10% but are commonly misread in the ED (normal conduction intervals, size of the QRS complex, and features of the ST segment and T wave vary with age and may differ greatly from those in adults), and only 2% to 3% of abnormalities found arc clinically relevant.

REFERENCES[www]

Berezin S, Medow MS, Glassman MS, Newman LJ: Chest pain of gastrointestinal origin, *Arch Dis Child* 63:1457, 1988.

Kaden GG, Shenker IR, Gootman N: Chest pain in adolescents, *J Adolesc Health* 12:251, 1991.

Rowe BH, Dulberg CS, Peterson RG, et al: Characteristics of children presenting with chest pain to a pediatric emergency department, *Can Med Assoc J* 143:388, 1990.

Selbst SM: Chest pain in children, *Pediatr Rev* 18:169, 1997.

Sclbst SM, Ruddy RM, Clark BJ, et al: Pediatric chest pain: a prospective study, *Pediatrics* 82:319, 1988.

[www]Additional references are available on the following web site: www.signsandsymptoms.com.

CHAPTER 8

Dizziness (Vertigo)

STEPHEN EPSTEIN

Dizziness is one of the more difficult diagnostic dilemmas an emergency physician faces. In particular, vertigo, the illusory sense of motion, must be distinguished from syncope or near-syncope (See Chapter 31, Syncope and Near-Syncope). Vertigo is most often caused by an inner ear process, but the emergency physician must be alert to the possibility of a CNS cause. Central causes of vertigo may be only minimally symptomatic, in contrast to the generally severe symptoms attributable to peripheral causes. Particular attention must be given to elderly patients, who more frequently have a serious cause of their dizziness.

In addition to a thorough examination, including a detailed neurologic examination (with particular attention to cranial nerve and cerebellar function), attention should be paid to the features of nystagmus, which tend to have characteristic patterns when vertigo is attributable to central or peripheral causes. If not already present at rest, nystagmus can generally be induced by moving a patient quickly from a seated to a lying position and then turning the head gently to the side (Nylen-Barany test).

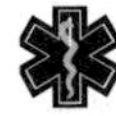

CENTRAL VERTIGO

CEREBELLAR HEMORRHAGE AND INFARCTION

Vertigo can be the initial symptom of a CNS process including cerebellar bleed or infarction. An intracranial process should be suspected in older patients, particularly those at risk for vertebrobasilar artery disease. Neurologic findings should further this suspicion, since their presence is specific, but not sensitive, for a CNS process. Symptoms may vary little with position. A complete neurologic exam that includes gait testing is essential.

Symptoms

- Vertigo may be minimal and be the only symptom ++, generally not significantly positional.
- Symptoms associated with pathologic conditions of the posterior circulation (clumsiness, weakness, change in speech) are variably present.
- Altered level of consciousness is uncommon.

Signs

- Neurologic findings are variably present and may indicate neurologic dysfunction in vertebrobasilar arterial distribution (e.g., dysmetria, dysarthria, facial palsy, ataxia).
- Nystagmus that has no latency period with lateral gaze, is nonfatiguing, or multidirectional suggests a central process.

Workup

- MRI is the test of choice for imaging the posterior fossa.
- CT demonstrates most bleeding and large lesions.

Comments and Treatment Considerations

One study found a 25% rate of cerebellar infarction in elderly patients who had nystagmus and had been dizzy for more than 2 days. ED consultation with a neurologist or neurosurgeon should be arranged for patients with a central cause of vertigo.

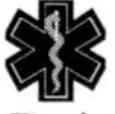

PERIPHERAL VERTIGO

Peripheral vertigo is generally very symptomatic, with prominent nausea and vomiting. Positioning may dramatically increase the severity of symptoms. History or physical examination may reveal otitis media, recent upper respiratory tract infection, previous exposure to ototoxic drugs, or recurrent episodes with progressive tinnitus and deafness (Ménière's disease). Often a precipitant cannot be found, and a diagnosis of benign positional vertigo is made.

Symptoms

- Profound vertigo ++++
- Nausea and vomiting

Signs

- Neurologic examination is normal.
- Nystagmus is typically horizontal or rotary, never vertical, and typically brought about by changes in head position. Generally, after the patient is asked to look laterally, a brief period elapses before nystagmus occurs. The nystagmus should be time limited. Nystagmus is suppressed by visual fixation.

Workup

No ancillary tests are required in the ED if peripheral vertigo is diagnosed.

Comments and Treatment Considerations

Treatment of peripheral vertigo consists of vestibular suppressant drugs. Meclizine (25 mg po q6-8h) remains the cornerstone of treatment. Although the phenothiazines (prochlorperazine), benzodiazepines (diazepam), and scopolamine also have efficacy, they can cause significant side effects. Head positioning maneuvers are sometimes used successfully in benign positional vertigo. Rapid resolution over the course of several days is the norm, although symptoms occasionally are persistent. Patients should be directed for follow-up, since rarely a cranial nerve VIII lesion or other condition requiring treatment is the cause of persistent peripheral vertigo.

REFERENCES[www]

Cohen NL: The dizzy patient: update on vestibular disorders, *Med Clin North Am* 75:6, 1991.

Froehling DA, Silverstein MD, Mohr DN, Beatty CW: Does this dizzy patient have a serious form of vertigo? *JAMA* 271:385, 1994.

Herr RD, Zun L, Matthews JJ: A directed approach to the dizzy patient, *Ann Emerg Med* 18:664,1989.

Norrving B, Magnusson M, Holtas S: Isolated acute vertigo in the elderly: vestibular or vascular disease? *Acta Neurol Scand* 91:43, 1995.

[www]Additional references are available on the following web site: www.signsandsymptoms.com.

CHAPTER 9

Ear Pain

STEPHEN EPSTEIN and JEREMY BROWN

Ear pain is a frequent complaint of patients in the ambulatory setting. The cause of ear pain is most commonly otitis media (OM) or otitis externa (OE). Although antibiotics are usually prescribed (often amoxicillin for initial treatment; trimethoprim-sulfamethoxazole (amoxicillin–clavulanic acid, or cefaclor for bacterial resistance or treatment failure), most cases of acute OM in children resolve spontaneously. Inflammation of the external auditory canal (OE) is caused by a number of bacterial agents including *Pseudomonas aeruginosa.* Uncomplicated OE is usually treated with an antibiotic ear drop solution (e.g., polymyxin B–neomycin–hydrocortisone qid).

Most cases of OM and OE are self-limited or effectively treated by oral antibiotics; however, serious complications occasionally occur. Mastoiditis and malignant otitis are rare diseases that are diagnosed based on the findings at physical examination. Patients at higher risk include those who are immunosuppressed as a result of diabetes, chemotherapeutics, or steroids, as well as those at extremes of age.

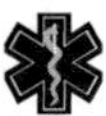

MASTOIDITIS

Mastoiditis is a rare condition usually seen in children. The diagnosis is made on clinical examination and occasionally may be subtle in patients being treated with antibiotics. Other coexisting or complicating conditions include neck abscess (Bezold abscess), facial nerve palsy, cavernous sinus thrombosis, meningitis, and intracranial abscess.

Symptoms

- Ear pain +++++
- Fever ++++
- Pain and fever lasting more than 4 days ++++
- Discharge +++
- Headache
- Irritability or gastrointestinal upset may be the only symptoms in infants.

Signs

- Postauricular swelling with erythema and tenderness +++++
- Mastoid tenderness, especially posterior and superior to the level of the external canal (Macewen's triangle)
- Pinna may be displaced outward and forward by the swelling ++++.
- Signs of otitis media

Workup

- Clinical diagnosis without need for laboratory studies
- CT scan is indicated if abscess is a concern.
- Blood cultures are generally low yield.

Comments and Treatment Considerations

Patients with mastoiditis should be admitted for intravenous antibiotics (e.g., ceftriaxone). ENT consultation should be obtained, because mastoidectomy or surgical drainage of a subperiosteal abscess may be indicated. Approximately 90% resolve with conservative therapy alone.

REFERENCES[www]

Adams G, Boies L, Hilger P, editors: *Fundamentals of otolaryngology*, Philadelphia, 1989, WB Saunders.

Harley E, Sdralis T, Berkowitz RG: Acute mastoiditis in children: a 12-year retrospective study, *Otolaryngol Head Neck Surg* 116:29,1997.

[www]Additional references are available on the following web site: www.signsandsymptoms.com.

Hawkins DB, Dru D, House JW, Clark RW: Acute mastoiditis in children: a review of 54 cases, *Laryngoscope* 93:568, 1983.
Khafif A, Halperin D, Hochman I, et al: Acute mastoiditis: a 10-year review, *Am J Otol* 19:170, 1998.

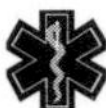

MALIGNANT OTITIS EXTERNA

Malignant otitis externa is a rare extension of otitis externa to surrounding tissues and is most commonly seen in diabetics and other immunocompromised patients.

Symptoms

- Severe unrelenting pain +++++
- Discharge ++++
- Prior history of otitis externa
- Fever and trismus (less common)

Signs

- Erythema and edema of the pinna and periauricular tissues
- Exacerbation of pain with movement of the pinna
- Cranial nerve palsies (most frequently VII) in advanced cases ++

Workup

- Clinical diagnosis without need for laboratory studies
- Glucose to rule out diabetes

Comments and Treatment Considerations

Patients who are immunocompromised or have significant infection should be admitted for intravenous antibiotics (e.g., imipenem, meropenem, or ciprofloxacin). *Pseudomonas* is the most common pathogen, but *Streptococcus, Staphylococcus,* and *Proteus* are also seen. ENT consultation is required.

For less severe cases in immunocompetent patients, treatment with fluoroquinolones (e.g., ciprofloxacin 500 mg po bid) and ear drops (e.g., polymyxin B–neomycin–hydrocortisone qid; place wick in auditory canal if edema) with ENT follow-up within 24 hours may be considered.

REFERENCES

Rubin J, Yu VL: Malignant external otitis: insights into pathogenesis, clinical manifestations, diagnosis, and therapy, *Am J Med* 85:391, 1988.

Santamaria JP, Abrunzo TJ: Ear and nose emergencies. In American College of Emergency Physicians: *Pediatric emergency medicine: a comprehensive study guide,* New York, 1995, McGraw-Hill.

CHAPTER 10

Extremity Pain and Numbness

STEVEN GO

Nontraumatic extremity pain is not a particularly common nor dangerous-sounding complaint. However, this symptom may arise in several disorders that are virtually impossible to diagnose unless the emergency physician's clinical suspicion for them is very high. Thus emergency physicians must consider spinal or vascular emergencies as possible causes of local extremity complaints.

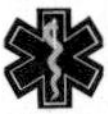

ACUTE ARTERIAL OCCLUSION

Acute arterial occlusion generally presents with an abrupt onset of pain. Classic findings—such as a cold, blue extremity, and the 5 p's (pain, pallor, paresthesia, pulselessness, and paralysis)—generally occur late. Ischemic tissue death can begin within 4 hours. Chronic arterial insufficiency also can cause ischemic changes. Worsening claudication or rest claudication may be the presenting symptom in the lower extremities that have collateral flow.

It is important to determine the cause of the obstruction because treatment can vary on the basis of whether the obstruction is due to in situ thrombosis or an embolus. Thrombosis is likely in the face of preexisting peripheral vascular disease as a result of local stasis. Embolic disease frequently occurs in patients without preexisting symptoms of peripheral arterial occlusive disease and is associated with atrial fibrillation or recent cardioversion.

Symptoms

Severity of symptoms depends on the location of the occlusion and on the level of collateral flow that had developed previously.

- Pain +++++
- Coldness
- Paresthesia
- Numbness
- Paralysis
- Acute embolic occlusion in digits may present rapidly with sudden pain and coldness.

Signs

- Tenderness
- Pallor
- Ischemic pain (typically worsens with passive stretch of ischemic muscles)
- Sensory deficit
- Paralysis (late)
- Pulse deficit
- Livedo reticularis (a fishnet appearance of the skin), coldness, and cyanosis
- Bruits may be heard in the presence of fistulas or aneurysms.

Workup

- Bedside Doppler examination should be used to determine the presence or absence of pulses, given previous studies showing physicians' inaccuracy in determining the presence of pulses by palpation alone.
- Ankle brachial indices (ABI), defined as the highest Doppler-derived systolic ankle blood pressure in either the dorsalis pedis or posterior tibial artery in each leg divided by the highest brachial artery systolic pressure, may indicate severity of disease (<50% indicates severe insufficiency).
- Allen's test (measuring the number of seconds of capillary refill in the hand by the ulnar and radial arteries) should be done if upper extremity occlusion is suspected.
- ECG (and/or echocardiography) should be obtained if an embolic cause is suspected.

Comments and Treatment Considerations

Once an acute arterial occlusion is suspected, an emergent vascular surgical consultation is warranted before other investigative studies are begun. Decisions about which confirmatory studies, if any, to be ordered should be made in consultation with a vascular surgeon. These may include color flow Doppler studies, arteriography, or magnetic resonance angiography. Once arterial occlusion has occurred, loss of muscle viability soon follows.

REFERENCES

Kazmers A, Koski ME, Groehn H, et al: Assessment of noninvasive lower extremity arterial testing versus pulse exam, *Am Surg* 62:315, 1996.

O'Donnell TF Jr: Arterial diagnosis and management of acute thrombosis of the lower extremity, *Can J Surg* 36:349, 1993.

Strandness DE Jr: Acute arterial occlusion, *Heart Dis Stroke* 2:322, 1993.

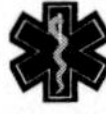

COMPARTMENT SYNDROME

Compartment syndrome (CS) occurs when the intracompartmental pressure compresses the neurovascular structures in an osseofascial space. It can occur in the leg (most common), foot, hand, forearm, arm, shoulder, thigh, and buttocks, with or without fractures. Some diseases predispose to compartment syndrome, including hemophilia, sickle cell disease, and anticoagulant use. The majority of cases occur after trauma (acute or repetitive).

Symptoms

- Pain +++++ (may be out of proportion to injury)
- Tightness and swelling
- Throbbing
- Paresthesias
- Weakness (late)
- Numbness (late)

Signs

- Swollen, tense compartment +++++

- Pain ++++ is exacerbated by passive stress of the compartment in question, although the severity of pain on passive stretch or palpation does not predict the amount of pressure.
- Diminished two-point discrimination +++
- Hyperesthesia
- Anesthesia
- Skin may be shiny and warm.
- Weakness (late)
- Loss of pulse (late)

Workup

- Compartment pressure measurement +++++
- Serial measurements should be performed by the same operator using the same method when possible.
- Nerve stimulation studies, arteriography, and Doppler studies have been described as diagnostic adjuncts but have limited use in an emergent setting.
- Laboratory testing is not useful.

Comments and Treatment Considerations

The level of pressure at which fasciotomy is indicated is controversial. Many cite a threshold from 30 mm Hg to 45 mm Hg. Alternatively, compartment pressure as a percentage of diastolic pressure has been used as a threshold. In general, elevated compartment pressures (30 mm Hg or greater) or a strong clinical suspicion of neurovascular compromise should prompt emergency orthopedic or surgical consultation. Failure to diagnose CS can have devastating consequences, and serial measurements may be required; the patient may need to be admitted for reevaluation. CS should always be suspected in extremity injuries.

REFERENCES

Abramowitz AJ, Schepsis AA: Chronic exertional compartment syndrome of the lower leg, *Orthop Rev* 23:219, 1994.

Good LP: Compartment syndrome: a closer look at etiology, treatment, *AORN J* 56:904, 1992.

Mabee JR: Compartment syndrome: a complication of acute extremity trauma, *J Emerg Med* 12:651, 1994.

McGee DL, Dalsey WC: The mangled extremity: compartment syndrome and amputations, *Emerg Med Clin North Am* 10:783, 1992.

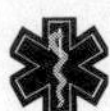

DEEP VENOUS THROMBOSIS

Risk factors for deep venous thrombosis (DVT) include prolonged venous stasis, advanced age, pregnancy (postpartum state), premenopausal estrogen use, obesity, malignancy, hypercoagulable states, congestive heart failure, trauma, long bone fractures, paralysis, dehydration, and polycythemia. A scoring system has been proposed to characterize pretest probability of disease to be used in association with ultrasound imaging (Table 10-1).

Symptoms

- Pain
- Swelling
- Erythema

Signs

- Normal examination +++
- Swelling (measured difference between lower extremities)
- Warmth
- Erythema
- Tenderness of thigh or calf
- Fever
- Homans' sign (frequently mentioned, but rare)
- Palpable venous "cord" in the popliteal fossa

Workup

- Duplex scanning (real-time ultrasound plus Doppler ultrasound). *Advantages:* Noninvasive; sensitivity for proximal DVT greater than Doppler alone; can diagnose conditions other than DVT; relatively inexpensive. *Disadvantages:* Operator dependent; inaccurate for DVT below the knee; frequently negative in patients with proven PE.
- Contrast venography. *Advantages:* Considered the "gold standard"; can view entire deep system of lower extremity. *Disadvantages:* Invasive; contrast dye load; can rarely cause DVT; cannot be done in 10% of patients (inability to acquire venous access, infection, renal insufficiency, previous allergy); observer disagreement (10%).

Table 10-1 Scoring System For Pretest Probability of Deep Vein Thrombosis

Clinical Feature	Score
Active cancer	+1
Paralysis, paresis, or recent casting of lower extremities	+1
Recently bedridden for more than 3 days or major surgery within 4 weeks	+1
Localized tenderness along the distribution of the deep venous system	+1
Entire leg swollen	+1
Calf swelling greater than 3 cm when compared with asymptomatic leg	+1
Pitting edema	+1
Collateral superficial veins (nonvaricose)	+1
Alternative diagnosis as likely or greater than that of DVT	−2

From Wells SP, Anderson DR, Bormanis J, et al: *Lancet* 350:1795, 1997.
Pretest probabilities based on Table 10-1: high ≥3; moderate 1-2, low ≤ 0 (see also Pulmonary Embolus in Chapter 7, Chest Pain).

- Impedance plethysmography. *Advantages:* Noninvasive; may be useful for serial examinations for propagation of calf vein thrombosis. *Disadvantages:* Poor performance below the knee; cannot distinguish between thrombotic and non-thrombotic obstruction of venous flow (e.g., CHF can lead to a positive result); poor in obese or uncooperative patients; variable sensitivity and specificity for proximal DVT have been reported. Not commonly available in the United States.
- MRI. *Advantages*: High accuracy reported in small trials to date. *Disadvantages*: High cost, limited data.

Comments and Treatment Considerations

Proximal DVT requires anticoagulation and admission to prevent pulmonary embolism. Administration of intravenous heparin following a weight-based nomogram is suggested, although subcutaneous low-molecular-weight heparin may provide an outpatient alternative in some cases. Calf DVT may propagate to proximal DVT. Management of calf DVT is controversial. Treatment options include admission for intravenous heparin and outpatient treatment with subcutaneous low-molecular-weight heparin or nonsteroidal antiinflammatory drug treatments. If outpatient management is elected, close follow-up is essential.

REFERENCES

Koopman MMW, van Beek EJ, ten Cate JW: Diagnosis of deep vein thrombosis, *Prog Cardiovasc Dis* 37:1, 1994.

Richlie DG: Noninvasive imaging of the lower extremity for deep venous thrombosis, *J Gen Intern Med* 8:271, 1993.

Stephen JM, Feied CF: Venous thrombosis: lifting the clouds of misunderstanding, *Postgrad Med* 97:36, 1995.

Wells SP, Anderson DR, Bormanis J, et al: Value of assessment of pretest probability of deep-vein thrombosis in clinical management, *Lancet* 350:1795, 1997.

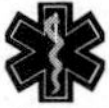

SUPERIOR VENA CAVA SYNDROME

Superior vena cava syndrome (SVCS) is a process characterized by obstruction of venous return in the thoracic portion of the SVC and is associated with facial or upper extremity swelling. This condition is most commonly seen in patients with malignancy due to hypercoagulable state or in patients with intrathoracic neoplasms that compress the SVC. The diagnosis is established clinically, with imaging studies performed to identify the causal lesion. In an immunocompromised host, tuberculosis or histoplasmosis should be considered. Less common causes include goiter, fibrosis, and aortic valve replacement. Iatrogenic causes include pacer wires, catheters, and central lines. Although symptoms may have a gradual onset, they may rapidly progress to become life threatening.

Symptoms

- Swelling of face, upper extremities, upper chest
- Dyspnea
- Cough

- Chest pain
- Difficulty swallowing
- Hoarseness
- Stridor
- Headache
- Nasal stuffiness
- Tongue swelling
- Nausea
- Light headedness
- Can be occult

Signs

- Facial edema ++++
- Jugular venous distention +++
- Distention of thoracic veins +++
- Dyspnea +++
- Facial plethora ++
- Upper extremity edema ++
- Cyanosis ++
- Paralysis of true vocal cords
- Papilledema
- Syncope
- Horner's syndrome (rare)

Workup

- Chest x-rays ++++
- Computed tomography +++++
- MRI +++++
- Venography not generally required
- Nuclear flow studies (using nonthrombogenic tracers) recommended by some authors

Comments and Treatment Considerations

Early consultation is important. The most common treatment is radiation therapy. Emergent stabilization measures may include elevation of the head of bed, oxygen, steroids, and occasionally diuretics.

REFERENCES

Abner A: Approach to the patient who presents with superior vena cava obstruction, *Chest* 103(suppl):394, 1993.

Baker GL, Barnes HJ: Superior vena cava syndrome: etiology, diagnosis, and treatment, *Am J Crit Care* 1:54, 1992.

Uaje C, Kahsen K, Parish L: Oncology emergencies, *Crit Care Nurs Q* 18:26, 1996.

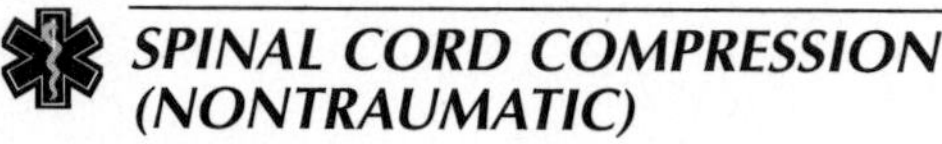

SPINAL CORD COMPRESSION (NONTRAUMATIC)

See Chapter 4, Back Pain, Lower.

CHAPTER 11

Eye Pain and Redness

JOSEPH S. ENGLANOFF

A chief complaint of an irritated, red eye is a common occurrence in the ED. The majority of cases typically involve viral or bacterial conjunctivitis, but vision-threatening causes and infections must always be considered. Global conjunctival injection should be distinguished from perilimbic injection, which is commonly seen in iritis.

True eye pain is a concerning symptom, as conjunctival irritation alone generally causes itching or a gritty sensation, but not pain. Pain is caused by pathologic conditions of other structures, such as the cornea, iris, and deeper eye tissues, or by inflammation of tissues surrounding the eye.

If topical anesthesia (used only for diagnostic and not prescribed for therapeutic purposes) does not provide pain relief, pathologic conditions deep to the cornea should be suspected. Consensual pain (eye pain elicited by shining a light in the opposite, unaffected eye) suggests iritis. Pain with eye movement is suggestive of bulbar or retrobulbar neuritis in the absence of orbital cellulitis, which causes similar symptoms. Eye pain with systemic symptoms raises the concern of glaucoma.

A complete ophthalmologic examination including visual acuity, lid eversion to rule out foreign body, and pupillary, slit-lamp, and funduscopic examinations are necessary in most cases in which typical conjunctivitis is not obvious. Measurement of intraocular pressure (IOP) and indirect ophthalmoscopy should also be performed when indicated.

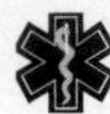

ACUTE ANGLE-CLOSURE GLAUCOMA

In acute angle-closure glaucoma, onset of symptoms is usually sudden and is often secondary to rapid pupillary dilation (e.g., after entering a darkened room or after use of anticholinergic or sympathomimetic [mydriatic] ophthalmic medications). Patients may appear systemically ill and report nausea and vomiting, as well as headache and eye pain. Most patients with angle-closure glaucoma are older than 50 years of age.

Symptoms

- Monocular eye pain usually of sudden onset
- Diffuse blurred vision (almost always)
- Nausea and vomiting secondary to vagal stimulation
- Frontal headache usually of sudden onset
- Colored halos around bright objects

Signs

- Closed angle or a shallow anterior chamber that may be seen by illuminating the iris temporally and failing to see the light reflection on the nasal aspect of the iris
- Corneal haziness or cloudiness almost always seen secondary to corneal edema
- Conjunctival injection
- Fixed mid-dilated pupil (very common)

Workup

- IOP measurement is necessary to rule out glaucoma. Pressure can be measured by Schiøtz tonometer, applanation method, Tono-Pen, or air-puff tonometer.
- Slit-lamp examination may show a shallow anterior chamber; glycerin eye drops may be needed to temporarily rid the cornea of edema and allow visualization of the anterior chamber.
- Palpation of the globe is a crude and unreliable method for assessing increased IOP.
- Funduscopic examination may be difficult, but mydriatic drops should not be used.

Comments and Treatment Considerations

Acute angle-closure glaucoma is an emergency that requires immediate ophthalmologic consultation. Outcome depends on the duration of the attack as opposed to the level of IOP, with total and permanent loss of vision usually occurring in about 12 hours. The goal of therapy is to decrease IOP as quickly as possible by instituting measures to both decrease production and increase removal of aqueous humor. While awaiting emergent ophthalmologic consultation, consider administering pilocarpine 2% every 15 minutes until pupillary constriction, then every 4 hours as needed (treat opposite eye prophylactically every 6 hours); topical timolol maleate 0.5% one drop; acetazolamide (carbonic anhydrase inhibitor) 500 mg po/IV; isosorbide or glycerin 1 ml/kg po (if no nausea or vomiting) or mannitol 20% IV (2.5 to 10 ml/kg) over 30 to 60 min. Antiemetics are also useful. Definitive treatment is a peripheral iridotomy.

REFERENCES

Fingeret M: Glaucoma medications, glaucoma therapy, and the evolving paradigm, *J Am Optom Assoc* 69:115, 1998.

Hillman JS: Acute closed-angle glaucoma: an investigation into the effects of delay in treatment, *Br J Ophthalmol* 63:817, 1979.

Sivalingam E: Glaucoma: an overview, *J Ophthalmic Nurs Technol* 15:15, 1996.

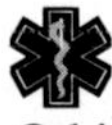

ORBITAL CELLULITIS

Orbital cellulitis must be distinguished from less severe infections including periorbital (preseptal) cellulitis. Orbital cellulitis must always be considered in any case of eyelid inflammation because of the devastating sequelae of brain abscess, cranial nerve palsies, and possibly blindness or death from sepsis. Orbital cellulitis may complicate ethmoid sinusitis.

Symptoms

- Eye pain
- Pain with eye movement
- Intense eyelid swelling
- Vision may be normal but blurred

- Double vision (common)
- Fever
- Headaches

Signs

- Eyelid inflammation with edema, erythema, and tenderness (Fig. 11-1)
- Proptosis and restricted eye movement or pain with movement (very common)
- Conjunctival injection, chemosis, and subconjunctival hemorrhages (common)
- Afferent pupillary defect (APD) with or without papilledema possible with orbital apex involvement (uncommon)
- Fifth cranial nerve sensory deficits (uncommon)

Workup

- CT scan of the orbits and sinuses rules out orbital cellulitis in equivocal cases and delineates infection margins if positive.
- Complete ophthalmologic evaluation is essential, checking for restrictive eye movement, APD, proptosis, and papilledema.
- CBC and ESR are not useful.
- Blood cultures may be helpful in patients who appear toxic.

Comments and Treatment Considerations

The most common causative organisms are *Staphylococcus aureus, Streptococcus pyogenes, S. pneumonia,* and *Haemophilus influenzae.* Treatment for orbital cellulitis begins with broad-spectrum intravenous antibiotics (e.g., antistaphylococcal agents and third-generation cephalosporin). ED consultation, followed by hospital admission, is required.

REFERENCES

Seah LL, Fu ER: Acute orbital cellulitis—a review of 17 cases, *Ann Acad Med Singapore* 26:409, 1997.

Tole DM, Anderton LC, Hayward JM: Orbital cellulitis demands early recognition, urgent admission, and aggressive management, *J Accid Emerg Med* 12:151, 1995.

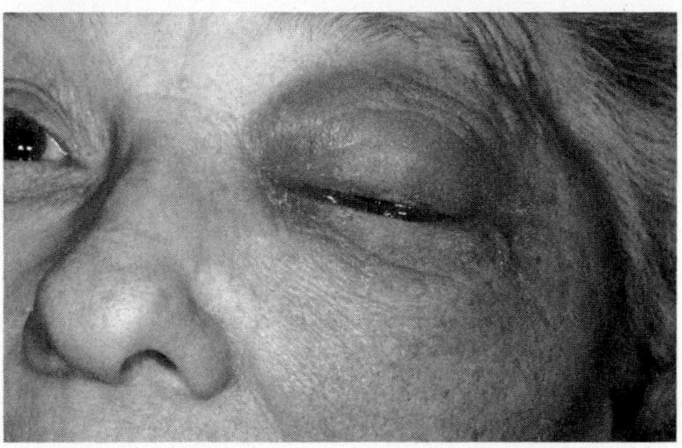

Fig. 11-1 Orbital cellulitis. Deep orbital infection is more commonly seen in children. (From Palay DA, Krachmer JH: *Ophthalmology for the primary care physician,* St Louis, 1997, Mosby.)

Uzcategui N, Warman R, Smith A, Howard CW: Clinical practice guidelines for the management of orbital cellulitis, *J Pediatr Ophthalmol Strabismus* 35:73, 1998.

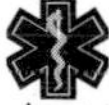

ANTERIOR UVEITIS AND IRITIS

Anterior uveitis and iritis can be caused by a number of systemic and local processes including juvenile rheumatoid arthritis, ulcerative colitis, ankylosing spondylitis, Reiter's syndrome, tuberculosis, syphilis, herpes, leukemia, lymphoma, and ocular trauma.

Symptoms

- Photophobia (almost always)
- Unilateral gradual onset of eye pain
- Red eye without discharge
- Blurred vision (common)
- Excessive tearing
- Other symptoms of primary medical condition

Signs

- Perilimbal injection
- Consensual photophobia—pain in the involved eye when light is shined in the uninvolved eye (very common)
- Miosis may be present.
- Cornea may be normal.

Workup

- Slit-lamp examination: cells and flare (WBC and RBC) in the anterior chamber are the hallmark signs. Posterior synechiae (iris adherent to the lens) may be seen.
- IOP may be low.
- Evaluation for possible primary disorder may include CBC, ESR, RPR, ANA, HLA-B27, FTA-ABS, PPD, CXR, Lyme titer.

Comments and Treatment Considerations

Anterior uveitis and iritis are ophthalmologic urgencies that once diagnosed need very close follow-up with an ophthalmologist. The initial treatment consists of topical cycloplegic agents and topical steroids (e.g., prednisolone [Pred-Forte] 1% q4-6h). This regimen rids the patient of the photophobia and suppresses the inflammatory response. The majority of cases resolve in 2 to 4 weeks, with long-term complications being permanent synechiae and glaucoma.

REFERENCES

Nishimoto JY: Iritis: how to recognize and manage potentially sight-threatening disease, *Postgrad Med* 99:255, 1996.

Suttorp-Schulten MS, Rothova A: The possible impact of uveitis in blindness: a literature survey, *Br J Ophthalmol* 80:844,1996.

Talley DK: Traumatic anterior uveitis, *Optom Clin* 3:21, 1993.

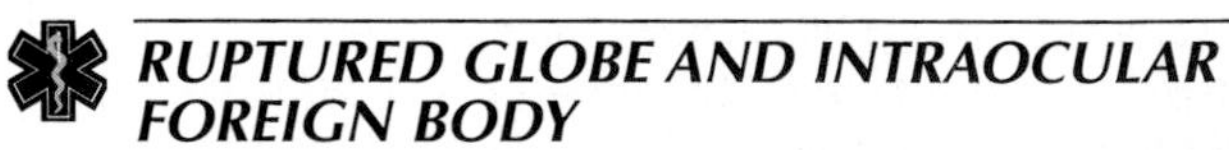

RUPTURED GLOBE AND INTRAOCULAR FOREIGN BODY

A ruptured globe is caused by a penetrating or blunt blow to the eye that results in a full-thickness scleral or corneal disruption. The patient's history may include exposure to a high-velocity projectile (including hammering metal) or blunt trauma (including air bag). A high index of suspicion is paramount, since up to 50% of ruptures are occult.

Symptoms

- Decreased vision
- Nausea and vomiting
- Eye pain

Signs

Examine *both* eyes for comparison

- Decreased visual acuity ++++
- No obvious evidence of rupture +++
- Decreased IOP ++++, although in obvious rupture it is prudent to *avoid* tonometry.
- Hyphema ++++, limited specificity. Ruptured globe must be ruled out when hyphema is present.
- Hemorrhagic chemosis ++++, if subconjunctival hemorrhage of > 180 degrees
- Afferent pupillary defect ++++, limited specificity
- Ovaling or pear-shaped tenting of the pupil is a subtle but specific sign.
- Fluorescein streaming indicates a full-thickness corneal laceration.
- Increased or decreased depth of anterior chamber ++++
- Vitreal hemorrhage ++++, specificity limited

Workup

- Orbital x-ray to rule out metallic foreign body
- Orbital CT, with coronal, sagittal, and axial cuts of 1.5 mm, is best for localizing rupture site and foreign body and for evaluating other associated injuries, such as orbital fractures and hemorrhage.
- Ultrasound, which requires some ocular manipulation, appears to be less useful for diagnosing rupture.

Comments and Treatment Considerations

Place a metallic protective shield over the eye and keep the patient NPO while awaiting ED ophthalmologic consultation. Avoid manipulation of the globe; do not perform tonometry or patching.

Due to the high risk of rebleeding, avoid salicylates and NSAIDs in hyphemas. Consider prophylactic antibiotics (e.g., IV vancomycin and either gentamicin or a second- or third-generation cephalosporin) to prevent endophthalmitis. Avoid topical antibiotics. Administer tetanus prophylaxis if indicated.

REFERENCES

Coles WH: Indirect global ruptures and sharp scleral injuries. In Fraunfelder FT, Roy FH, editors: *Current ocular therapy*, ed 4, Philadelphia, 1995, WB Saunders.

Navon SE: Management of the ruptured globe, *Int Ophthalmol Clin* 35:71, 1995.

Shingleton BJ: Eye injuries, *N Engl J Med* 325:408, 1991.

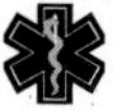

CONJUNCTIVITIS, KERATITIS, AND OPHTHALMIA NEONATORUM

Most cases of conjunctivitis have bacterial, viral, or allergic etiologies and are easily treated. Allergic conjunctivitis is usually seasonal, recurrent, and bilateral and presents with pruritus and watery discharge.

Bacterial conjunctivitis is neither pruritic nor seasonal and presents with a purulent discharge, early morning crusting of the eyelid, and a beefy red conjunctiva. *Staphylococcus* spp., *Streptococcus pneumoniae,* and *Haemophilus influenzae,* the most common causes of bacterial conjunctivitis, rarely bring about significant sequelae and are treated with topical antibiotics. However, infection with *Pseudomonas aeruginosa* and *Neisseria gonorrhoeae* are considered medical emergencies, since both can penetrate and perforate the cornea within 24 hours. Contact lens wearers are prone to *Acanthamoeba* and *P. aeruginosa.*

Viral conjunctivitis presents with a watery discharge and follicular hypertrophy. Although adenovirus remains the leading viral cause of viral conjunctivitis, herpes simplex 1 and 2 and herpes zoster can lead to scarring and blindness with recurrence. In the elderly, ocular complications occur in 50% with recurrent V_1 distribution herpes zoster (always consider with vesicular rash around the eye or tip of nose).

N. gonorrhoeae, Chlamydia trachomatis, and herpes simplex 1 and 2 must be considered as a cause of ophthalmia neonatorum. *N. gonorrhoeae* generally occurs within 2 to 4 days of life and *Chlamydia* within 5 to 13 days. Neonatal *C. trachomatis* carries a 50% risk of pneumonia over the ensuing 2 to 3 months. Herpetic infections develop in half of neonates exposed to genital herpes during birth, and of these, ocular herpes develops in 20%.

A fungal cause should be considered in patients who are immunocompromised and those with a history of trauma involving organic matter.

Symptoms

Bacterial and viral etiologies present similarly.

- Ocular pain and redness
- Photophobia (with keratitis)
- Foreign body sensation
- Crusting, discharge
- Decreased vision

N. gonorrhoeae

- Initially unilateral +++++
- Thick discharge

C. trachomatis

- Watery discharge +++
- Mucopurulent discharge +++

Herpes simplex

- Unilateral +++++
- Watery discharge, less with recurrence
- Risk factors: immunosuppression, sunlight, local trauma, stress

Signs

N. gonorrhoeae

- Hyperpurulent discharge
- Severe chemosis

C. trachomatis

- Lid edema ++++
- Conjunctival hyperemia
- Hypertrophic papillae without follicles

Primary herpes simplex keratitis

- Punctate lesions (more common in primary infection) on fluorescein staining, often *not* typical dendritic pattern (Fig. 11-2)
- Lid lesions, periocular dermatitis ++++
- Decreased corneal sensitivity +++
- Uveitis (very rare)
- Isolated ocular involvement in neonates (rare); search for disseminated disease

Herpes zoster ophthalmicus

- Punctate lesions or dendritic ulcers on fluorescein staining ++++
- Lesions along nasociliary branch of trigeminal nerve (tip of the nose) +++

Workup

- Full ophthalmologic examination including search for foreign bodies and slit-lamp examination with fluorescein staining of cornea
- Gram stain and culture: patients <1 month of age; *or* if >1 month of age, or adult, and systemic evidence of STD (usually adolescents and older), immunocompromised, thick purulent discharge, or no improvement after 48 hours of antibiotic therapy

Special Considerations

Corneal ulcer

- Gram stain and culture (may require debridement by ophthalmologist)

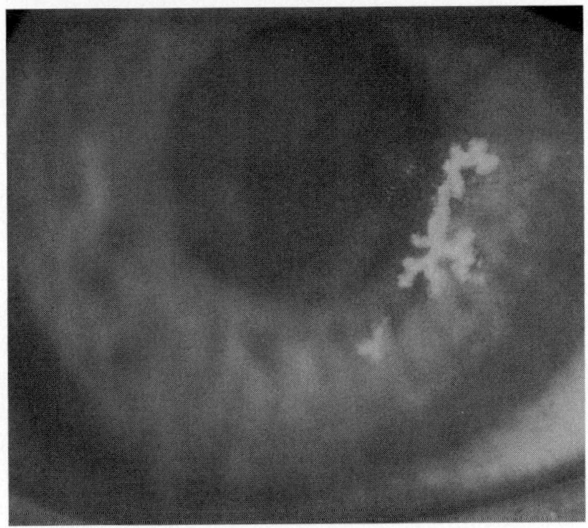

Fig. 11-2 Herpes keratitis. Dendritic pattern with fluorescein uptake. (From Palay DA, Krachmer JH: *Ophthalmology for the primary care physician,* St Louis, 1997, Mosby.)

N. gonorrhea

Gram stain and culture
Genital and pharyngeal cultures

C. trachomatis

- ELISA and immunofluorescent studies for *C. trachomatis* ++++ (very high specificity)
- Gram stain has poor sensitivity.
- Genital culture
- PCR more sensitive than culture for *C. trachomatis.*

Herpes simplex, herpes zoster

- Serologies not helpful

Comments and Treatment Considerations

All routine cases of bacterial keratitis should be treated with broad-spectrum topical antibiotics and referred for ophthalmologic follow-up. Patients with corneal ulcers (especially if contact lens wearers) or those infected with *N. gonorrhoeae, C. trachomatis,* and herpes need aggressive care and generally a ED ophthalmologic consultation. Patients with suspected *N. gonorrhoeae* and *C. trachomatis* conjunctivitis may have concomitant oral or genital infections that are often asymptomatic +++.

N. gonorrhoeae

If < 1 month of age with mild disease, treat with single dose ceftriaxone 125 mg IM or cefotaxime 100 mg IM in close consultation and follow-up with an ophthalmologist. In adults with mild infection, use ceftriaxone 125 mg IM/IV. The presence of a hypopyon (a layered infiltrate in the anterior chamber suggesting endophthalmitis), severe purulent conjunctivitis with corneal involvement, or large or multiple ulcers suggests more serious disease that requires ED ophthalmologic consultation and possible hospital admission.

C. trachomatis

In pediatric or pregnant patients, treat with erythromycin 50 mg/kg/day, divided in four doses, po for 2 to 3 weeks. In other adults, treat with doxycycline 100 mg po bid for 2 weeks.

Herpetic keratitis

Herpes simplex

Consider ED ophthalmologic consultation. Treatment often includes topical antivirals (e.g., trifluridine 1% 1 gtt 9 times/day). Cycloplegics to reduce pain and topical antibiotics for secondary bacterial infection may be prescribed. Consider admission for neonates with herpes because of the risk of disseminated disease.

Herpes zoster

Consider ED ophthalmologic consultation. Famciclovir 500 mg tid po for 10 days early in the course of herpes zoster may lessen the severity of the disease.

In general
Avoid topical steroids and topical anesthetics until ophthalmologic consultation. Avoid atropine for cycloplegia because of its long-lasting effect.

REFERENCES[www]

Liesegang TJ: Bacterial keratitis, *Infect Dis Clin North Am* 6:815, 1992.
Mader TH, Stulting RD: Viral keratitis, *Infect Dis Clin North Am* 6:831, 1992.
Ng EW, Golledge CL: The management of ocular infections, *Aust Fam Physician* 25:1831, 1996.
Stonecipher KG, Jensen H: Diagnosis, laboratory analysis, and treatment of bacterial corneal ulcers, *Optom Clin* 4:53, 1995.

[www]Additional references are available on the following web site: www.signsandsymptoms.com.

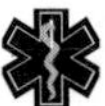

OCULAR CHEMICAL BURNS

Both acidic and alkaline substances can cause serious corneal and conjunctival damage. While all but the most trivial of exposures require copious (liters) of irrigation, alkaline substances are particularly notable for causing deep burns. Ammonia (fertilizer and household cleaners) is one of the most aggressive alkaline substances, followed by lye (drain cleaners), lime (plaster, cement), and magnesium hydroxide. A detailed ophthalmologic examination is generally deferred until after irrigation has normalized the eye pH.

Symptoms

- Pain following history of exposure
- Decreased vision (depending on extent of injury)

Signs

- Conjunctival erythema, edema
- Decreased visual acuity
- Corneal clouding in severe burns
- Stromal whitening in severe burns
- Increased IOP in alkali burns

Workup

- Baseline and post-irrigation eye pH measurements (normal tears pH approximately 7.3 to 7.6)

Comments and Treatment Considerations

There are no specific antidotes. Any solid or particulate matter should be removed. After topical anesthesia, copious lavage using normal saline or lactated Ringer should be started immediately until eye pH is approximately 7.4 (Consider use of specialized lenses attached to IV fluid bags and deliver several liters of fluid.) Patients are generally given topical antibiotics following irrigation and a full examination. Cycloplegics and systemic analgesics may be necessary to relieve pain; avoid atropine for cycloplegia because of its long-lasting effects. Obtain ophthalmologic consultation for significant alkali exposure and deep corneal acid burns. Administer tetanus prophylaxis if indicated.

REFERENCES

Mead M: Evaluation and initial management of patients with ocular and adnexal trauma. In Albert DM, Jakobiec FA, editors: *Principles and practice of ophthalmology,* Philadelphia, 1994, WB Saunders.

Pfister RR: Alkaline injury. In Fraunfelder FT, Roy FH, editors: *Current ocular therapy*, ed 4, Philadelphia, 1995, WB Saunders.

Slansky HH: Acid burns. In Fraunfelder FT, Roy FH, editors: *Current ocular therapy*, ed 4, Philadelphia, 1995, WB Saunders.

Wagoner MD: Chemical injuries of the eye: current concepts in pathophysiology and therapy, *Surv Ophthalmol* 41:275, 1997.

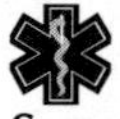

CORNEAL ABRASION

Symptoms

- Significant eye pain +++++
- Foreign body sensation
- Photophobia
- Tearing
- Irritable infant without other condition

Signs

- Eyelid edema
- Conjunctival injection may be present

Workup

- Slit-lamp examination: hallmark sign is an epithelial defect noted with fluorescein +++++ (if a surrounding infiltrate is seen then it is infected and by definition is now a corneal ulcer).
- Eversion of the eyelids for evaluation of any possible foreign body (suspect a foreign body especially if vertical linear abrasions are noted on the cornea.)

Comments and Treatment Considerations

Corneal abrasions are extremely painful, but if treated properly will heal in 24 to 72 hours. Treatment consists of topical antibiotics, topical cycloplegic medications with oral analgesics, and daily follow-up until the epithelial defect resolves. Patching is no longer recommended except to provide patient comfort or for very large abrasions. No contact lenses should be worn until complete resolution.

REFERENCES

Kaiser PK: A comparison of pressure patching versus no patching for corneal abrasions due to trauma or foreign body removal, *Ophthalmology* 102:1936, 1995.

Patterson J, Fetzer D, Krall J, et al: Eye patch treatment for the pain of corneal abrasion, *South Med J* 89:227, 1996.

Poole SR: Corneal abrasion in infants, *Pediatr Emerg Care* 11:25,1995.

CHAPTER 12

Fever (Elevated Temperature)

VIRGINIA M. RIBEIRO

Temperature elevation can occur through two general mechanisms: (1) the hypothalamic set point (typically 37° C) can be adjusted upward because of infections, toxins, or drugs or (2) the body's mechanisms to adequately compensate for heat stress can be overwhelmed (increased heat load or decreased heat dissipation). Important historical clues to the cause of hyperthermia include associated symptoms, duration and magnitude of fever, occupational exposures, travel, recreational history, and presence of an immunocompromised state. Any suggestion of an infectious cause for elevated temperature should lead to appropriate evaluation and antibiotic therapy. Important physical examination clues suggesting a possible infectious source of fever include altered mental status, stiff neck, rash, lymphadenopathy, abnormal lung examination findings, joint effusions, heart murmurs, or other localizing findings. *This chapter focuses on noninfectious causes of hyperthermia.* Other emergent causes of fever are addressed in other chapters.

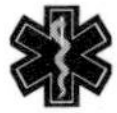

HEATSTROKE

Heatstroke is a life-threatening condition in which the patient's thermoregulatory mechanisms are unable to adequately respond to heat stress. This results in an increase in body temperature leading to organ dysfunction and failure. Temperatures are usually very high, often in excess of 41° C (106° F). In classic heatstroke, precipitants include exposure to high ambient temperature in a patient with a preexisting disease (coronary artery disease, diabetes, alcohol, and obesity) or medication (phenothiazines, anticholinergics, sedatives, diuretics) that limits thermoregulation. This may occur, for example, in older patients who are confined to a hot environment. Care must be taken to rule out infectious causes of fever in these patients.

In exertional heatstroke, precipitants include physical exertion, high temperature, humidity approaching 100% (evaporation ceases), and incomplete acclimatization. Heatstroke patients are hot, usually, though not always, anhydrotic, and have CNS abnormalities. Rapid and aggressive cooling measures are imperative in all heatstroke patients.

Heat exhaustion is a less emergent form of heat illness that is treated primarily by cooling and oral or IV fluid replacement. Heat cramps may also occur and seem to be related to salt depletion. Treatment consists of oral or IV fluid and NaCl repletion.

Symptoms

- Fever +++++
- Altered mental status (agitation, confusion) +++++
- Headache
- Dizziness
- Weakness
- Anorexia
- Stupor
- "Sense of impending doom"

Signs

- Hyperthermia +++++
- Altered mental status (coma, stupor, agitation) +++++
- Hot, dry skin (not universal) ++++
- Neurologic deficits in severe cases
- Oliguria (may be sign of rhabdomyolysis in exertional heat stroke)
- Hypotension
- ECG changes
- Disseminated intravascular coagulation (DIC)

Workup

- Rule out other causes of elevated temperature (e.g., cultures, CT, and LP when indicated)
- Urinalysis, CPK, creatinine to rule out rhabdomyolysis
- Electrolytes
- Evaluate for multiorgan dysfunction (e.g., liver function tests and chest x-rays)
- PT and PTT (anticipation of DIC)
- ECG (may show ST depression, T wave changes, SVT)

Comments and Treatment Considerations

Treatment consists of rapid cooling with evaporative methods (water sprayed on disrobed patient along with use of fans). This is preferred over applying ice packs to axilla and groin, which promotes vasoconstriction peripherally. Cooling should exceed 0.1° to 0.2° C/min with aggressive treatment until temperature reaches 39° C (102° F); do not overshoot. Use continuous rectal probe monitoring. Oxygenation and hemodynamic support are provided as needed. Empiric antibiotics are given when uncertain of infection. Benzodiazepines should be given for shivering (phenothiazines may decrease ability to cool patient). Treat hypokalemia if also acidotic, since it represents a true deficit. No aspirin or acetaminophen should be given because their effects depend on a normally functioning hypothalamus. Admit the patient to the intensive care unit. If rhabdomyolysis is present, fluids should be alkalinized and furosemide administered to keep urine output at 100 ml/hr.

In classic heatstroke, intravenous fluids are generally indicated but should be used with care to avoid pulmonary edema. Many heatstroke victims are normovolemic and peripherally vasodilated with distributive shock and high output failure; cooling will redistribute from periphery to core. In exertional heatstroke, intravenous fluids and electrolyte replacement are required. Complications include cardiovascular dysfunction (including CHF), DIC, acute renal failure, rhabdomyolysis, seizure, liver injury (very common), ARDS, electrolyte disorders, and death.

REFERENCES[www]

Clowes GHA, O'Donnell TF: Heatstroke, *N Engl J Med* 291:564, 1974.

Graham BS, Lichtenstein MJ, Hinson JM, Theil GB: Nonexertional heatstroke, *Arch Intern Med* 146:87, 1996.

Olson KR, Benowitz NL: Environmental and drug-induced hyperthermia, *Emerg Med Clin North Am* 2:459, 1984.

Tek D, Olshaker JS: Heat illness, *Emerg Med Clin North Am* 10:299, 1992.

[www]Additional references are available on the following web site: www.signsandsymptoms.com.

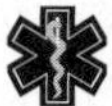

NEUROLEPTIC MALIGNANT SYNDROME

DSM-IV criteria for the diagnosis of neuroleptic malignant syndrome (NMS) include elevated temperature with muscular rigidity accompanied by two or more of the following: diaphoresis, dysphagia, tremor, incontinence, altered consciousness, tachycardia, blood pressure changes, leukocytosis, or elevated creatine kinase. It usually occurs 3 to 9 days after initiation of neuroleptic therapy or addition of second neuroleptic medication.

Precipitants

- Neuroleptic drug use (phenothiazines, butyrophenones, thioxanthenes)
- Withdrawal of dopaminergic stimulants in Parkinson's disease (amantadine, levodopa/carbidopa, bromocriptine)
- Dopamine antagonist use (metoclopramide, tetrabenazine, promethazine, prochlorperazine, amoxapine, reserpine, droperidol)
- Lithium combined with clozapine, carbamazepine, phenelzine, chlorpromazine, doxepin
- Tetracyclic antidepressants
- Monoamine oxidase inhibitors

Symptoms

- Elevated temperature +++++ (by definition)
- Rigidity +++++

- Dyspnea ++
- Tremor ++
- Urinary incontinence
- Dysphagia
- Diaphoresis
- Drowsiness
- Confusion
- Agitation

Signs

Tetrad:

- Elevated temperature (usually 38.5° to 42° C)
- Rigidity (classic lead pipe, which may be localized, trismus, masked facies ++, and dyskinesia)
- Altered level of consciousness (from confusion and agitation to lethargy, stupor, coma ++, and mutism +++)
- Autonomic dysfunction (tachycardia ++++, labile blood pressure +++, diaphoresis +++, tachypnea +++, hyperreflexia ++, pallor, and dysrhythmias/cardiac arrest).

Workup

- Diagnosis is established clinically and by exclusion (i.e., one must be sure that no infectious or metabolic processes are responsible for the increased temperature)
- Urinalysis (check for myoglobinuria) and creatinine phosphokinase to rule out rhabdomyolysis
- BUN, creatinine, LFTs, electrolytes, calcium, and magnesium
- Drug levels are typically normal.

Comments and Treatment Considerations

The key to treatment of NMS is recognition of the syndrome, withdrawal of the offending medication, and intensive symptomatic care. If infection is suspected, antibiotic administration is reasonable pending culture results. Treatment is focused on the alleviation of symptoms and prevention of complications and consists of hydration, fever reduction, benzodiazepine sedation, and maintenance of appropriate fluid and electrolyte balance. There is no good evidence that any specific treatment alters outcome. Among those that have been proposed: bromocriptine 2.5 to 5.0 mg po tid; dantrolene sodium 2.5 mg/kg/d IV, maximum of 10 mg/kg/d (if muscle relaxation required); amantadine 100 mg bid (preferred for NMS in Parkinson's disease); and electroconvulsive therapy +++ (may be indicated if no response for 2 days). One study reported that patients receiving pharmacologic therapy do worse and have more complications.

Differential Diagnosis

- CNS infection
- Sepsis
- Encephalitis
- Strychnine poisoning
- Tetanus
- Serotonin syndrome
- Environmental heat disorder
- Drug fever
- Thyrotoxicosis
- Extrapyramidal syndrome
- Anticholinergic toxicity
- Lethal catatonia

See also Chapter 32, Toxic Ingestion, Approach to.

REFERENCES[www]

Bristow MF, Kohen D: Neuroleptic malignant syndrome, *Br J Hosp Med* 55:517, 1996.

Guze BH, Baxter LR: Neuroleptic malignant syndrome, *N Engl J Med* 313:163, 1985.

Kellam AMP: The neuroleptic malignant syndrome, so-called: a survey of the world literature, *Br J Psychiatry* 150:752, 1987.

Rosebush PI, Stewart T, Mazurek MF: The treatment of neuroleptic malignant syndrome: are dantrolene and bromocriptine useful adjuncts to supportive care? *Br J Psychiatry* 159:709, 1991.

Schneider SM: Neuroleptic malignant syndrome: controversies in treatment, *Am J Emerg Med* 9:360, 1991.

[www]Additional references are available on the following web site: www.signsandsymptoms.com.

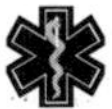 *DRUG-INDUCED HYPERTHERMIA*

Drug-induced hyperthermia is a rare cause of increased body temperature. Signs and symptoms of drug-induced hyperthermia depend on the activity of the drug. The following classes of drugs should be considered.

Drugs That Cause Muscular Hyperactivity

- Amphetamines
- Designer amphetamines
- Monoamine oxidase inhibitors
- Cocaine
- Methaqualone
- Lithium
- Antipsychotics
- Tricyclic antidepressants
- Halothane, cocaine, succinylcholine (malignant hyperthermia)
- Lysergic acid diethylamide (LSD)
- Phencyclidine (PCP)
- Strychnine
- Isoniazid (INH)
- Sympathomimetics (theophylline, ephedrine, pseudoephedrine)
- Serotonin syndrome (MAOIs + SSRIs, TCAs, meperidine, dextromethorphan, tryptophan)

Drugs That Cause Hypermetabolism

- Salicylate
- Thyroid hormone
- Dinitrophenol
- Sympathomimetics
- Ethanol withdrawal
- Sedative-hypnotic withdrawal

Drugs That Impair Thermoregulation

- Ethanol
- Antipsychotics (phenothiazines)

Drugs That Impair Heat Dissipation

- Anticholinergics
- Skeletal muscle relaxants
- Antipsychotics
- Sympathomimetics

Symptoms, signs, and workup vary with intoxication. See Chapter 32, Toxic Ingestion, Approach to.

REFERENCES

Burns MJ: Drug-associated hyperthermias: a rational approach to treatment, *Progress Notes* (American Society of Clinical Psychopharmacology), in press.

Callaway CW, Clark RF: Hyperthermia in psychostimulant overdose, *Ann Emerg Med* 24:68, 1994.

Rosenberg J, Pentel P, Pond S, et al: Hyperthermia associated with drug intoxication, *Crit Care Med* 14:964, 1986.

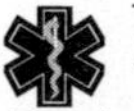

SEROTONIN SYNDROME

Precipitants of serotonin syndrome include the following:

1. Drug combinations—serotonin precursors or agonists (tryptophan, LSD, lithium, L-dopa, buspirone [BuSpar]), serotonin-release agents, SSRIs (paroxetine [Paxil], fluoxetine [Prozac], sertraline [Zoloft], fluvoxamine [Luvox]), nonselective serotonin reuptake inhibitors (clomipramine [Anafranil], imipramine, dextromethorphan, meperidine, venlafaxine [Effexor], nefazodone [Serzone], pentazocine [Talwin], trazodone, fenfluramine), nonspecific inhibitors of serotonin metabolism (cocaine, MAOIs)
2. Increased serotonin precursors or agonists
3. Increased release of serotonin (3,4-methylenedioxymethamphetamine [Ecstasy], fenfluramine)

Symptoms

- Altered mental status +++: mania, hallucinations, and confusion
- Autonomic dysfunction: diaphoresis ++, diarrhea ++, lacrimation, and shivering ++
- Neuromuscular abnormalities: akathisia +++ and fever +++

Signs

- Altered mental status: coma, delirium, mutism, and agitation
- Autonomic dysfunction: mydriasis, hyperthermia, tachycardia, and alteration in blood pressure
- Neuromuscular abnormalities: myoclonus +++, hyperreflexia ++, tremor ++, incoordination ++, clonus, nystagmus, rigidity

- Seizure
- Headache

Workup

- Diagnosis is made clinically and requires taking an appropriate drug history and excluding other causes (infectious, metabolic, primary neurologic, and other drug-induced syndromes).
- Urinalysis and CPK if muscle rigidity is present to rule out rhabdomyolysis

Comments and Treatment Considerations

Complications include hypertension, arrhythmias, rhabdomyolysis, myoglobinuria, renal failure, hepatic failure, DIC, and ARDS. Mild to moderate cases usually resolve in 24 to 72 hours. Treatment is mostly supportive, involving aggressive cooling, intravenous fluids, sedatives, cardiac monitoring, anticonvulsants, antihypertensives, and rarely paralytics (reduce hyperthermia secondary to muscle hyperactivity). If the patient is moderate to severely symptomatic and conventional supportive therapy fails, including benzodiazepine treatment (which decreases muscle hyperactivity and decreases sympathetic response), treatment with nonspecific inhibitors of serotonin (cryptoheptadine 8 mg po, then 4 mg po q4h for 24 hours or methysergide 2 mg po bid) has been successful in case reports. Consultation with a toxicologist is recommended. Bromocriptine (increases brain serotonin) and dantrolene (may increase central serotonin metabolism and increase serotonin) are not recommended.

REFERENCES[www]

Brown TM, Skop BP, Mareth TR: Pathophysiology and management of the serotonin syndrome, *Ann Pharmacother* 30:527, 1996.

Martin TG: Serotonin syndrome, *Ann Emerg Med* 28:520, 1996.

Sporer KA: The serotonin syndrome: implicated drugs, pathophysiology, and management, *Drug Saf* 13:94, 1995.

[www]Additional references are available on the following web site: www.signsandsymptoms.com.

CHAPTER 13

Fever in Children Under 2 Years of Age

MAUREEN MCCOLLOUGH

Most fevers in children are the result of benign viral conditions, but the emergency physician must identify those children whose fever is caused by a life-threatening illness. Meningitis and other serious infections may be occult or produce only nonspecific symptoms in children under 2 years of age.

Febrile infants of any age who are ill appearing (e.g., weak cry, inconsolable by parent, decreased alertness and responsiveness) should receive a full "septic workup," including lumbar puncture (LP), unless another significant source is identified and meningitis is not suspected. Blood and urine cultures should be obtained as a part of this evaluation for sepsis. Rapid and limited attempts should be made to obtain cultures before administering antibiotics, but treatment should *never* be substantially delayed in order to accomplish diagnostic procedures (including LP). These patients should be given intravenous antibiotics early in their ED course and be admitted to the hospital after an appropriate evaluation.

Children brought to the ED with a fever should receive a thorough physical examination. All their clothes should be removed to allow for a complete examination of the skin for petechiae, purpura, and cellulitis. Their level of alertness and activity should be documented. An 8-month-old who is grabbing for a stethoscope and smiling but has a temperature of 104° F is of lesser concern than an 8-month-old with a temperature of 101.8° F who is lethargic and ill appearing on the gurney. "Playful," "interactive," "smiling," "cooing," and "consolable" are useful descriptions of children who appear well. Children who are "lethargic," "irritable," "sleepy," and "inconsolable" are more likely to have a serious cause of fever, such as meningitis.

Any child with a fever who has an abnormal mental status should have antibiotics administered and an LP performed. A chest x-ray to screen for pneumonia should be considered in any child who has signs of lower respiratory tract disease, such as tachypnea, grunting, nasal flaring, or retractions. Urinary tract infection, more common in female children, can present with fevers and vomiting. If the cause of the fever cannot be identified, both a urinalysis and urine culture are recommended in male infants under 6 months old and in female infants under 1 year, since urinalysis alone may miss an infection in this age group.

This chapter is directed toward the diagnosis and treatment of previously healthy infants. Those who are immunocompromised or have other significant medical problems need special consideration.

REFERENCES

American College of Emergency Physicians: Clinical policy for the initial approach to children under the age of 2 years presenting with fever, *Ann Emerg Med* 22:628, 1993.

INFANTS UNDER 4 WEEKS OF AGE

Physical examination cannot reliably rule out serious disease in infants younger than 4 weeks. Therefore most authorities agree that such infants should receive intravenous antibiotics, a full septic workup, and be admitted to the hospital.

Workup

- Blood culture
- Catheterized or suprapubic tap for urinalysis and urine culture
- Chest x-ray
- LP
- Stool culture, if history of diarrhea

Comments and Treatment Considerations

Intravenous antibiotics (e.g., ampicillin 50 mg/kg IV for infants less than 7 days old; 50 to 100 mg/kg for infants older than 7 days plus gentamicin 2.5 mg/kg for patients in both age groups) should be given. These patients should be admitted to the hospital and treated with antibiotics pending culture results (see Meningitis, below).

INFANTS BETWEEN 4 AND 12 WEEKS OF AGE

Until recently most (in many cases all) infants between 4 and 12 weeks of age were admitted to the hospital because they may present with only subtle signs of serious disease. A high index of suspicion for the possibility of meningitis or other serious infection is critical, and LP should be performed in children who do not appear well. Overt signs such as meningismus are frequently absent. However, careful clinical and social evaluation allows for many patients who appear well to be discharged with follow-up in 24 hours. Some authorities advise routine laboratory studies for these patients; however, significant controversy exists regarding the need to conduct tests in well-appearing infants for whom close follow-up is available.

Workup

- Full physical examination
- LP, if clinically indicated
- Chest x-ray, if clinically indicated
- Urinary catheter or suprapubic tap for urinalysis and urine culture if no source of fever is identified
- Stool for WBC and culture, if history of diarrhea
- Blood culture
- CBC, controversial (see Occult Bacteremia)

Comments and Treatment Considerations

Ill-appearing infants should have a full septic workup for sepsis and be treated with intravenous antibiotics (e.g., ampicillin 100 mg/kg IV divided plus cefotaxime 50 mg/kg or ceftriaxone 50 mg/kg) pending culture results. If the risk of meningitis is high and drug-resistant *Streptococcus pneumoniae* is a concern, then vancomycin can be used instead of ampicillin.

Currently, well-appearing children with fever and no identifiable source are frequently evaluated for occult bacteremia, although the significance of the evaluation is debatable (see Meningitis and Occult Bacteremia, below).

INFANTS OLDER THAN 12 WEEKS AND LESS THAN 2 YEARS OF AGE

Fever in children in this age range is common, and serious conditions are generally more clinically apparent. However, early presentations of life-threatening disease processes can be subtle. Older infants and children may show signs of focal diseases, which are addressed in other chapters.

Comments and Treatment Considerations

Treatment should be directed toward underlying conditions when possible. Decisions regarding admission are generally based on clinical appearance and underlying disease process. Ill-appearing children with a fever but without a source of infection should receive a full septic workup and antibiotic treatment without delay (e.g., ceftriaxone 50 to 100 mg/kg IV). If the risk of meningitis is high and drug-resistant *Streptococcus pneumoniae* is a concern, then vancomycin can be added (see also Meningitis and Occult Bacteremia, below).

REFERENCES

Chiu CH, Lin TY, Bullard MJ: Identification of febrile neonates unlikely to have bacterial infections, *Pediatr Infect Dis J* 16:59, 1997.

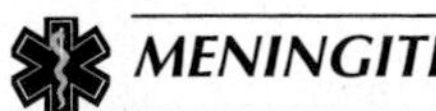

See also Chapter 15, Headache.

Symptoms

- May be variable and subtle
- Altered responsiveness ranging from irritability to lethargy
- Vomiting and decreased oral intake
- Fever is common but not universal, especially in the neonate.

Signs

- May be irritability alone or nonspecific
- May not have nuchal rigidity (especially in infants under 1 year)

- Seizures
- Altered mental status and signs of circulatory collapse, such as mottling or decreased capillary refill
- Disseminated intravascular coagulation can be sequela of septic shock.

Comments and Treatment Considerations

Treatment should not be delayed to obtain specimens. Antibiotics should be chosen on the basis of age and underlying disease. In the few cases where it may be appropriate to delay LP in order to do CT first, blood should be drawn for blood cultures, and antibiotics then given *before* CT. LP should then be performed if not contraindicated by CT findings. This strategy identifies the cause of bacterial meningitis in most cases, even when LP is performed 1 to 2 hours after the initiation of antibiotics. Younger infants, less than 4 to 8 weeks old, should be treated with ampicillin for *Listeria* coverage and either gentamicin or a third-generation cephalosporin, such as cefotaxime. Vancomycin should be added for infants with a positive gram stain or in whom bacterial meningitis is highly suspected, since streptococcal resistance is increasing. Ceftriaxone or cefotaxime (plus vancomycin if indicated) is used in older children. Dexamethasone 0.15 mg/kg IV may be given before antibiotics when meningitis is strongly suspected.

REFERENCES

Barkin R, editor*: Pediatric emergency medicine:concepts and clinical practice,* St Louis, 1992, Mosby.

Talan DA, Hoffman JR, Yoshikawa TT, Overturf GD: Role of empiric parenteral antibiotics prior to lumbar puncture in suspected bacterial meningitis: state of the art, *Rev Infect Dis*10:365,1988.

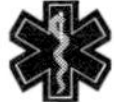

MENINGOCOCCEMIA

Neisseria meningitidis, a gram-negative diplococcus, can cause occult bacteremia, meningitis, and sepsis. Meningococcemia is characterized by a classic petechial rash (see Fig. 25-6). A significant proportion of patients with a fever and petechial rash have a bacterial infection. Of these, half are caused by *N. meningitidis.* Even with antibiotics and supportive care, the mortality rate for meningococcemia is still significant. Because meningococcemia is often fulminant in its presentation, and patients can deteriorate dramatically over minutes to hours, IV antibiotics should be given immediately when meningococcemia is suspected (fever and petechiae or purpura).

See Chapter 25, Rash.

REFERENCES

Salzman MB, Rubin LG: Meningococcemia, *Infect Dis Clin North Am* 10:709, 1996.

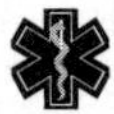

OCCULT BACTEREMIA

Occult bacteremia is considered a possibility in any child who does not have a source for a significant fever (usually considered >39.0 C, increased rates of bacteremia as temperature rises) on physical examination laboratory tests, or radiographs. Occult bacteremia occurs in approximately 3% of such patients. The evaluation and treatment of possible occult bacteremia in young children who appear clinically well and who have good medical follow-up remain controversial. Algorithms using ED WBC testing, blood cultures, and antibiotic prophylactic treatment are frequently followed, although their sensitivity and specificity are limited in predicting occult bacteremia. The clinical significance of occult bacteremia itself remains unclear, as most patients will clear the bacteremia without treatment. Some experts worry that, if left untreated, bacteremia may cause a serious bacterial infection, such as septic arthritis or meningitis, although this is rare.

The causes of occult bacteremia in young children are multiple, with *Streptococcus pneumoniae* now the most common owing to the *Haemophilus influenzae* vaccine.

Symptoms

- Fever
- Nonspecific symptoms

Signs

- Fever
- Nonfocal examination

Workup

What constitutes an appropriate workup for these patients is a subject of debate.

- Blood culture; although considered the definitive test, most patients have either cleared the organism or have returned for treatment before results are available.
- CBC (controversial)
- Catheter or suprapubic tap for urinalysis and culture in male infants less than 6 months old and female infants less than 1 year old
- LP should be performed in those for whom meningitis is a clinical concern and generally in all patients 4 to 8 weeks old before antibiotics are given to treat a possible occult bacteremia.
- Urinalysis and urine culture, if indicated
- Chest x-rays, if indicated

Comments and Treatment Considerations

Management of children older than 4 to 8 weeks old who have a fever without a source and who appear clinically well may be managed in four general ways:

1. Draw blood cultures and administer intramuscular antibiotics (ceftriaxone 50 mg/kg IM) for all children.
2. Draw blood cultures and provide antibiotics only for those children more likely to have occult bacteremia, i.e., those with WBC >15,000, neutrophils >500, ANC >10,000, temperature >41.0° C, or those with unreliable parents.
3. Draw blood cultures and administer po antibiotics.
4. No WBC testing or antibiotic prophylaxis.

Follow-up within 24 hours (sooner if any changes) is necessary for all these children regardless of treatment strategy.

REFERENCES

American College of Emergency Physicians: Clinical policy for the initial approach to children under the age of 2 years presenting with fever, *Ann Emerg Med* 22:628, 1993.

Baraff LJ, Bass JW, Fleisher GR, et al: Practice guideline for the management of infants and children 0 to 36 months of age with fever without source, *Ann Emerg Med* 22:1198, 1993.

Harper MB, Bachur R, Fleisher GR: Effect of antibiotic therapy on the outcome of outpatients with unsuspected bacteremia, *Pediatr Infect Dis J* 14:760, 1995.

Isaacman DJ, Karasic RB, Reynolds EA, Kost SI: Effect of number of blood cultures and volume of blood on detection of bacteremia in children, *J Pediatr* 128:190, 1996.

Rothrock SG, Harper MB, Green SM, et al: Do oral antibiotics prevent meningitis and serious bacterial infections in children with *Streptococcus pneumoniae* occult bacteremia? A meta-analysis, *Pediatrics* 99:438, 1997.

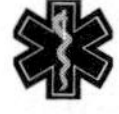

KAWASAKI'S SYNDROME

See Chapter 25, Rash.

REFERENCES

Durongpisitkul K, Gururaj VJ, Park JM, Martin CF: The prevention of coronary artery aneurysm in Kawasaki disease: a meta-analysis on the efficacy of aspirin and immunoglobulin treatment, *Pediatrics* 96:1057, 1995.

CHAPTER 14

Fractures Not To Miss

SCOTT RODI

Missed fractures are a significant cause of morbidity in ED patients and account for a significant percentage of malpractice suits against emergency physicians. The subject of this chapter is limited to extremity fractures of clinical significance that may be diagnostically subtle. Some fractures may not be apparent on initial x-ray examination. In some circumstances (such as possible scaphoid fracture of the wrist), patients should be treated as if they have a fracture, even if x-rays are "negative," and should receive appropriate treatment and referral for reexamination.

Signs

Most fractures are suggested by clinical examination findings (swelling, deformity, and bony tenderness.) Examination should include peripheral pulses, capillary refill, and distal sensation, motor function, and palpation of and range of motion (ROM) of joints proximal and distal to the suspected injury. Assessment of possible rotatory deformity is also important in metacarpal and finger injuries. Any cutaneous disruption in the area of injury should be noted and treated as a possible open fracture. Associated injuries and evidence of a compartment syndrome should also be sought (see Chapter 10, Extremity Pain and Numbness).

Workup

Most fractures can be identified on plain radiographs in the ED. The simplest way to identify a fracture is to trace the cortical lines, looking for abnormalities including lucencies, stepoffs, acute angulations, buckles, or sclerotic lines. Effusions, soft tissue swelling, and bone fragments should be noted. Patients who sustain traumatic injuries in certain conditions (e.g., osteoporosis) or locations (e.g., wrist) have notoriously subtle signs, and presumptive treatment or additional imaging techniques may be necessary if clinical suspicion of fracture is sufficient.

At least two perpendicular views should be obtained when assessing any fracture. Additional oblique views should be considered for periarticular fractures. Joints proximal and distal to the suspected injury should also be x-rayed *when clinically indicated.* Comparison views of the contralateral, asymptomatic extremity are sometimes helpful, particularly in children. Groups of bones effectively forming a ring (pelvis, forearm, wrist, tibia-fibula, mandible) typically break at two points, and both lesions should be sought. In some fractures, however, the second "break" is in a ligament or joint, rather than bone, and may not be visible on x-ray.

Accurate fracture description is important for charting and consultation. Fractures are described by anatomic location (intraarticular, proximal, middle or distal third of a long bone, and so forth), direction of fracture line (transverse, oblique, spiral), and degree of comminution (i.e., fragmentation) or impaction (i.e., compression). The relationship of the axes of the distal and proximal fragments is described in degrees of angulation, and the amount of contact between fractured ends as opposition. *Dislocation* refers to a total disruption of joint surfaces, with the position of the distal fragment described relative to the proximal one. *Subluxation* refers to partial disruption and diastasis to a disruption of the interosseous membrane. Children may have special x-ray presentations of fracture due to their increased bone compliance and growth plate activity. These are described as the following:

- Greenstick: bowing of a bone without distinct fracture line
- Torus: buckling of the bony cortex
- Salter-Harris: scheme for characterization of growth plate fractures (Fig. 14-1)

Comments and Treatment Considerations

As always, airway, breathing, and circulation should be addressed first. Significant blood loss can occur with many fractures, up to 500 ml with tibial fractures, 1000 ml with femur

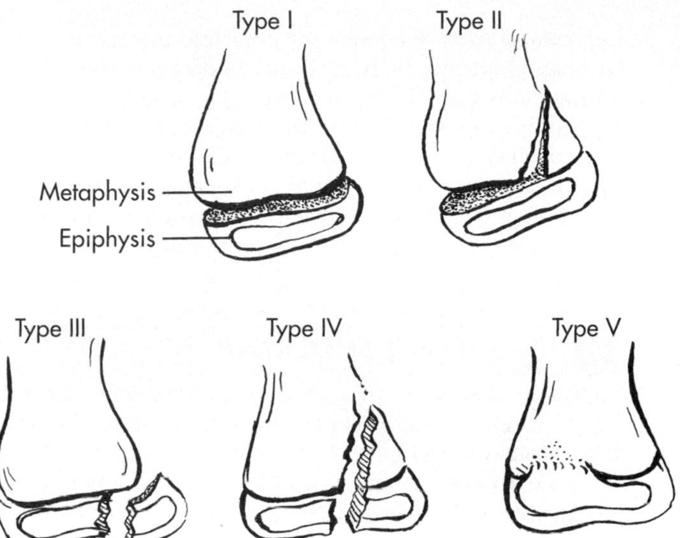

Fig. 14-1 Salter-Harris classification of growth plate fractures in children.

fractures, and 3000 ml with pelvic fractures. Intravenous access and close observation for hypovolemia should be considered with relevant injuries.

When a fracture or dislocation leads to vascular compromise at the site or distal to the lesion, immediate relocation/reduction should be initiated. This is generally accomplished by applying in-line traction followed by exaggeration of the mechanism of injury, and then distraction to reduce the bony deformity. An arteriogram is necessary for detecting signs of vascular impairment despite reduction, as well as for knee dislocations and perhaps other high-energy injuries near blood vessels.

Patients with open fractures should be given a tetanus booster and begin a regimen of broad-spectrum antibiotics (e.g., cefazolin and gentamicin). Wounds should be covered with a moist, sterile dressing; cultures are not indicated.

If compartment syndrome is suspected, pressures must be measured in all potentially involved compartments (see Chapter 10, Extremity Pain and Numbness).

Most fractures should be splinted to provide comfort, maintain reduction, and minimize the risk of fat embolization. Bony injuries are painful, and appropriate analgesia is required. Evidence of a pathologic fracture, intraarticular fracture, or physeal injury should prompt orthopedic consultation.

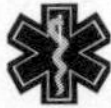

THE PAINFUL SHOULDER

Evaluation of shoulder pain after trauma should be guided by the mechanism of injury and include consideration of possible thoracic and cervical injuries. In addition to humeral, clavicular, and other more obvious fractures, the possibility of scapular fractures and glenohumeral dislocations must be investigated.

SCAPULAR FRACTURES

Scapular fractures are uncommon (0.5% to 1% of all fractures, 5% of shoulder fractures) and occur most often in 40- to 60-year-olds as a result of major trauma.

Signs

- Local tenderness
- Usually resist abduction, as the first 90 degrees of abduction is largely scapulothoracic

Workup

- X-rays: AP shoulder view initially; if not apparent, then add transscapular views
- CT scan if necessary

Comments and Treatment Considerations

The significance of a scapular fracture is primarily as a marker for major injuries (+++ have associated fractures). Head injury (++), hemopneumothorax (++), cervical spine fracture (++), rib fracture (+++), and brachial plexus injury should be sought.

Approximately 10% involve the glenoid and are associated with a high rate of osteoarthritis. Mortality is approximately 10%.

GLENOHUMERAL DISLOCATIONS

Anterior dislocation is the most common shoulder dislocation and is generally caused by abduction with external rotation.

Posterior dislocation is rare and is the most commonly missed major dislocation. It may be caused by a sudden, forceful muscle contraction (e.g., epilepsy or electric shock) or direct blow. Luxatio erecta is a rare dislocation that occurs when the superior aspect of the humeral head lies below the inferior rim of the glenoid fossa.

Signs

- Anterior: may feel mass anterior, inferior, or medial to normal glenohumeral joint with posterior sulcus. Internal rotation is restricted.
- Posterior: note a prominent coracoid with an anterior sulcus. External rotation is restricted.
- Luxatio erecta: patient may have arm locked overhead in abduction (Fig. 14-2).

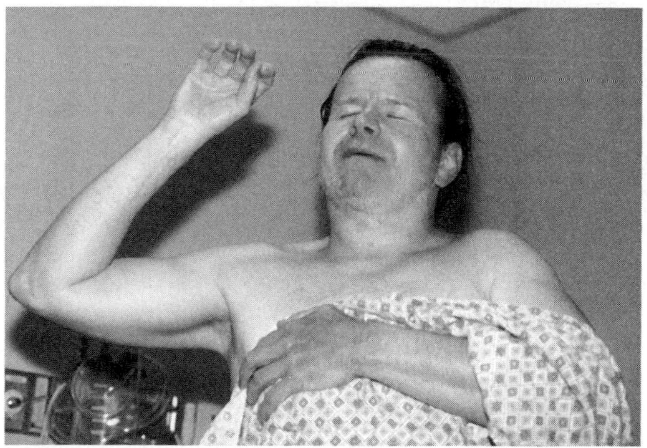

Fig. 14-2 Luxatio erecta, a rare form of shoulder dislocation.

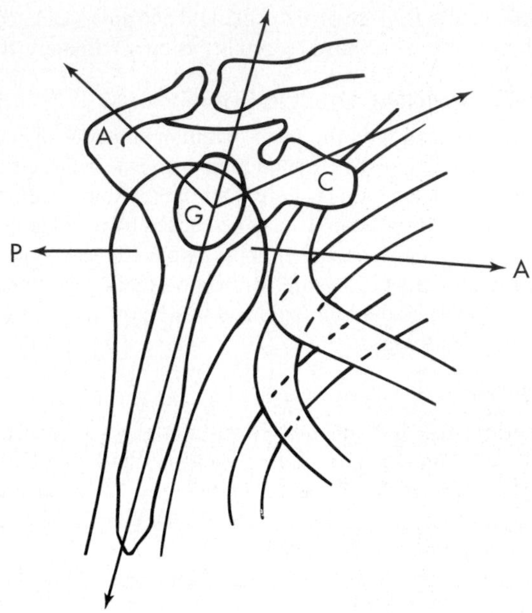

Fig. 14-3 Y, or transscapular, views of the shoulder to identify possible dislocation. *A,* Acromion; *C,* coracoid; *G,* glenoid; *P,* direction of posterior dislocation; *A,* direction of anterior dislocation. (Courtesy Michael F. Rodi, MD.)

Workup

- X-ray: AP and a scapular Y view. Anterior: humeral head may overlap glenoid or be inferior to coracoid on AP and will not lie in center of Y on scapular Y view (Fig. 14-3). Posterior: head may appear more symmetric ("light bulb" sign) and will not be centered on Y.
- Axillary view or CT if suspicious (Figs. 14-4 and 14-5)

Comments and Treatment Considerations

Treatment consists of early ED reduction with appropriate sedation and analgesia. Associated injuries to the axillary nerve (10% to 15%), cervical spine, and chest wall should be considered.

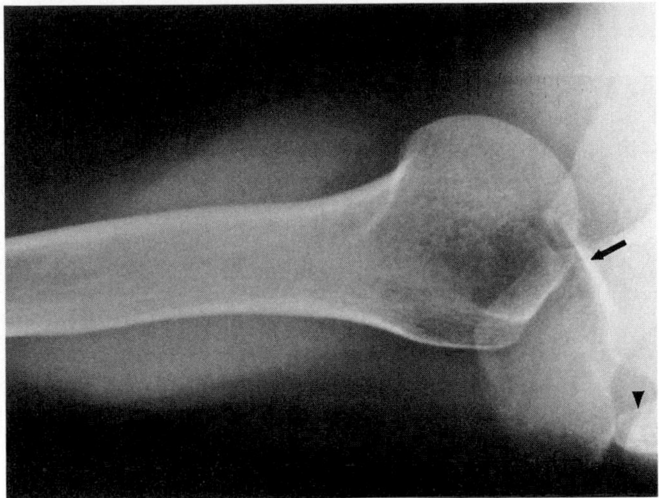

Fig. 14-4 Axillary shoulder view of anterior dislocation of the glenohumeral joint. Coracoid process is anterior *(arrowhead)*. Glenoid fossa *(arrow)*. (Courtesy Michael Zucker, MD, Los Angeles.)

Humeral head fractures should be noted; posterolateral fractures (Hill-Sachs) (Fig. 14-6) are associated with anterior dislocations, and anterolateral (reverse Hill-Sachs) are associated with posterior dislocations. Glenoid lip fractures (Bankart lesions) are noted in 80% of patients with recurrent dislocations.

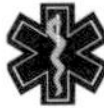

THE PAINFUL ELBOW IN CHILDREN

In children, many injuries that involve elbow pain are radiographically subtle; "sprain" is a dangerously conservative diagnosis in this setting. If doubt exists, the elbow should be immobilized and an ED orthopedic consultation obtained. Comparison views of the asymptomatic elbow may be helpful but are often not required.

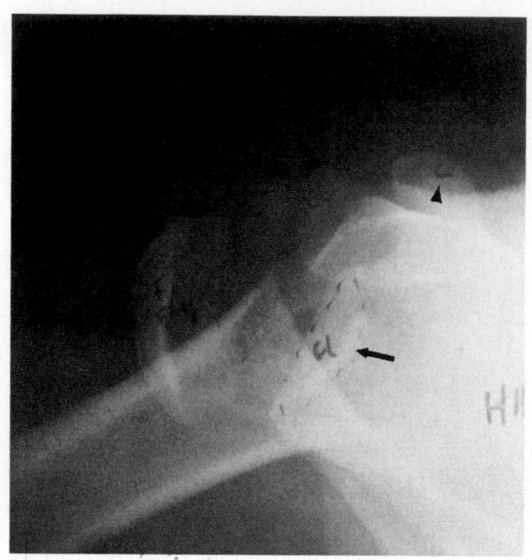

Fig. 14-5 Axillary shoulder view of posterior dislocation of glenohumeral joint. The humeral head is posterior to the glenoid. Coracoid is anterior *(arrowhead)*. Glenoid fossa *(arrow)*. (Courtesy Michael Zucker, MD, Los Angeles.)

SUPRACONDYLAR HUMERAL FRACTURE

Supracondylar humeral fractures represent 3% of all fractures in children and 85% of elbow fractures in children. They are generally caused by a fall on the outstretched hand (FOOSH), usually with hyperextension of the elbow. The male:female ratio is 9:1, with a bimodal age distribution: 2 to 8 and 11 to 15 years old.

Signs

- Tenderness at distal humerus and resistant to motion in all planes
- Neurologic deficit ++, most commonly anterior interosseous nerve

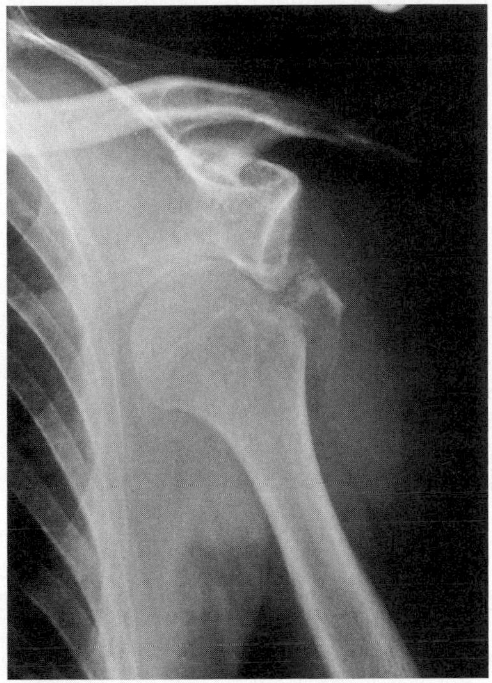

Fig. 14-6 AP view of shoulder demonstrates anterior dislocation of the glenohumeral joint. Hill-Sachs fracture with avulsion of greater tubercle. (Courtesy Michael Zucker, MD, Los Angeles.)

Workup

- X-ray: AP and lateral views of the elbow. Occult fracture is suggested by fat pad displacement, especially posterior (Fig. 14-7), and displacement of the anterior humeral line (greater than one third of capitellum normally lies anterior to anterior cortex of distal humerus [Fig. 14-8]); less than this suggests fracture).

Comments and Treatment Considerations

Supracondylar humeral fractures are associated with significant morbidity including brachial artery and nerve injury and compartment syndrome. Volkmann's contracture or cubitus varus deformity (10%) are possible sequelae. Moderate flexion should be attempted if pulse deficit is noted. Orthopedic consultation is necessary, and patients are generally admitted for observation.

Other significant causes of elbow pain in children include the following.

Medial epicondylar avulsion fracture

Represents 5% to 10% of elbow injuries in children, usually occurring in those 9 to 15 years of age. To diagnose radiographically, if the trochlear ossification center is visible, then the medial epicondyle ossification center should appear normal; if not, then a displaced fracture should be suspected. This frac-

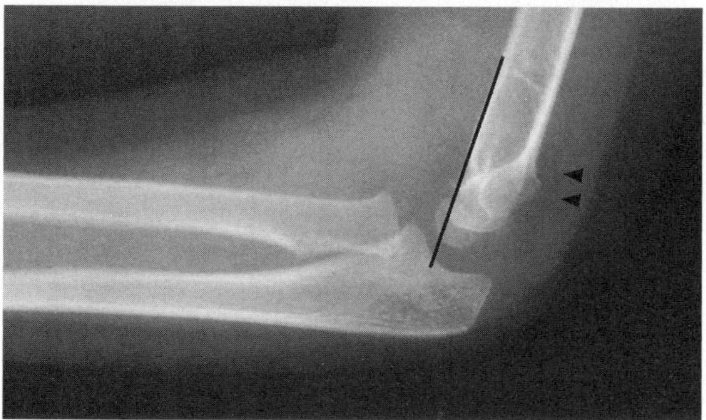

Fig. 14-7 Lateral view of elbow shows supracondylar fracture in a child. The posterior fat pad is displaced *(arrowheads)* indicating hemarthrosis. The anterior humeral line is abnormal, indicating posterior displacement of the distal humerus *(line).* (Courtesy Michael Zucker, MD, Los Angeles.)

ture is associated with elbow dislocation and loss of forearm flexor attachment, and the prognosis is guarded.

Lateral condyle fracture

Usually type IV Salter fractures that require operative repair. An orthopedist should be consulted even if the fracture appears radiographically nondisplaced. Complications include nonunion, cubitus valgus, ulnar nerve palsy, and osteonecrosis.

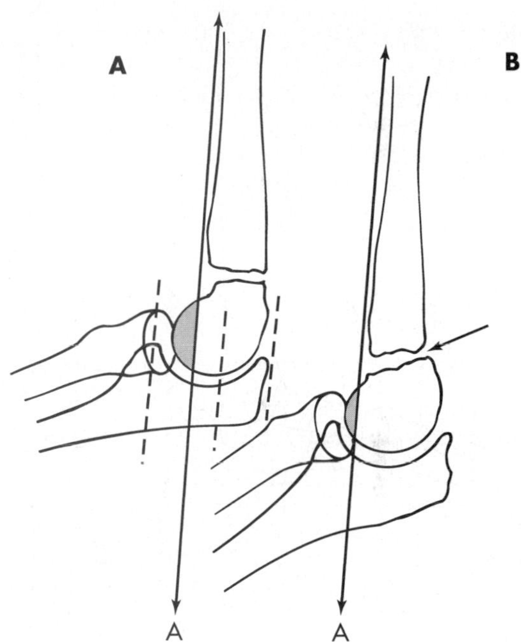

Fig. 14-8 Depiction of "true" lateral view to assess possible supracondylar fracture. **A,** Normal—one third of capitellum lies anterior to anterior humeral line. **B,** Less than one third of capitellum lying anterior to anterior humeral line indicates a probable supracondylar fracture *(arrow)*. *A,* Anterior humeral line. (Courtesy Michael F. Rodi, MD.)

Nursemaid's elbow

This elbow injury is common in 2- to 5-year-olds and is usually caused by sudden traction of the hand, pulling the radial head out of the annular ligament. Children with this injury usually hold the elbow stiffly in flexion and pronation. The diagnosis is generally made by a typical history and physical examination. X-rays may be considered in unusual cases to exclude fracture; the radiocapitellar line is inspected for

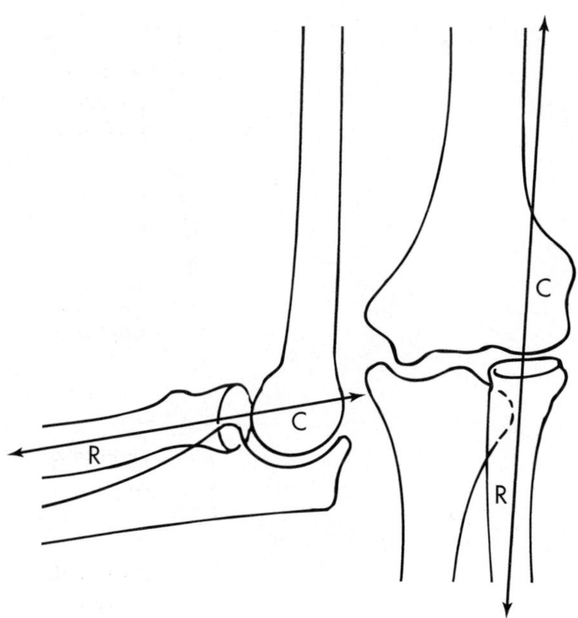

Fig. 14-9 Depiction of "true" AP and lateral views of the elbow to assess possible dislocation of the radial head. *R,* Radius; *C,* capitellum. Arrows represent the radiocapitellar line drawn through the shaft of the radius; if the line does not pass through the capitellum, the radial head is likely dislocated. (Courtesy Michael F. Rodi, MD.)

radial head subluxation (Fig. 14-9) and evidence of fracture. Subluxations are reduced by supination and flexion (or extension) of the elbow while applying pressure over the radial head with the thumb.

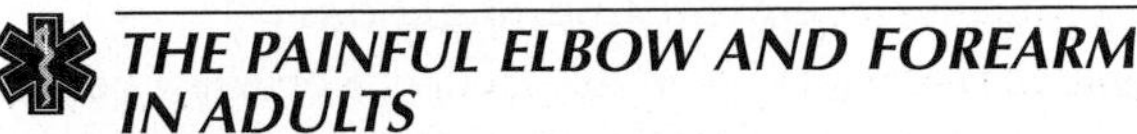

THE PAINFUL ELBOW AND FOREARM IN ADULTS

Even if an obvious forearm fracture is noted, associated elbow and wrist injuries must be suspected.

GALEAZZI FRACTURE

A Galeazzi fracture is fracture of the distal third of the radius with associated dislocation or subluxation of the distal radioulnar joint (DRUJ) caused by an axial load on a pronated forearm.

Signs

- Tenderness at DRUJ in addition to fracture site

Workup

- X-ray: AP/lateral forearm including elbow and wrist. Widened DRUJ, ulnar styloid fracture, or radius >5 mm shorter than ulna suggests the diagnosis.

Comments and Treatment Considerations

Patients should be observed for compartment syndrome while an orthopedic consultation in the ED is obtained.

MONTEGGIA FRACTURE

A Monteggia fracture involves the proximal third of the ulna and is associated with radial head dislocation caused by a direct blow to the forearm ("nightstick" injury) or fall on pronated hand.

Signs

- Tenderness at fracture site and radial head
- Decreased ROM

Workup

- X-ray: AP lateral forearm (with wrist and elbow). Displacement of the radiocapitellar line should be sought; normally, a line through the proximal radius intersects with the capitellum in all views (see Fig. 14-9).

Comments and Treatment Considerations

An orthopedic consultation in ED should be obtained because the fracture may require surgical reduction.

RADIAL HEAD FRACTURE

Radial head fracture is generally caused by FOOSH with the elbow extended and the hand pronated or by a fall backward with the hand supinated.

Signs

- Pain and swelling over the radial head, which can be elicited by palpation of the elbow laterally with the thumb during supination and pronation. A concomitant wrist injury or mechanical block to supination should be investigated (may need surgery).

Workup

- X-ray: Frequently occult. If fracture is not visible, look for signs of effusion including elevated anterior fat pad ("sail sign") or visible posterior fat pad.

Comments and Treatment Considerations

A small minority of patients with radial head fracture have associated elbow dislocation, and a few have DRUJ injury. If <30% of the head is involved and is nondisplaced (Mason I), fracture may be treated with a sling and early ROM (vast majority of cases); if >30% (Mason II) with poor ROM or comminuted (Mason III), surgery may be necessary.

CORONOID PROCESS FRACTURE

Coronoid fracture is present is 2% to 15% of elbow dislocations.

Signs

- Painful elbow
- Possible instability or decreased ROM

Workup

- X-ray: AP/lateral radiographs of elbow. Type I: tip avulsion; type II: $< 50\%$ fractured; type III: $>50\%$. Prognosis worse and associated injuries greater with increasing grade.

Comments and Treatment Considerations

Significance is as marker of possible dislocation

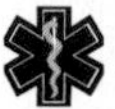

THE PAINFUL WRIST

Many wrist injuries are subtle and a diagnosis of sprain should not be made until a careful evaluation has eliminated other possibilities. A zone of vulnerability has been described (Fig. 14-10); tenderness or x-ray abnormality in this arc should prompt careful evaluation.

SCAPHOID FRACTURES

Scaphoid fractures are the most commonly missed fractures and represent 60% to 70% of carpal fractures. They typically occur as a result of FOOSH.

Signs

- Tenderness with or without swelling in anatomic snuff-box (++++, 40% specific), or at scaphoid tubercle (++++, 57% specific).

Workup

- X-ray: four-view series (AP, lateral, and AP in radial and ulnar deviation) with specific scaphoid views. On follow-up films, 2% to 20% reveal a fracture, and 2% to 5% remain false negatives (Fig. 14-11).

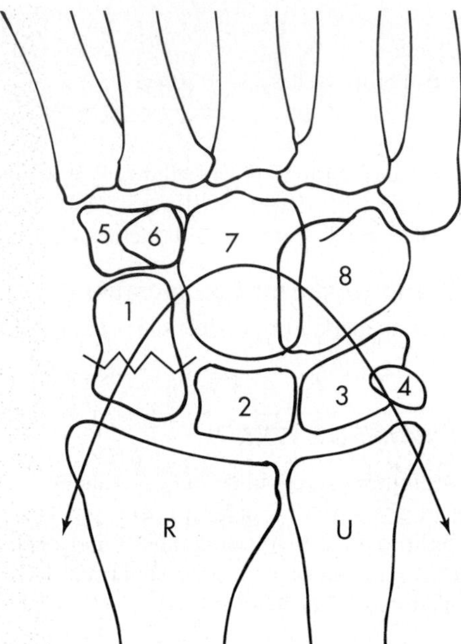

Fig. 14-10 Zone of vulnerability *(arrow)* on AP view of the wrist to evaluate possible combination fractures or injuries. *1,* Scaphoid (navicular); *2,* lunate; *3,* triquetrum; *4,* pisiform; *5,* trapezium (greater multangular); *6,* trapezoid (lesser multangular); *7,* capitate; *8,* hamate; *R,* radius; *U,* ulna. (Courtesy Michael F. Rodi, MD.)

Comments and Treatment Considerations

If no fracture is seen but an occult fracture is suspected because of snuff-box tenderness, a thumb-spica splint is applied and x-rays repeated in 14 days. Earlier reexamination by an orthopedist may facilitate earlier discontinuation of the splint if the patient has a normal examination. Primary concern is nonunion or avascular necrosis (with subsequent chronic pain) because blood supply may enter through the distal pole only. If fracture

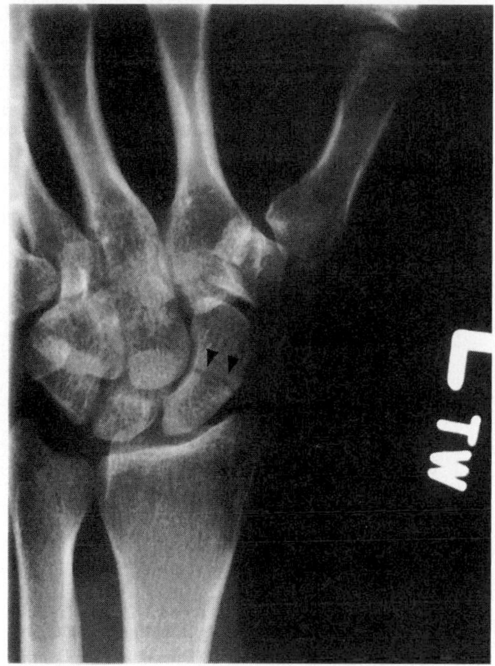

Fig. 14-11 AP view of wrist demonstrates scaphoid fracture *(arrowheads)*. (Courtesy Michael Zucker, MD, Los Angeles.)

is displaced (>1 mm) and angulated, an orthopedic consultation should be obtained for possible early surgery. No associated injuries are present in most cases.

Wrist tenderness can be caused by other carpal bone fractures including a triquetrum fracture, which is often apparent only on a lateral wrist x-ray.

LUNATE AND PERILUNATE DISLOCATIONS

Lunate dislocation is an uncommon injury in which the lunate alone is dislocated while the rest of the carpals remain in place; *perilunate dislocation* (also uncommon) occurs when all carpals except the lunate dislocate posteriorly and usually occurs with FOOSH.

Signs

- Swollen, tender wrist with decreased ROM and pain with axial compression of third metacarpal. Tenderness of the lunate itself should be examined. This is elicited by compression over the depression present just proximal to the third metacarpal, and is exacerbated when the wrist is flexed, which brings the lunate up into the "empty space."

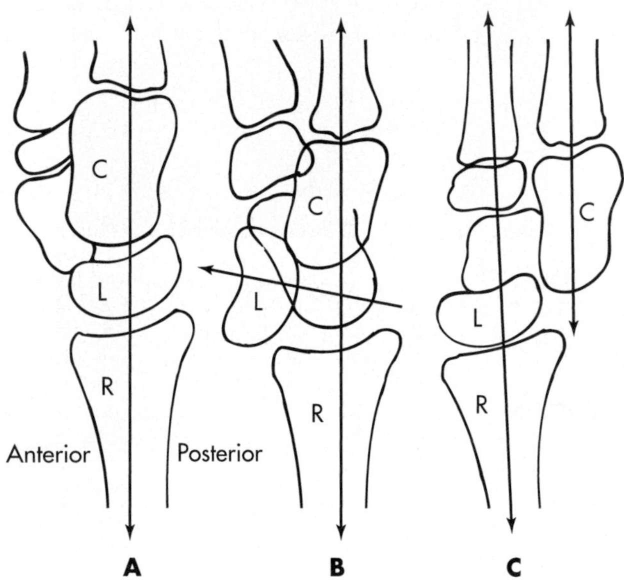

Fig. 14-12 Depiction of "true" lateral view of the wrist to assess lunate and perilunate dislocations. Normal **(A),** lunate dislocation **(B),** perilunate dislocation **(C).** *R,* Radius; *L,* lunate; *C,* capitate. (Courtesy Michael F. Rodi, MD.)

Workup

- X-ray: AP/lateral of wrist. On AP, uniform space between carpals (1 to 2 mm) is noted (see Fig. 14-10) in the normal wrist. Widening, or a triangular-appearing lunate, suggests ligamentous disruption or dislocation. On lateral x-rays, the radius, lunate, and capitate should line up, appearing like multiple cups seated in saucers. If the lunate appears empty, a dislocation is suspected. If the capitate and radius are still aligned, a lunate dislocation is most likely; if the radius and capitate are not aligned, a perilunate dislocation is likely (Figs. 14-12 to 14-14).

Comments and Treatment Considerations

An urgent orthopedic consultation for reduction is necessary. The prognosis is guarded and ROM limited. Evidence of median nerve compression should be sought.

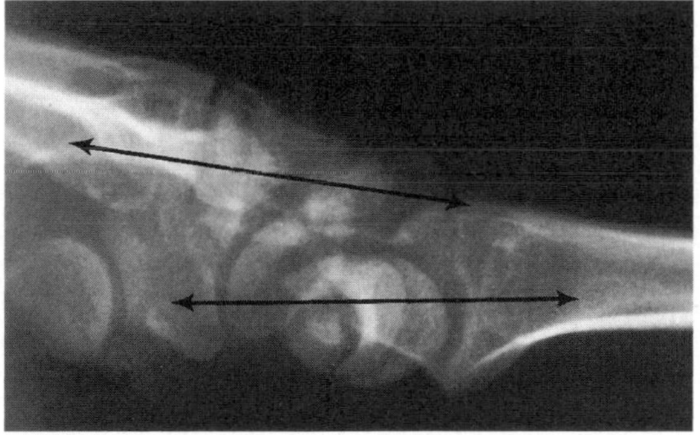

Fig. 14-13 Lateral view of wrist shows perilunate dislocation. The radiolunate line *(bottom arrow)* is intact, but the lunate-capitate relationship is disrupted with dorsal dislocation of the capitate *(top arrow)*. (Courtesy Michael Zucker, MD, Los Angeles.)

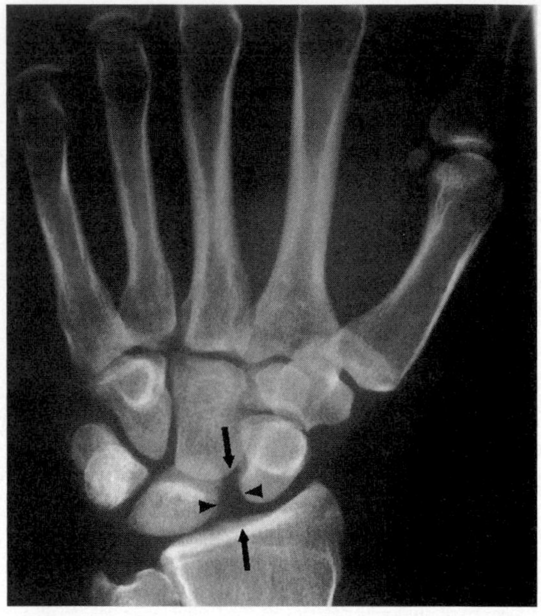

Fig. 14-14 AP view of wrist shows scapholunate dissociation. The gap between the lunate and scaphoid is greater than 4 mm *(arrowheads)*. (Courtesy Michael Zucker, MD, Los Angeles.)

THE PAINFUL HIP

Pelvic fractures from high-energy mechanisms are diagnostically straightforward but are associated with high morbidity and mortality and have a high risk of hemorrhagic shock. In reviewing pelvic films, sacroiliac joints and pubic symphysis should be checked for symmetry, and sacral foramina arcuate lines and acetabular lines for irregularities (Fig. 14-15). Hip fractures in the elderly are similarly associated with high morbidity and mortality but may be radiographically occult on plain films and require CT or MRI for diagnosis.

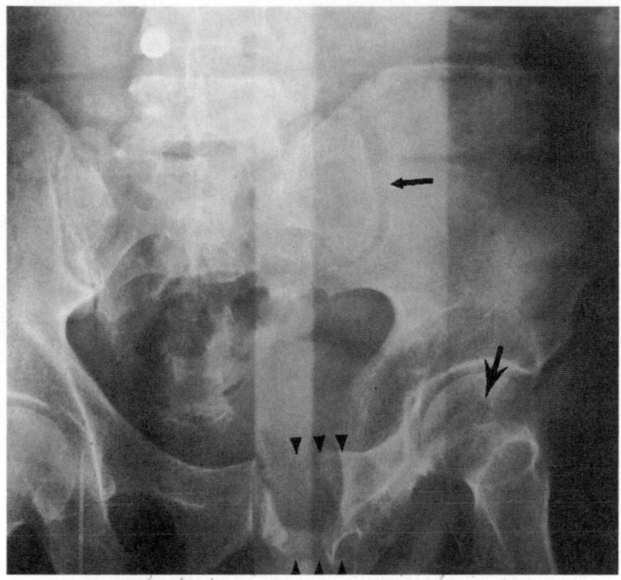

Fig. 14-15 AP view of pelvic fractures. Disruption of symphysis pubis and fractures of left rami *(arrowheads)* and disruption of the anterior ligaments of the left sacroiliac joint *(small arrow)*. Also note left acetabular fracture *(large arrow)*. (Courtesy Michael Zucker, MD, Los Angeles.)

PROXIMAL FEMUR FRACTURES

Hip fractures are common (250,000/year in the United States), particularly among elderly women (74% >65 years old; female:male, 4:1). They occur commonly after falls, and it is important to elicit any antecedent symptoms such as chest pain or dizziness that may indicate a primary medical or surgical condition that caused the fall.

Signs

- Thigh, knee, or groin pain
- Affected extremity may appear shortened and externally

rotated if displaced; however, alignment may be normal, and the patient may even be ambulatory if there is no displacement.

Workup

- X-ray: AP, lateral, and internal rotation views of affected hip and an AP pelvic view to check that cortices are unbroken, trabecular pattern is smooth, and there are no sclerotic lines (Fig. 14-16). Shenton's line and neck-shaft angle (normal, 120 to 130 degrees) are traced (Fig. 14-17). MRI or CT may be considered if no fracture is identified and there is clinical concern of hip fracture.

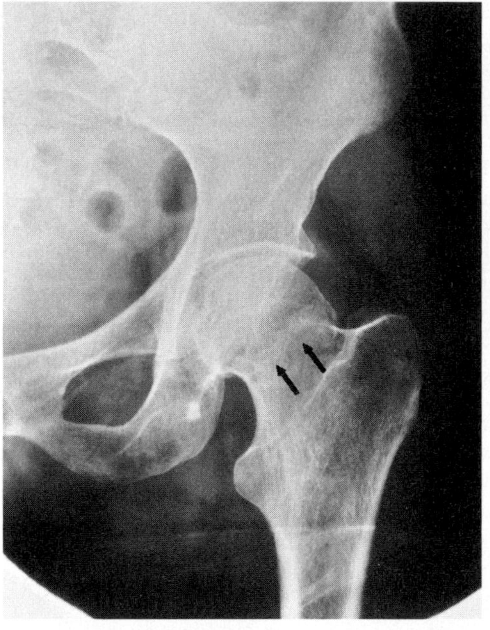

Fig. 14-16 AP hip radiograph shows femoral fracture. Impacted fracture of the neck of the femur, Garden I type *(arrows)*. (Courtesy Michael Zucker, MD, Los Angeles.)

Comments and Treatment Considerations

Associated conditions to check include ipsilateral upper extremity fracture (1% to 2%) and cervical spine injury. Morbidity and mortality are high; less than one half regain prefracture level of function, and mortality is 15 times greater than in age-matched controls in the first month after injury. Medical complications are minimized by early surgery. Consider pathologic fracture in younger patients.

PEDIATRIC HIP PAIN

In addition to fractures, considerations in a child complaining of hip (or knee) pain should include transient synovitis, avascular necrosis, slipped capital femoral epiphysis, and septic hip (see Chapter 21, Limping Child/Child Won't Walk). Avulsion fractures should be considered in adolescents, specifically ASIS (sartorius origin), AIIS (rectus femoris origin), and ischial tuberosity (hamstrings origin).

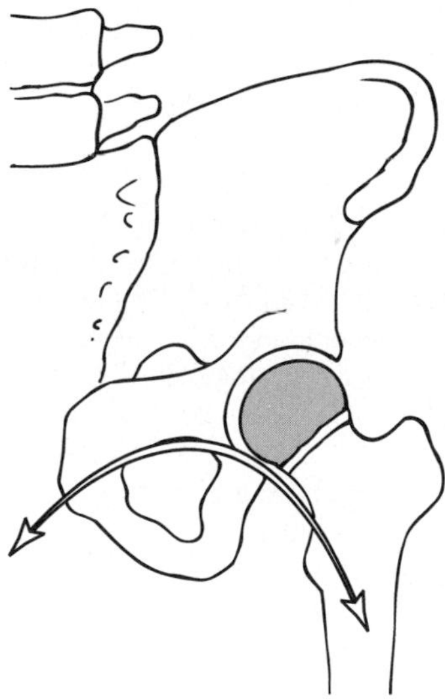

Fig. 14-17 AP view of the pelvis with Shenton's line to assess fracture, dislocation, or subluxation of the acetabulum and femoral head. (Courtesy Michael F. Rodi, MD.)

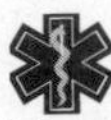

THE PAINFUL KNEE

Most fractures and dislocations about the knee are radiographically obvious. Clinical criteria have been developed for determining which patients may not need x-ray examination. An apparently isolated fibular fracture should prompt careful evaluation of the ankle, and a fat-fluid level on a lateral radiograph or a lipohemarthrosis on arthrocentesis should prompt an evaluation for an intraarticular fracture. Soft tissue injuries to the knee can generally be managed with a knee immobilizer, crutches, and outpatient follow-up. Nontraumatic knee pain may represent septic arthritis (see Chapter 20, Joint Pain).

KNEE DISLOCATION

Dislocation of the knee usually is caused by motor vehicle accidents, sports injuries, or falls. Dashboard injuries cause posterior dislocations (i.e., posterior translation of tibia), and hyperextension injuries cause anterior dislocations. Popliteal artery injury is common after knee dislocation and requires emergent vascular surgical consultation for repair.

Signs

- May be obviously dislocated or grossly unstable, which may indicate dislocation with spontaneous reduction
- Popliteal fossa may be full owing to vascular injury or may appear normal if decompressed by capsular tear
- Diminished pulses or neurologic deficit

Workup

- If appears dislocated on examination, reduce immediately
- Surgery if diminished pulses
- X-ray and angiography (some centers prefer observation with selective angiography)
- If grossly unstable, treat as a spontaneously reduced dislocation (angiography)

Comments and Treatment Considerations

Generally, traction-countertraction with conscious sedation

effectively reduces knee dislocations. Between 30% and 40% of dislocations are associated with popliteal artery injury, most of which require amputation if surgical repair is delayed >8 hours.

TIBIAL PLATEAU FRACTURE

Tibial plateau fracture may occur in younger individuals when valgus stress (e.g., bumper injury) causes lateral plateau fracture. The injury may be more subtle in the elderly, in whom axial compression can cause fracture.

Signs

- Local tenderness, usually decreased ROM
- Possible varus or valgus laxity

Workup

- X-ray: AP, lateral, and oblique views. Only sclerotic line below articular surface may be seen. Fracture should be suspected if AP view shows lateral margin of tibia is >5 mm beyond lateral cortex of femur.
- CT or MRI is confirmatory.

Comments and Treatment Considerations

Fractures of the medial plateau (20% of cases) should be treated as high-energy injuries or as possible spontaneous relocations; angiograms may be helpful. Patients should be observed for compartment syndrome while an orthopedic consultation in the ED is obtained.

MARKERS OF ANTERIOR CRUCIATE INJURY

Anterior cruciate injury is the most common ligamentous knee injury. A rapid effusion may develop following twist, rapid deceleration, or hyperextension; 35% report an audible "pop."

Signs

- Lachman ++++, gentle traction, since can be falsely negative if patient resists with muscles because of pain
- Laxity with anterior drawer +++

Workup

- X-rays: AP and lateral. Note Segond fracture (vertical fracture of lateral plateau), tibial spine avulsion, or "kissing contusion" (fracture of lateral condyle and lateral tibial plateau).

Comments and Treatment Considerations

Orthopedic consultation is necessary. Surgical results are especially favorable with bony avulsions.

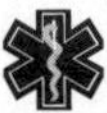

THE PAINFUL ANKLE AND FOOT

Most injuries to the foot and ankle are clinically and radiographically obvious. The mortise view should always be assessed for uniform joint space around the talus, and the lateral view to check calcaneus and posterior tibial integrity. The base of the fifth metatarsal should be checked in all patients with tenderness in this area after ankle inversion.

MAISONNEUVE FRACTURE

Maisonneuve fracture is a disruption—bony or ligamentous—of the medial ankle and proximal fibula and is usually caused by external rotation of the ankle.

Signs

- Tenderness at medial malleolus and proximal fibula

Workup

- X-ray: ankle series and AP and lateral views of proximal fibula. Only widening (i.e., no ankle fracture) may be noted if the deltoid ligament is ruptured.

Comments and Treatment Considerations

The instability of fibular fractures often necessitates surgical treatment. Fibular shortening predisposes to early arthritis.

LISFRANC FRACTURE-DISLOCATION

Lisfranc fracture-dislocation is a tarsometatarsal dislocation due to hyperplantar flexion over fixed forefoot; 20% are missed.

Signs

- Midfoot pain
- Midfoot swelling
- Difficulty ambulating

Workup

- X-ray: AP, lateral, and oblique. Suspect if bony fragment is seen at any metatarsal base. On normal AP, medial border of second metatarsal (MT) and middle cuneiform are aligned, and on normal oblique, medial border of third MT and lateral cuneiform are aligned (Figs. 14-18 and 14-19). On lateral, no MT should appear dorsal to cuboid. May confirm by CT.

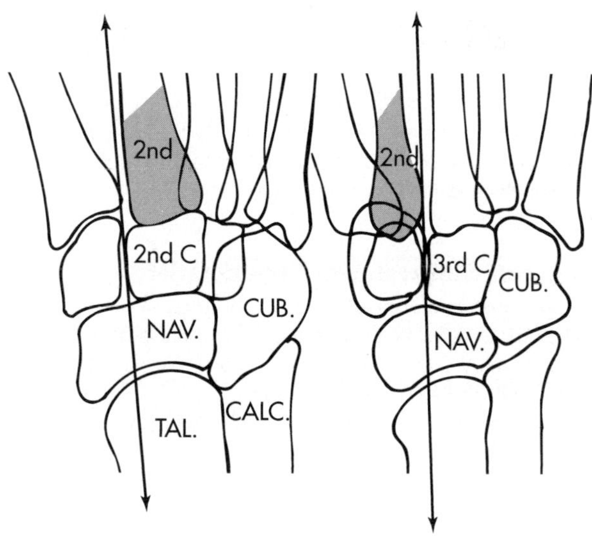

Fig. 14-18 AP and oblique views of the normal foot to assess fractures, dislocations, and subluxations in the foot (note the normal alignment of the tarsometatarsal joints–Lisfranc joints). (Courtesy Michael F. Rodi, MD.)

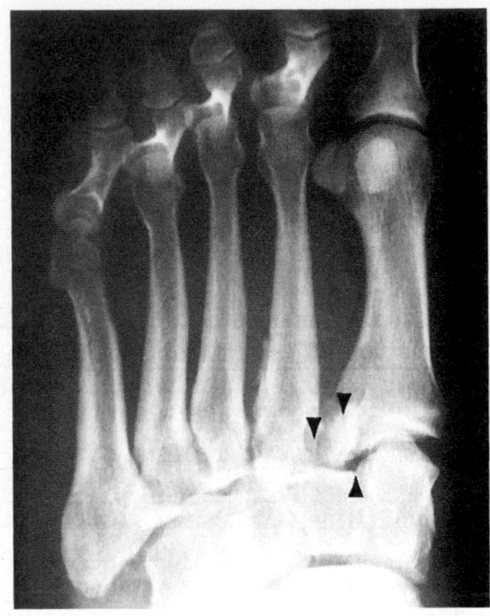

Fig. 14-19 AP view of foot shows Lisfranc fracture-dislocation. All tarsometatarsal joints are involved. Note malalignment of first and second metatarsals *(arrowheads)*. (Courtesy Michael Zucker, MD, Los Angeles.)

Comments and Treatment Considerations

Orthopedic consultation should be obtained in the ED. Surgery is often necessary. Posttraumatic arthritis is common.

CALCANEUS FRACTURE

Calcaneus fracture is usually caused by a fall or jump and may result from twisting.

Signs

- Local swelling and tenderness
- Unable to bear weight

Workup

- X-ray: Bohler's angle (Figs. 14-20 and 14-21) <30 degrees

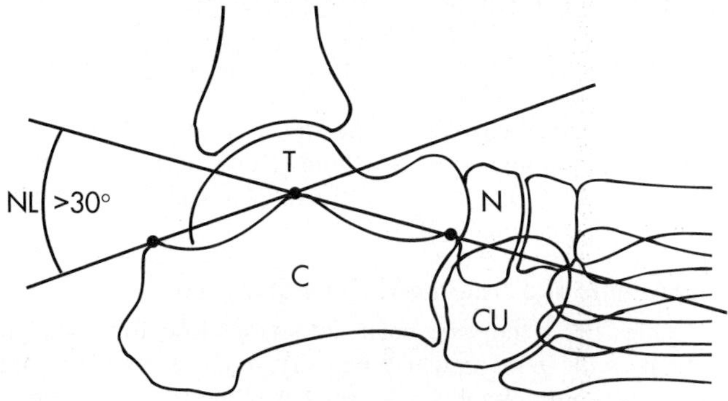

Fig. 14-20 Lateral view of the foot to assess fractures of the calcaneus. Note Bohler's angle; if less than 30 degrees, then suspect fracture of the calcaneus. *T,* Talus; *C,* calcaneus; *N,* navicular; *CU,* cuboid. (Courtesy Michael F. Rodi, MD.)

suggests a fracture, as do sclerotic lines in the calcaneal body, disruption of trabeculae, increased density (overlapping bone), and cortical lucencies. Also consider axial views or CT.

Comments and Treatment Considerations

Associated injuries should always be considered, especially to the axial skeleton; 10% have dorsolumbar compression fractures and compartment syndrome. The x-ray needs to be inspected closely to rule out talar dome fractures, which may have a similar clinical presentation.

FIFTH METATARSAL FRACTURE

There are three general fracture types of the fifth metatarsal: ankle twist causes avulsion fracture of the tuberosity at the base of the fifth metatarsal by contraction of the plantar fascia (dancer's); landing on the lateral border of the foot causes fracture at the metaphyseal-diaphyseal junction (Jones); and repetitive impact causes fatigue fracture at the diaphyseal base ("stress").

Signs

- Local tenderness at base of fifth metatarsal

Workup

- X-ray: AP, lateral, oblique
- Bone scan if negative and concern for stress fracture
- Normal apophysis in children (long axis parallel to metatarsal) should not be confused with avulsion fracture (usually perpendicular).

Comments and Treatment Considerations

Consider ED orthopedic consultation or close follow-up for patients with intraarticular tuberosity fractures or diaphyseal fractures. Posterior splint and crutches with orthopedic referral are necessary in most other cases.

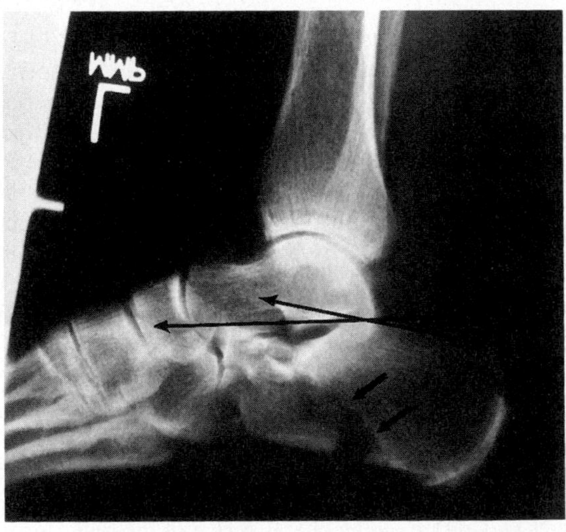

Fig. 14-21 Lateral view of foot shows calcaneus fracture. Intraarticular fracture *(short arrows)*. Bohler's angle is abnormal *(long arrows, arrowhead)*. (Courtesy Michael Zucker, MD, Los Angeles.)

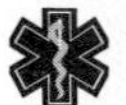 CHILD ABUSE

Many fractures are especially associated with abuse. Multiple fractures at different stages of healing are seen in 23% to 85% of abuse cases. Subperiosteal bone formation, "bucket-handle" fractures (i.e., fractures at the metaphyseal corners of long bones, Fig. 14-22), and fractures of the ribs, femur (especially in the nonambulatory), fingers, humerus, pelvis, spine, and skull are all suggestive of possible abuse.

See Chapter 18, The Irritable Child and Vomiting.

REFERENCES

Armstrong CP, Van der Spuy J: The fractured scapula: importance and management based on a series of 62 patients, *Injury* 15:324,1984.

Browner BD, Jupiter JB, Alan M. Levine AM, Trafton PG : *Skeletal trauma: fractures, dislocations, ligamentous injuries*, Philadelphia, 1992, WB Saunders.

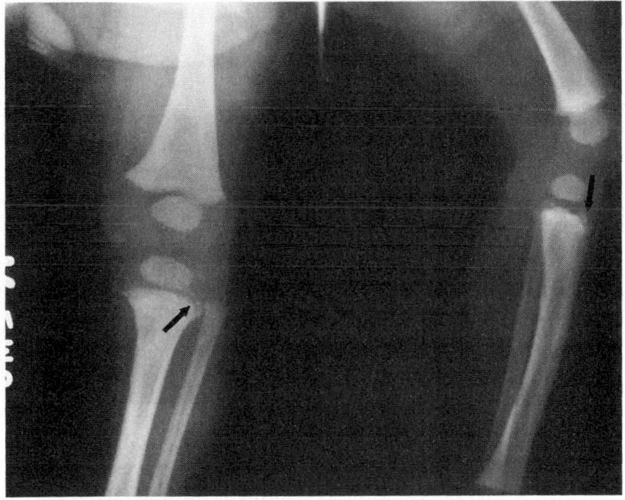

Fig. 14-22 AP and lateral knee radiographs demonstrate corner, or "bucket-handle," fracture of the proximal tibia *(arrows)* as a result of nonaccidental trauma (child abuse) (Courtesy Michael Zucker, MD, Los Angeles.)

Calandra JJ, Goldner RD, Hardaker WT Jr: Scaphoid fractures: assessment and treatment, *Orthopedics* 15:931, 1992.

Carty HM: Fractures caused by child abuse, *J Bone Joint Surg* 75B:849, 1993.

Council on Scientific Affairs: AMA diagnostic and treatment guidelines concerning child abuse and neglect, *JAMA* 254:796, 1985.

Englanoff G, Anglin D, Hutson HR: Lisfranc fracture-dislocation: a frequently missed diagnosis in the emergency department, *Ann Emerg Med* 26:229, 1995.

Freeland P: Scaphoid tubercle tenderness: a better indicator of scaphoid fractures? *Arch Emerg Med* 6:46, 1989.

Hoppenfeld S: *Physical examination of the spine and extremities,* London, 1976, Appleton-Century-Crofts.

Kaufman SL, Martin LG: Arterial injuries associated with complete dislocation of the knee, *Radiology* 184:153, 1992.

Kezdi-Rogus PC, Lomasney LM: Radiologic case study: plain film manifestations of ACL injury, *Orthopedics* 17:967, 1994.

Lawrence SJ, Botte MJ: Jones' fractures and related fractures of the proximal fifth metatarsal, *Foot Ankle* 14:358, 1993.

Leventhal JM, Thomas SA, Rosenfield NS, et al: Fractures in young children: distinguishing child abuse from unintentional injuries, *Am J Dis Child* 147:87, 1993.

Miller MD: Commonly missed orthopedic problems, *Emerg Med Clin North Am* 10:151, 1992.

Raby N, de Lacy G, Berman L: *Accident and emergency radiology—a survival guide*, Philadelphia, 1995, WB Saunders.

Regan W, Morrey BF: Classification and treatment of coronoid process fractures, *Orthopedics* 15:845, 1992.

Rockwood C, Green D: *Fractures in adults,* Philadelphia, 1984, JB Lippincott.

Rockwood C, Wilkins K, King R: *Fractures in children,* Philadelphia, 1984, JB Lippincott.

Simon R: *Emergency orthopedics—the extremities,* Norwalk, Conn, 1987, Appleton & Lange.

Treiman GS, Yellin AE, Weaver FA, et al: Examination of the patient with a knee dislocation: the case for selective arteriography, *Arch Surg* 127:1056, 1992.

Waeckerle JF: A prospective study identifying the sensitivity of radiographic findings and the efficacy of clinical findings in carpal navicular fractures, *Ann Emerg Med* 16:733, 1987.

Waizenegger M, Barton NJ, Davis TR, et al: Clinical signs in scaphoid fractures, *J Hand Surg* 19B:743, 1994.

CHAPTER 15

Headache

JONATHAN EDLOW and LAURA MACNOW

Headache is a common chief complaint of patients seeking care in the ED. Studies indicate that in only a few percent of these patients can headache be attributed to serious causes (life, limb, or vision threatening and treatable). Care must be taken not to draw unwarranted conclusions from either the degree of pain or measures required for its relief. Patients can be in a great deal of pain yet have a relatively benign condition; conversely, others may have only mild pain yet have a life-threatening illness. Even nonnarcotic analgesics have been reported to relieve the pain of subarachnoid hemorrhage, pseudotumor cerebri, and brain tumor. Therefore careful attention must be given to the cornerstone of diagnosis—a careful history and physical examination.

Besides the standard questions asked of a patient with any painful condition (onset, duration, alleviating factors, and so forth), some aspects of the history warrant special emphasis. Headache with acute onset should always raise the concern for subarachnoid hemorrhage, as headache with fever does for meningitis. Some patients, especially the elderly, can have a subdural hematoma weeks after relatively minor trauma. Therefore this history must be actively elicited. If the patient suffers from regular headaches, it is important to establish if the current episode deviates from the normal pattern.

Age is important; up to 15% of patients over 65 years with new onset of headache have a serious medical condition. Even the season may be significant; during the winter months, carbon monoxide poisoning should be considered as a possible diagnosis.

Prior history of or risks for HIV infection, malignancy, and neurosurgery should be obtained. Drug history, especially of anticoagulants, MAO inhibitors, and cocaine, should be sought. With the caveat that a complete physical examination be done, key elements include vital signs, sinuses, tympanic membranes, optic fundi, cornea, temporal arteries, neck, and skin (rash and color) and a detailed neurologic examination. Components that are commonly omitted are bedside visual field and gait testing. Both of these can be performed quickly and cover a lot of neuroanatomic territory. It is noteworthy that patients with intracranial masses occasionally have a completely normal examination.

Laboratory tests, neuroimaging studies, and examination of the cerebrospinal fluid must be tailored to the individual situation. Neuroimaging of unselected patients with headache yields a very low incidence of significant abnormalities. The high availability of CT scanners has encouraged physicians to routinely perform a scan before doing a lumbar puncture (LP). This practice is unnecessary in many cases, and obtaining a CT scan should never delay treatment of suspected bacterial meningitis. Post–spinal tap headache is more common in younger, thinner females and is reduced by using smaller-gauge needles that split rather than transect the dural fibers. Other variables have not correlated with post-LP headache.

Although this chapter focuses on the diagnosis and treatment of emergent conditions, it is equally important to relieve pain in the vast majority of patients with less serious illnesses.

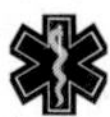

BACTERIAL MENINGITIS

Bacterial meningitis typically presents with headache, stiff neck, and photophobia in its more advanced stages. Early in the course the presentation may be more subtle. Meningitis should always be considered in patients with fever and altered mental status. Early treatment with antibiotics is imperative and should not be delayed in order to perform any test (including LP). In the few cases when it may be appropriate to delay LP in order to do CT first, blood should be drawn for blood cultures, and antibiotics then given *before* CT. LP should then be performed if not contraindicated by

CT findings. This strategy identifies the cause of bacterial meningitis in most cases, even when LP is performed 1 to 2 hours after the initiation of antibiotics.

Symptoms

- Fever ++++
- Headache +++
- Stiff neck ++
- Vomiting +++
- Photophobia
- Altered mental status

Signs

- Temperature >38° C ++++
- Classic triad +++: fever, nuchal rigidity, change in mental status
- Meningismus +++: nuchal rigidity, Brudzinski's sign, Kernig's sign
- Mental status changes: irritable +++, confused, lethargic +++, decreased responsiveness to pain ++, coma ++, normal
- Seizures ++, much more common with *Streptococcus pneumoniae* than with *Neisseria meningitidis*
- Focal CNS findings: cranial nerve palsies, gaze preference, aphasia, hemiparesis ++
- Rash: maculopapular, petechial, purpuric (+++ of *N. meningitidis*)

Workup

- Antibiotics should not be delayed for evaluation. Blood and urine cultures, if indicated, should be obtained immediately and antibiotic treatment initiated (also consider steroid treatment) if any delay in obtaining CSF is likely.
- CT scan before LP if coma, papilledema, focal neurologic deficit, or AIDS
- Lumbar puncture for cerebrospinal fluid analysis: cell count and differential, glucose, protein, gram stain, culture (+/− special tests only if indicated: India ink, latex agglutination [if negative gram stain], cryptococcal Ag, Ab studies for histoplasmosis, coccidioidomycosis, blastomycosis,

VDRL, Lyme serology, cultures for tuberculosis, fungi, anaerobes, and so on)

Comments and Treatment Considerations

Antibiotic administration must not be delayed. Meningismus does not often develop in infants, who may have only fever, irritability, lethargy, poor feeding, or vomiting. Similarly, elderly patients may be lethargic and obtundent, have no fever, and show variable meningeal signs. Patients (especially children) with recent antibiotic treatment may have masked symptoms, and there should therefore be a low threshold for performing an LP (CSF cell count, differential, glucose, protein should not be affected, but gram stain and cultures are often negative in partially treated patients). Treatment should target the most likely organism. Vancomycin may be added to cover emerging strains of resistant *S. pneumoniae.*

- Age <3 months: group B streptococcus, *E. coli*, *Listeria monocytogenes* (ampicillin plus broad-spectrum cephalosporin, e.g., cefotaxime or ceftriaxone)
- Age 3 months to <18 years: *N. meningitidis*, *S. pneumoniae*, *H. influenzae* (broad-spectrum cephalosporin, e.g., cefotaxime or ceftriaxone)
- Age 18 to 50: *S. pneumoniae*, *N. meningitidis* (broad-spectrum cephalosporin, e.g., cefotaxime or ceftriaxone)
- Age >50: *S. pneumoniae*, *L. monocytogenes*, gram-negative bacilli (ampicillin plus broad-spectrum cephalosporin, e.g., cefotaxime or ceftriaxone)
- Immunocompromised: ampicillin plus ceftazidime
- Head trauma, neurosurgery, CSF shunt: vancomycin plus ceftazidime

Adjuvant dexamethasone use is controversial, although it is recommended for bacterial meningitis in children younger than 2 months, especially those who are likely infected by *H. influenzae* (i.e., children not vaccinated). It may possibly benefit adults who have a high concentration of bacteria in the CSF (i.e., positive gram stain) and evidence of increased intracranial pressure (ICP). Dose: 0.15 mg/kg q6h for 4 days. Anticonvulsants may be added if necessary.

REFERENCES

Quagliarello VJ, Scheld WM: Treatment of bacterial meningitis, *N Engl J Med* 336:708, 1997.

Sigurdardottir B, Bjornsson OM, Jonsdottir KE, et al: Acute bacterial meningitis in adults: a 20-year overview, *Arch Intern Med* 157:425, 1997.

Tunkel AR, Scheld WM: Acute bacterial meningitis, *Lancet* 346:1675, 1995.

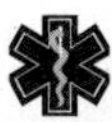

SUBARACHNOID HEMORRHAGE

Subarachnoid hemorrhage (SAH) is bleeding in the subarachnoid space that can be caused by rupture of a cerebral aneurysm or by arteriovenous malformation. Although aneurysmal SAH typically begins abruptly, produces a headache that is most severe at onset, and is described by patients as the worst headache of their life, a minority has less severe (though generally very distinctive) symptoms. Prompt evaluation with CT scan and LP excludes this condition. SAH may present with a large bleed and an abnormal neurologic examination or with minimal headache at the time of ED presentation and a normal neurologic exam (in the case of a "sentinel bleed"). It is critical to make the diagnosis of cerebral aneurysm at the time of a sentinel bleed, since debilitating hemorrhage may follow if neurosurgical intervention is delayed.

Symptoms

- Headache +++++: often abrupt onset of severe headache ("worst headache of life"). Headache is usually global; can be associated with nausea, vomiting, and transient loss of consciousness, classically during exercise but can be at rest.
- Warning headache +++: a distinctive "thunderclap" headache, also referred to as a sentinel bleed, preceding the major SAH by days to weeks; thought to be caused by a minor leak of blood, bleeding into the wall of the aneurysm, or thrombosis at the site of the aneurysm
- Neck pain: from blood irritating the meninges (can be the only presenting complaint)

- Back and radicular pain: occurs later in some patients from irritation as the blood settles into the lumbar thecal sac
- Altered mental status with severe bleeds

Signs

- May have normal examination
- Meningismus (frequent)
- Retinal subhyaloid hemorrhage ++ : significant bleeding often with a fluid level seen on funduscopic examination
- Focal or generalized neurologic abnormalities (variable)

Workup

- CT scan: generally considered primary screening test ++++ in first 24 hours, although is likely much less sensitive for warning leak. Sensitivity continues to decline over time (Fig. 15-1)
- LP: the definitive test; indicated after negative CT. It can occasionally be negative during first several hours. Xanthochromia takes hours to develop; can be negative by visual inspection, but by spectrophotometry is almost always is present from 12 hours to 2 weeks.
- Angiography/MR angiography: once diagnosed by CT or LP, used to identify the source of bleeding
- MR angiography: in thunderclap headache with normal CT and LP results, the vast majority of patients have a benign course; in the occasional patient with high clinical suspicion of SAH, MR angiography may be indicated.
- MRI: not as sensitive as CT

Comments and Treatment Considerations

Emergent neurosurgical consultation is required after the diagnosis of SAH is made. Nonspecific treatment includes bed rest, isotonic fluids to prevent hyponatremia (which could cause or worsen cerebral edema), and nimodipine within the first 12 hours (to decrease vasospasm).

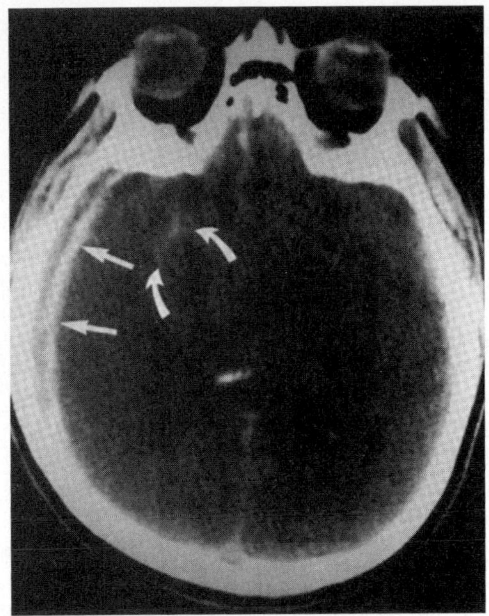

Fig. 15-1 Noncontrast CT scan of subarachnoid hemorrhage. High-density areas within the sylvian fissure represent subarachnoid hemorrhage. An acute subdural hematoma on the right is also present. (From Rosen P, Doris PE, Barkin RM, et al: *Diagnostic radiology in emergency medicine,* St Louis, 1992, Mosby.)

REFERENCES

Adams HP, Jergenson DD, Kassell NF, Sahs AL: Pitfalls in the recognition of subarachnoid hemorrhage, *JAMA* 244:794, 1980.

Edlow JA: Diagnosis of subarachnoid hemorrhage: avoiding the pitfalls and expediting assessment, *Emerg Med Reports* 19:15, 1998.

Hauerber J, Anderson BB, Eskesen V, et al: Importance of the recognition of a warning leak as a sign of a ruptured intracranial aneurysm, *Acta Neurol Scand* 83:61, 1991.

Schievink WI: Intracranial aneurysms, *N Engl J Med* 336:28, 1997.

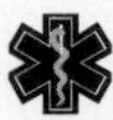 *BRAIN OR PARAMENINGEAL ABSCESS*

Careful attention to risk factors is crucial in diagnosing brain and parameningeal abscess, since patients can have a normal examination, no fever, and no leukocytosis. *Patients who are immunocompromised may look well or may be clinically very ill appearing.* Predisposing factors include the following:

- Infectious focus: otitis media, mastoiditis, sinusitis, skin infection (with bacteremia), endocarditis and congenital heart disease, pulmonary infection, dental infection
- Prior head injury
- Steroid use and immunosuppression
- Surgical procedure

Symptoms

- Headache ++++
- Focal neurologic deficit +++
- Nausea and vomiting +++
- Diffuse neurologic symptoms ++: coma, seizures, behavioral disturbances
- Subtle personality changes (with frontal lobe abscesses)

Signs

- Fever +++
- Toxic appearing ++ (variable)
- Meningismus ++: (variable, especially with occipital or temporal lobe)
- Papilledema +++
- Focal neurologic deficit +++: mild hemiparesis most common

Workup

- CT *with contrast* is very sensitive. Antibiotics should be started before scan.
- LP: only if signs of meningismus or diffuse neurologic symptoms are present and CT scan is negative
- CBC: WBC >10,000 (50%)
- Blood culture before starting antibiotics

Comments and Treatment Considerations

Generally patients have rapidly progressing symptoms. Infection is polymicrobial in almost half of the cases. Treatment consists of high-dose intravenous antibiotics to cover likely organisms. If cutaneous source is likely, coverage needs to include *S. aureus*. Corticosteroids are given to treat symptomatic cerebral edema.

REFERENCES

Harrison MJ: The clinical presentation of intracranial abscesses, *Q J Med* 51:461, 1982.

Seydoux C, Francioli P: Bacterial brain abscesses: factors influencing mortality and sequelae, *Clin Infect Dis* 15:394, 1992.

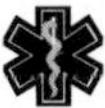

SUBDURAL AND EPIDURAL HEMATOMA

Epidural and subdural hematomas (EDH and SDH) manifesting shortly after acute head trauma generally, although not always, lead to neurologic deficits. These entities (commonly SDH) can also present some time after the traumatic event, especially in the elderly, in whom headache may be the only finding.

Symptoms

- Decreased level of consciousness (LOC) following head injury
- Headache (common in conscious and chronic SDH patients)
- Seizures ++
- Focal neurologic symptoms
- Confusion, personality changes (chronic SDH)

Signs

- Diminished LOC including coma
- Focal neurologic signs including dilated pupil and hemiparesis. Classically the dilated pupil is ipsilateral to the hematoma and the hemiparesis is contralateral; however, the pupil may be contralaterally dilated ++, and the hemiparesis can be ipsilateral ++. This is caused by either direct injury of the third nerve or midbrain or by compression of the contralateral

cerebral peduncle. (Patients with dilated pupils from this mechanism have severely diminished LOC; anisocoria in a conscious patient nearly always represents local eye injury or installation of mydriatic drops.)

- May have normal examination or subtle deficits

Workup

- CT scan should be done promptly to define size, location, and presence of associated injuries (e.g., cerebral contusion). CT scan in SDH between 10 to 20 days may appear isodense, hypodense thereafter (Figs. 15-2 and 15-3).
- Careful evaluation for signs of noncranial trauma

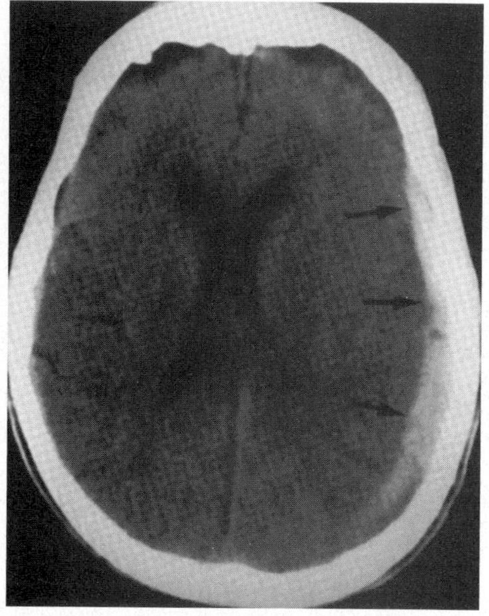

Fig. 15-2 Noncontrast CT scan of subdural hematoma. High-density region conforming to the convexity of the skull. (From Rosen P, Doris PE, Barkin RM, et al: *Diagnostic radiology in emergency medicine,* St Louis, 1992, Mosby.)

Comments and Treatment Considerations

Most patients with SDH or EDH arrive at the ED shortly after trauma. Careful attention must be paid to the airway, breathing, and circulation (ABCs), especially ventilation. Hyperventilation significantly decreases ICP but should not be too aggressive (probably PCO_2 in low thirties). Neurosurgeons should be consulted early for decompression and possible use of mannitol.

Rarely, (as high as 8% in one series) an EDH has a delayed presentation (after an initially normal CT scan), usually within 12 to 24 hours; thus an initially normal CT scan does not exclude EDH, so caution is appropriate when the clinical suspicion is high.

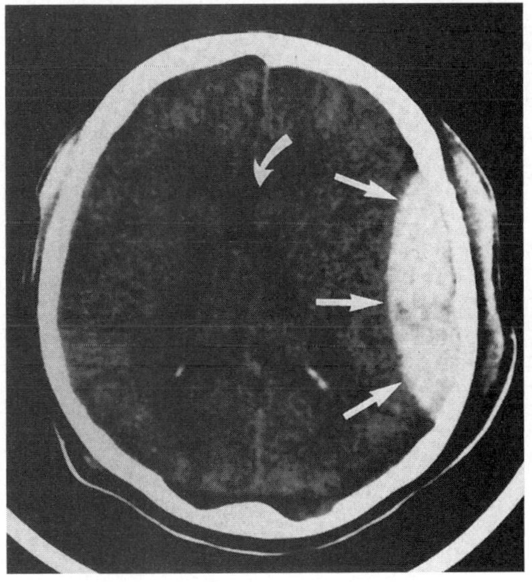

Fig. 15-3 Noncontrast CT scan of epidural hematoma. Biconvex high-density lesion. (From Rosen P, Doris PE, Barkin RM, et al: *Diagnostic radiology in emergency medicine*, St Louis, 1992, Mosby.)

Chronic SDHs are far more common, especially in the elderly, in whom they can present weeks after injury (which may be minor) with headache (+++), focal weakness, confusion, personality changes, anisocoria, seizures, and changes in LOC. These symptoms and signs can be transient.

REFERENCES

Fink M: Emergency management of the head-injured patient, *Emerg Clin North Am* 5:783, 1987.

Obana WG, Pitts LH: Extracerebral lesions (in the management of head injury), *Neurosurg Clin North Am* 2:351, 1991.

Springer MFB, Baker FJ: Cranial burr hole decompression in the emergency department, *Am J Emerg Med* 6:640, 1988.

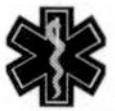

TEMPORAL ARTERITIS

Giant cell arteritis (GCA) is a systemic vasculitis of large and medium arteries that usually, though not exclusively, involves the temporal artery. The diagnosis should be considered in every patient over the age of 50 with headache. This is one cause of headache in which a laboratory test—the erythrocyte sedimentation rate—is quite useful in increasing or decreasing the likelihood of the diagnosis, although false positive and negative ESR results do occur. GCA is frequently associated with polymyalgia rheumatica (PMR).

Symptoms

- Headache ++++: unilateral temporal ++, nontemporal (>30%)
- Jaw claudication and facial pain +++
- Decreased visual acuity, sudden loss of vision
- Constitutional symptoms (malaise, weight loss)
- Muscle pain and stiffness ++: large proximal muscle groups, since may have PMR
- Visual disturbances +++ : including diplopia, visual field defect

Signs

- Scalp tenderness +++
- Abnormal palpable temporal artery +++: nonpulsatile, cord-like, nodular, tender
- Fever ++
- Cranial nerve palsy ++: diplopia, ptosis, rarely deafness
- Funduscopy: may reveal ischemic changes if retinal artery occlusion

Workup

- ESR: usually elevated >40 ++++ (often much higher). Normal ESR does not rule out diagnosis, nor does level correlate with severity of disease.
- CBC: decreased hematocrit +++, mild leukocytosis (30%)

Comments and Treatment Considerations

Giant cell arteritis is extremely rare in black and Asian individuals. Incidence increases with age >55. Female-to-male ratio is 2:1. GCA is a clinical diagnosis, and immediate treatment should be initiated to prevent significant morbidity (e.g., blindness and cerebral infarction). Therefore, in a patient with high clinical probability of GCA, steroid treatment should be initiated and urgent temporal artery biopsy arranged. A temporal artery biopsy can be performed to establish a definitive diagnosis, but a negative biopsy does not rule out GCA. Treatment consists of prednisone 45 to 60 mg/day for 4 days, with the course tapering by 5 mg every 2 weeks until a maintenance dose of 15 mg/day is reached. Close follow-up is required.

REFERENCES

Karanjia ND, Cawthorn SJ, Giddings AEB: The diagnosis and management of arteritis, *J R Soc Med* 86:267, 1993.

Nordborg E, Nordborg C, Malmvall BE, et al: Giant cell arteritis, *Rheum Dis Clin North Am* 21:1013, 1995.

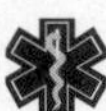

COMPLICATED SINUSITIS

The ED physician must distinguish common maxillary sinusitis from more severe infections in the ethmoid, sphenoid, and frontal sinuses, which, because of risk of serious complications, may require hospital admission for administration of intravenous antibiotics.

Acute ethmoiditis is most commonly seen in children. It may be complicated by periorbital cellulitis (swelling, erythema, and warmth) and orbital cellulitis (chemosis, proptosis, and gaze disturbance) (see Chapter 11, Eye Pain and Redness). Sphenoid sinusitis can be occult because of its lack of significant facial drainage and facial tenderness. Headache can be retro-orbital or at the vertex and can also produce infraorbital hypesthesia. Features of acute sphenoid sinusitis include severe, progressive headache (++++), often increasing with activity or coughing, nausea and vomiting (+++), and fever (+++). Patients may *not* complain of nasal discharge or congestion.

Patients with sphenoid sinusitis often present late with complications (57%), which often produce ophthalmologic symptoms (chemosis, proptosis, ptosis, diplopia, ophthalmoplegia, and decreased visual acuity) or neurologic symptoms (hypoesthesia of the first and second divisions of the fifth cranial nerve, hemiparesis, meningitis, and altered sensorium). Patients may have a vertex headache.

Frontal sinusitis is associated with intracranial abscess and meningitis. Osteomyelitis of the frontal bone (Pott's puffy tumor) is a rare complication of frontal sinusitis characterized by pain and pitting edema over the forehead. The risk of complications is high among immunocompromised patients, individuals with previous history of intracranial surgery, orbital cellulitis, recurrent outpatient failure, and previous inadequate treatment (may mask complications), and those unable to obtain follow-up. Other complications of frontal sinusitis include cavernous sinus thrombosis and brain or parameningeal abscess.

Symptoms

- Nasal discharge or congestion ++++
- Cough or recent upper respiratory tract infection ++++

- Headache +++
- Facial pain +++
- Tooth or palate pain (common in maxillary sinusitis)

Signs

- Fever +++
- Tenderness over sinuses +++
- Purulent rhinorrhea +++
- Abnormal transillumination of sinuses (frontal or maxillary)

Workup

- For routine sinusitis, diagnosis is clinical
- Sinus CT: especially for possible frontal, sphenoid, or ethmoidal sinusitis and orbital or cranial complications
- MRI: if concern of cavernous sinus thrombosis (rare)
- Sinus x-ray: low sensitivity +++ and specificity (36% to 76%)
- CBC: not helpful

Comments and Treatment Considerations

Acute uncomplicated sinusitis should be treated with a 10- to 14-day course of antibiotics directed against common pathogens (*S. pneumoniae* and *H. influenzae*); decongestants also should be used (oral or nasal; caution against overuse of nasal preparations >5 days). Treatment failures should be given a penicillinase-resistant drug (e.g., amoxicillin/clavulanic acid or a second- or third-generation cephalosporin). Chronic sinusitis (symptoms lasting more than 3 months) should be treated with broad-spectrum antibiotics to cover other pathogens (*S. aureus* and anaerobes, in addition to usual microbes), and, since antibiotic therapy is often ineffective, patients should be referred for ENT evaluation. Admission for intravenous antibiotic treatment should be considered for complicated sinusitis.

REFERENCES

Dolan RW, Chowdhury K: Diagnosis and treatment of intracranial complications of paranasal sinus infections, *J Oral Maxillofac Surg* 53:1080, 1995.

Kibblewhite DJ, Cleland J, Mintz DR: Acute sphenoid sinusitis: management strategies, *J Otolaryngol* 17:159, 1988.
Willett LR, Carson JL, Williams JW: Current diagnosis and management of sinusitis, *J Gen Intern Med* 9:38, 1994.

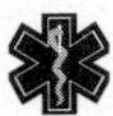

CARBON MONOXIDE POISONING

Headache is a common symptom of carbon monoxide poisoning. In addition to known exposures, winter presentation (heating systems), typical symptoms, and clustering of cases all suggest this diagnosis. There is a correlation with winter months; other people in the house being ill, problems with home heating, or use of kerosene or gas space heaters.

Symptoms

Symptoms correlate variably with the carboxyhemoglobin level (CoHb); levels up to 9% can be seen in smokers and 2% to 4% in patients in congested urban areas. In general, the CoHb levels listed below roughly correlate to the following symptoms:

- 10% to 20%—headache, dizziness, chest pain, dyspnea
- 20% to 30%—visual disturbances, confusion
- 30% to 40%—syncope
- 40% to 50%—seizures, coma, death at levels >55% or 60%
- Headache is very common.

Signs

- Physical examination is usually normal.
- Cutaneous and mucosal erythema, retinal hemorrhages, and bullae on the skin are all rare.

Workup

- CoHb level (use ABG kit)
- Arterial blood gases: may show metabolic acidosis. Readings of oxygen saturation will be falsely normal (if calculated from Po_2) unless directly measured by co-oximetry.
- Electrocardiogram: may show nonspecific repolarization

changes. May be useful in ruling out other pathologic conditions.

- Chest x-ray: ++ shows nonspecific findings of interstitial or alveolar edema, atelectasis, perivascular/bronchial cuffing, and peripheral opacities. May be useful in ruling out other pathologic conditions.

Comments and Treatment Considerations

The half-life of CoHb is 4 to 6 hours breathing room air, 90 minutes breathing 100% O_2, and 45 minutes with hyperbaric O_2 (hyperbaric oxygen, HBO) at 2.5 standard atmosphere. Do not rely on pulse oximetry. This technique measures CoHb the same as O_2-Hb and will be falsely normal. Treat immediately with 100% O_2. Indications for HBO (not universally agreed on) include CoHb level >25% (at the peak level), pregnancy, end-organ damage (neurologic, including mental status deficits, or cardiopulmonary), metabolic acidosis, age >50, and worsening or failure to improve on 100% O_2 for 4 hours.

REFERENCES

Ely EW, Moorehead B, Haponik EF: Warehouse worker's headache: emergency evaluation and management of 30 patients with carbon monoxide poisoning, *Am J Med* 98:145, 1995.

Hecherling PS, Leikin JB, Maturen A: Occult carbon monoxide poisoning: validation of a prediction model, *Am J Med* 84:251, 1988.

Sadovnikoff N, Varon J, Sternbach GL: Carbon monoxide poisoning—an occult epidemic, *Postgrad Med* 92:86, 1992.

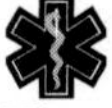

CAVERNOUS SINUS THROMBOSIS

The most common cause of cavernous sinus thrombosis is sphenoid or ethmoid sinusitis. Treatment consists of high-dose, broad-spectrum intravenous antibiotics and an ENT referral for surgical drainage. Careful attention to the HEENT examination often suggests this unusual entity. Rapid treatment and surgical consultation are key. The structures passing through the cavernous sinus include the third and fourth cranial nerves, ophthalmic and maxillary divisions of fifth and sixth cranial nerves, and the internal carotid artery with its sympathetic plexus.

Symptoms

- Headache: severe, frontal or retro-orbital pain
- Diplopia
- Vomiting, seizures, hemiplegia, dysarthria, and altered mental status are not as commonly seen as in other cerebral venous thromboses.

Signs

- Chemosis, proptosis, or ptosis ++++
- Periorbital or orbital edema: progressive unilateral or bilateral
- Isolated abducens nerve palsy or involvement of third, fourth, and fifth cranial nerves and paresthesia of V1/V2 distribution
- Fever
- Funduscopy: venous engorgement, papilledema
- Meningismus +++

Workup

- CT
- MRI
- Blood culture before starting antibiotics

REFERENCES

Ameri A, Bousser MG: Cerebral venous thrombosis, *Neurol Clin* 10:87, 1992.

Dolan RW, Chowdhury K: Diagnosis and treatment of intracranial complications of paranasal sinus infections, *J Oral Maxillofac Surg* 53:1080, 1995.

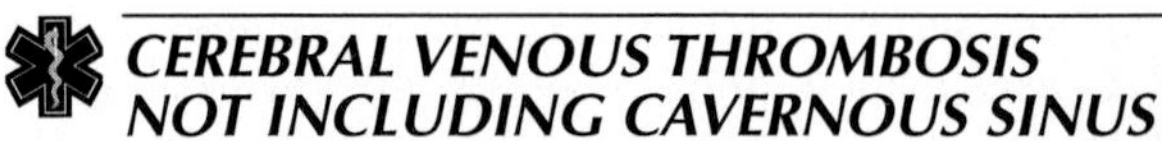

CEREBRAL VENOUS THROMBOSIS NOT INCLUDING CAVERNOUS SINUS

Cerebral venous thrombosis (CVT) is a rare entity that can be difficult to diagnose and for which imaging studies can be normal. Routine measurement of the opening pressure of spinal fluid is one safeguard for not missing the diagnosis. CVT should be considered in patients with severe headache without other explanation.

Symptoms

- Headache ++++, not location specific
- Vomiting +++
- Thunderclap headache +
- Focal neurologic deficit ++
- Seizures ++ focal or generalized

Signs

- Papilledema +++
- Mental status changes ++
- Cranial nerve palsies ++
- Dysarthria or dysphasia ++
- Hemiplegia

Workup

- Angiography: gold standard; next method if MRI is negative; four-vessel study needed; must visualize entire venous phase
- MRI: useful to distinguish CVT from pseudotumor cerebri
- CT with and without contrast; may be normal in up to 20% of CVT
- LP: may see increased opening pressure, increased protein, or increased RBCs
- Blood culture
- Coagulation studies

Comments and Treatment Considerations

Approximately 40% of patients have isolated intracranial hypertension (headache and papilledema) that can be confused with pseudotumor cerebri. The cause of CVT is diverse:

- Septic thrombosis usually from infections of middle third of face and sphenoid or ethmoid sinus; otitis media or mastoiditis; septicemia, endocarditis (especially with dehydration)

- Hypercoagulable states such as malignancies, inflammatory diseases, factor V Leiden mutation, hereditary antithrombin III, protein C, and protein S deficiencies
- Pregnancy, puerperium, and oral contraceptive use
- Local head trauma (open or closed, with or without fracture)

Treatment is controversial and may include anticonvulsants, high-dose, broad-spectrum intravenous antibiotics for septic CVT, anticoagulants (despite risk of intracranial hemorrhage with increased ICP, heparin has been shown to decrease morbidity and mortality in one randomized control trial), mannitol (to decrease ICP, but diuresis may worsen hypercoagulability), and repeated LPs if increased ICP.

REFERENCES

Ameri A, Bousser MG: Cerebral venous thrombosis, *Neurol Clin* 10:87, 1992.

Pannke TS: Cerebral dural sinus thrombosis, *Ann Emerg Med* 20:813, 1991.

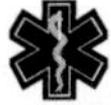

BENIGN INTRACRANIAL HYPERTENSION (PSEUDOTUMOR CEREBRI)

Pseudotumor cerebri is a rare condition that is most commonly seen in overweight females. The incidence in the general population is low (~0.9/100,000); however, in obese females weighing more than 20% of ideal body weight, the incidence rises to ~20/100,000. Associations with vitamin A, tetracycline, estrogen, and steroid use, steroid tapering, and various endocrine problems have been reported. Except for vitamin A use, these associations are based mostly on case reports and may not be universally applicable; their absence should by no means dissuade one from making the diagnosis. An imaging study followed by a lumbar puncture are required to establish diagnosis. The criteria for diagnosis include the following:

- Elevated ICP (>20 cm H_2O)
- Normal neurologic examination except papilledema (and sixth nerve palsy)

- Normal neuroimaging (no mass or ventricular enlargement)
- Normal CSF (except low CSF protein)
- No suspicion of cerebral venous sinus thrombosis or other cause for elevated ICP

Symptoms

- Headache ++++ can be constant or intermittent, often retrobulbar +++, and sometimes worse with eye movement
- Transient visual obscurations +++ defined as visual symptoms lasting seconds to minutes
- Nausea +++
- Visual loss ++
- Neck pain ++
- Vomiting ++
- Diplopia ++
- Tinnitus ++
- Radicular back and neck pain ++
- Diminished sense of smell ++

Signs

- Papilledema—very frequent, but precise figures are unavailable, since the diagnosis may be made less often in its absence.
- Sixth nerve palsy may occur by definition. To make the diagnosis, no other neurologic physical findings are allowed.

Workup

Establishing the diagnosis requires an imaging study (at least a CT scan) and a lumbar puncture. Evaluation may include MR or cerebral angiography to rule out other causes of increased ICP, such as venous sinus thrombosis.

Comments and Treatment Considerations

Papilledema may be unilateral or asymmetric. When the diagnosis is suspected on the basis of epidemiology, history, physical examination, and initial imaging, more than the usual amount of cerebrospinal fluid should be taken when performing the spinal tap.

Medical therapy consists of removing the inciting drug or endocrine condition (if one is present), repetitive LPs, acetazolamide, furosemide, or a short course of glucocorticoids. Controlled trials have not consistently shown surgical shunting procedures to be more effective than medical therapy.

REFERENCES

Durcan FJ, Corbett JJ, Wall M: The incidence of pseudotumor cerebri, *Arch Neurol* 45:875, 1988.

Giuseffi V, Wall M, Siegel PZ, Rojas PB: Symptoms and disease associations in idiopathic intracranial hypertension (pseudotumor cerebri): a case-controlled study, *Neurology* 41:239, 1991.

Wall M: The headache profile of idiopathic intracranial hypertension, *Cephalalgia* 10:331, 1990.

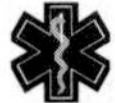

BRAIN TUMOR

To diagnose a brain tumor, the index of suspicion must be high, since there is no characteristic pattern of signs and symptoms. The classic combination of early morning headache and papilledema is uncommon. Emergent treatment is generally necessary only for symptoms or signs of an acute increase in ICP or bleeding. Most patients require only consultation with a neurologist or neurosurgeon and timely referral for full evaluation.

Symptoms

- Headache: +++ for both primary and metastatic brain tumors. The quality of headache is nondescript. In the majority, the quality is similar to a tension headache and is usually bifrontal. The headache may become worse on bending or with Valsalva maneuver ++, be associated with nausea and vomiting +++, or be the "worst headache ever" in the patient's life +++. However, it can also be mild or be relieved by nonnarcotic analgesics. The classic pattern of worse headache upon awakening in the early morning is uncommon.

- In patients with normal intracranial pressure (ICP), headache ++ and vomiting ++
- In patients with elevated ICP, headache ++++ and vomiting +++
- Focal neurologic symptoms depend on location and size of tumor.

Signs

- Any focal neurologic examination abnormality depends on the location and size of tumor.
- Papilledema: +++ in patients with elevated ICP (not seen in patients with normal ICP)
- Ataxia: +++ in patients with increased ICP (+ of patients with normal ICP)

Workup

Workup involves an imaging study, either a contrast-enhanced CT scan or an MRI. Emergently, a noncontrast CT scan provides enough information to safely discharge the patient, but it will not rule out tumor or abscess with certainty. Early follow-up is required.

Comments and Treatment Considerations

For patients with elevated ICP, neurosurgical consultation is mandatory. Consider intravenous dexamethasone (Decadron) and mannitol (after neurosurgical consultation). Anticonvulsants should be considered.

REFERENCES

Edgeworth J, Bullock P, Bailey A, et al: Why are brain tumors still being missed? *Arch Dis Child* 74:148, 1996.

Forsyth PA, Posner JB: Headaches in patients with brain tumors: a study of 111 patients, *Neurology* 43:1678, 1993.

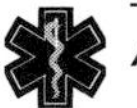

ACUTE ANGLE-CLOSURE GLAUCOMA

Although acute angle-closure glaucoma is a disease of the eye, it can cause severe systemic symptoms with, or without, eye pain. Patients may have headache, malaise, abdominal pain, or nausea and vomiting. Patients are generally elderly, and the diagnosis is made through eye examination including intraocular pressure measurement.

See Chapter 11, Eye Pain and Redness.

REFERENCES

Watson NJ, Kirkby GR: Acute glaucoma presenting with abdominal symptoms, *BMJ* 299:254, 1989.

Zimmerman TJ: The treatment of acute angle-closure glaucoma revisited, *Ann Ophthalmol* 16:1101, 1984.

CHAPTER 16

Hypertension

MARK LOUDEN and ATILLA UNER

Patients with elevated blood pressure frequently visit the ED. Their "hypertension" may be the result of essential hypertension, the effect of a specific pathologic process, a by-product of the stress of the ED visit, or an erroneous blood pressure reading. Hypertensive emergency is an elevation in blood pressure that causes end-organ dysfunction. True hypertensive emergency develops in only 1% to 2% of patients with hypertension. A good history, physical examination, and a few simple tests are all that are generally required to rule out end-organ damage that requires emergent intervention. In the absence of such a condition, hypertension generally requires only close follow-up, although one oral (not sublingual) dose of a low-strength antihypertensive agent may be considered.

Severe hypertension associated with myocardial ischemia, renal damage, CNS dysfunction, or other end-organ disease should be treated with easily titratable intravenous medications. Neither oral nor sublingual medications should be used in this circumstance. Blood pressure should generally not be lowered to a "normal" pressure because patients with a history of hypertension have elevated cerebral pressure requirements. Nitroprusside is an effective, short-acting, and titratable agent, and it requires moment-to-moment monitoring to prevent hypotension.

In some hypertensive patients, lowering blood pressure can be detrimental. For example, high blood pressure in patients with acute stroke may be "appropriate" as a homeostatic mechanism to maintain blood flow to threatened parts of the CNS. In addition, overly aggressive treatment of asymptomatic blood pressure elevations, without evidence of end-organ dysfunction, is unnecessary and can have deleterious effects, such as stroke, myocardial infarction (MI), or fetal distress.

Initial workup consists of ruling out other causes of the presenting signs and symptoms, such as stroke, infection, or toxicologic emergency (e.g., cocaine overdose), and evaluating for other coexistent end-organ damage or dysfunction.

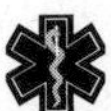

AORTIC DISSECTION

See Chapter 7, Chest Pain.

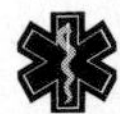

MYOCARDIAL INFARCTION

See Chapter 7, Chest Pain.

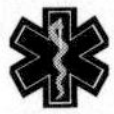

CONGESTIVE HEART FAILURE

See Chapter 29, Shortness of Breath.

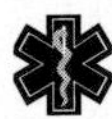

STROKE

For patients with ischemic stroke or intracerebral hemorrhage, acute pharmacologic reduction of blood pressure should be avoided. Initial blood pressure elevations usually resolve spontaneously in 12 to 72 hours (80% with significant improvement in 4 hours), and overly aggressive therapy may worsen ischemia. Active treatment should be employed in cases of persistent, extreme elevation of pressure (SBP >220, DBP >120, mean arterial pressure [MAP] >140). Pressure should then be reduced over 24 hours, with titrated intravenous therapy. If the patient is at risk for MI, congestive heart failure (CHF), or aortic dissection, more rapid reduction of pressure may be required. In subarachnoid hemorrhage, therapy may be needed to lessen the likelihood of rebleeding if analgesics, sedation, and rest do not reduce pressure to near prebleed levels.

See Chapter 15, Headache, and Chapter 36, Weakness and Fatigue.

REFERENCES

Adams HP Jr, Brott TG, Crowell RM, et al: Guidelines for the management of patients with acute ischemic stroke: a statement for healthcare professionals from a special writing group of the Stroke Council, American Heart Association, *Circulation* 90:1588, 1994.

Carlberg B, Asplund K, Hägg E: The prognostic value of admission blood pressure in patients with acute stroke, *Stroke* 24:1372, 1993.

Lisk DR, Grotta JC, Lamki LM, et al: Should hypertension be treated after acute stroke? A randomized controlled trial using single photon emission computed tomography, *Arch Neurol* 50:855, 1993.

Powers WJ: Acute hypertension after stroke: the scientific basis for treatment decisions, *Neurology* 43:461, 1993.

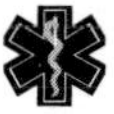

HYPERTENSIVE ENCEPHALOPATHY

Symptoms

- Severe headache
- Vomiting
- Confusion
- Lethargy

Signs

- Markedly elevated blood pressure and abnormal mental status are essential features (mental status may fluctuate).
- Papilledema is usually, if not always, present.
- Fever should suggest another cause, such as meningitis, encephalitis, thyroid storm, or neuroleptic malignant syndrome.

Workup

- Evaluate for other possible causes of signs and symptoms
- Head CT without contrast (or other neurologic imaging; MRI may be useful) is essential for ruling out hemorrhagic CNS lesions or a mass or large stroke with increased intracranial pressure.

- O_2 saturation to rule out hypoxia
- Glucose
- Urinalysis to look for protein or blood, indicating renal involvement
- Electrolytes, BUN, creatinine
- ECG to detect evidence of cardiac ischemia (may be masked or silent)
- Chest x-ray to detect CHF or investigate for evidence of dissection, if suspected
- Blood smear for detection of hemolysis, suggesting thrombotic thrombocytopenic purpura (TTP)

Comments and Treatment Considerations

Nitroprusside is the treatment of choice in most situations and should be titrated to produce symptomatic improvement to a maximum diastolic pressure reduction of 20% to 25% or to a diastolic pressure of 100, whichever is higher. Its use requires careful hemodynamic monitoring.

REFERENCES

Calhoun DA, Oparil S: Treatment of hypertensive crisis, *N Engl J Med* 323:1177, 1990.

Healton EB: Hypertensive encephalopathy and the neurologic manifestations of malignant hypertension, *Neurology* 32:127, 1982.

Katsumata Y, Maehara T, Noda M, et al: Hypertensive encephalopathy: reversible CT and MR appearance, *Radiat Med* 11:160, 1993.

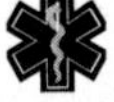

RETINAL HEMORRHAGE OR PAPILLEDEMA

Symptoms

- Headache and visual loss are frequent.
- No symptoms may be reported.

Signs

- Abnormal funduscopic examination
- Hypertension
- Other signs of other end-organ damage

Workup

- Urinalysis to look for protein or blood, indicating renal involvement
- Electrolytes, BUN, creatinine
- ECG to detect evidence of cardiac ischemia
- Chest x-ray to detect CHF or evidence of dissection, if suspected
- CBC to detect hemolysis, suggesting TTP
- Other tests should be tailored to detect evidence of end-organ damage.

Comments and Treatment Considerations

The priority is treatment of the underlying hypertension with ophthalmologic consultation to further evaluate acute versus chronic changes through indirect ophthalmoscopy. In the absence of other conditions (or of a specific cause of the hypertension) requiring different therapy, nitroprusside is the treatment of choice.

REFERENCES

Murphy C: Hypertensive emergencies, *Emerg Med Clin North Am* 13:973, 1995.

Rodgers A, MacMahon S, Gamble G, et al: Blood pressure and risk of stroke in patients with cerebrovascular disease: the United Kingdom Transient Ischaemic Attack Collaborative Group, *BMJ* 313:147, 1996.

Starkman S, Barron D: Stroke: emergency management and evaluation, *Emerg Med Reports* 15:75, 1994.

Zampaglione B, Pascale C, Marchisio M, Cavallo-Perin P: Hypertensive urgencies and emergencies: prevalence and clinical presentation, *Hypertension* 27:144, 1996.

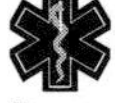

PREECLAMPSIA AND ECLAMPSIA

Preeclampsia is a complication of pregnancy characterized by hypertension, edema, and proteinuria. The diagnosis of eclampsia is made once seizures begin. The disease does not occur until after the twentieth week of gestation, except with hydatidiform mole. Some patients will not know (or admit) that they are or may be pregnant. Those without adequate prenatal care may not know the gestational age. Approximately 14% of cases occur in the postpartum period (25% of these in the 2- to 14-day range). HELLP syndrome (hemolysis, elevated liver function tests, and low platelets) occurs in up to 10% of cases of severe preeclampsia and carries a high risk of disseminated intravascular coagulation (DIC) (30%).

Symptoms

- Swelling of the hands, face, legs
- Abdominal pain (especially epigastric and right upper quadrant)
- Headache
- Visual disturbances
- Altered mental status
- Seizures may be among presenting complaints and is required for the diagnosis of eclampsia

Signs

- Hypertension is diagnosed at much lower pressures than in other situations. Blood pressure of 140/90, or an increase of 30/15 from baseline, is abnormal. Treatment is required for blood pressure 160/110 or higher.
- Edema, although isolated leg edema may be normal.
- Altered mental status
- Hyperreflexia
- Petechiae
- Bruising

Workup

- Urinalysis should be obtained for all patients who are beyond their twentieth week of pregnancy; any more than a trace of protein is abnormal.
- CBC with platelets
- Liver function tests
- PT, PTT, fibrin, and fibrin degradation products (DIC panel) should be obtained if HELLP is suspected.
- Chest x-ray or CT should not be delayed if indicated.
- Workup for possible infection should be considered if seizure might be caused by meningitis.

Comments and Treatment Considerations

Once the diagnosis is made or is strongly suspected, immediate obstetric consultation is essential. Delivery, usually by cesarean section, remains the treatment of choice for eclampsia. Hydralazine (10 mg IV) remains the antihypertensive treatment of choice (labetalol appears to be equally efficacious). Patients with end-organ dysfunction or microangiopathy should have their diastolic pressure reduced to less than 90 within 1 hour. Less severe cases may await emergency obstetric consultation. Overly aggressive therapy may cause hypotension, thus worsening uteroplacental ischemia. Seizure prophylaxis (usually with magnesium sulfate 4 g load over 20 min, then 2 g/hr; watch for respiratory depression) should be instituted in cases of severe preeclampsia, preeclampsia at term, or eclampsia. Seizure treatment may include benzodiazepines. Beware of common misdiagnoses (e.g., cholecystitis and hepatitis) and commonly missed diagnoses (e.g., TTP, hemolytic-uremic syndrome, and sepsis) (see Chapter 27, Seizure, Adult).

REFERENCES

Cunningham FG, Lindheimer MD: Hypertension in pregnancy, *N Engl J Med* 326:927, 1992.

Duldner JE, Emerman CL: Stroke: comprehensive guidelines for clinical assessment and emergency management. II. *Emerg Med Reports* 18:213, 1997.

Mabie WC, Gonzalez AR, Sibai BM, Amon E: A comparative trial of labetalol and hydralazine in the acute management of severe hypertension complicating pregnancy, *Obstet Gynecol* 70:328, 1987.

Miles JF, Martin JN Jr, Blake PG, et al: Postpartum eclampsia: a recurring perinatal dilemma, *Obstet Gynecol* 76:328, 1990.

Schobel HP, Fischer T, Heuszer K, et al: Preeclampsia—a state of sympathetic overactivity, *N Engl J Med* 335:1480, 1996.

Sibai BM, Taslimi MM, el-Nazer A, et al: Maternal-perinatal outcome associated with the syndrome of hemolysis, elevated liver enzymes, and low platelets in severe preeclampsia-eclampsia, *Am J Obstet Gynecol* 155:501, 1986.

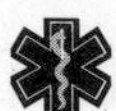

CATECHOLAMINE EXCESS

Catecholamine excess includes pheochromocytoma, sympathomimetic overdose (cocaine, amphetamines, decongestant or diet pills, and so forth), withdrawal from clonidine or sedative-hypnotics, or food interaction with monoamine oxidase inhibitors (MAOIs).

Symptoms

- Anxiety
- Abdominal discomfort
- Diaphoresis
- Headache
- Nausea
- Palpitations

Signs

- Hypertension
- Tachycardia
- Diaphoresis
- Pallor
- Signs of specific end-organ damage

Workup

- O_2 saturation to rule out hypoxia
- Glucose check to rule out hypoglycemia
- Urinalysis to look for protein or blood, indicating renal involvement
- Electrolytes, BUN, creatinine
- ECG to detect evidence of cardiac ischemia
- Chest x-ray to detect CHF or evidence of dissection, if suspected
- A drug screen may be informative if the history is considered unreliable, but it will not detect over-the-counter diet pills, some amphetamine derivatives, or MAOIs.
- Other tests should be tailored to detect evidence of end-organ damage.

Comments and Treatment Considerations

Benzodiazepine therapy may be adequate for reduction of blood pressure in cocaine overdose. In severe cases, alpha-blockade with phentolamine is the treatment of choice. Labetalol is, at best, a second-line choice, and beta-blockade without alpha-blockade is contraindicated, as this may worsen the hypertension. Nitroprusside is a reasonable alternative when the others are unavailable or ineffective.

Thyroid storm may mimic this syndrome.

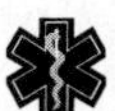

THYROID STORM

See Chapter 24, Palpitation and Tachycardia.

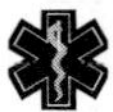

ASYMPTOMATIC HYPERTENSION

Asymptomatic hypertension may be due to situational ("white coat") or undiagnosed hypertension.

Symptoms

None; no chest pain, shortness of breath, headache, dizziness, or abdominal pain

Signs

- Normal blood pressure measured in legs of patients under 20 years old to rule out coarctation of the aorta

Workup

- Urinalysis to look for protein or blood, indicating renal involvement
- Pregnancy test if possibility of pregnancy
- Electrolytes, BUN, creatinine
- Consideration of ECG to rule out silent cardiac ischemia

Comments and Treatment Considerations

Because it is not possible to determine whether a patient's hypertension is situational or undiagnosed, close follow-up for a recheck is probably all that is required. If the patient is to be treated, a single, low-dose oral (not sublingual) antihypertensive medication should be prescribed. A single elevated blood pressure should not be "chased" with repeated doses of any medicine because this can lead to excessive blood pressure reduction.

REFERENCES

Grossman E, Messerli H, Groczicki T, Kowey P: Should a moratorium be placed on sublingual nifedipine capsules given for hypertensive emergencies and pseudoemergencies? *JAMA* 276:1328, 1996.

Kaplan NM, Gifford RW: Choice of initial therapy for hypertension, *JAMA* 275:1577, 1996.

Tach AM, Schultz PJ: Nonemergent hypertension: new perspectives for the emergency medicine physician, *Emerg Med Clin North Am* 13:1009, 1995.

Veterans Administration Cooperative Study Group on Antihypertensive Agents: Effects of treatment on morbidity in hypertension, *JAMA* 202:116, 1967.

Zeller KR, Kuhnert LV, Matthews CM: Rapid reduction of severe asymptomatic hypertension: a prospective, controlled trial, *Arch Intern Med* 149:2186, 1989

CHAPTER 17

Hypotension

MYLES GREENBERG

Low blood pressure is a common finding during initial patient evaluation, and the emergency physician must determine whether a life-threatening condition is causing the hypotension. Hypotension should prompt a thorough history and physical examination to search for serious conditions. The approach to hypotensive patients should be initiated in the same way as the approach to all emergency patients: airway and breathing first, then circulation. If patients are hemodynamically unstable, two large-bore peripheral intravenous lines should be started. Most patients should initially receive fluid resuscitation using isotonic crystalloid solutions.

After initial resuscitation, history and physician examination may indicate the need for emergent intervention despite the lack of a definitive diagnosis confirmed by ancillary tests.

Hypovolemia from bleeding (internal or external) or dehydration, limitation of cardiac output (e.g., cardiac tamponade, tension pneumothorax, massive pulmonary embolism, myocardial infarction, arrhythmia, sepsis, toxic ingestion, and metabolic emergencies are general categories to consider in the approach to hypotension.

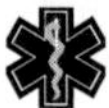

ACUTE HYPOVOLEMIA

Acute hypovolemia is a condition of decreased intravascular volume that may be caused by blood loss or dehydration. Hypovolemia is primarily a clinical diagnosis. Initial hematocrit in the setting of blood loss is normal until fluid equilibration has time to dilute the intravascular compartment.

See Chapter 33, Trauma, Approach to.

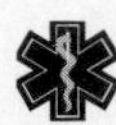

TENSION PNEUMOTHORAX

Tension pneumothorax is caused by a defect in the lung that allows air to escape and create pressure in the pleural space; this in turn causes compression of the heart or great vessels that limits venous return and cardiac filling, decreasing systemic blood pressure. This diagnosis often must be made clinically, since there may not be time for radiologic confirmation. Tension pneumothorax and cardiac tamponade have similar manifestations. Close attention must be paid to the chest, lung, heart, and trachea examinations to differentiate these two entities. Treatment of tension pneumothorax consists of immediate tube thoracostomy. If this is not immediately available, then the patient's chest should be decompressed using a large-bore intravenous catheter placed above the rib, in the midclavicular line, at the second intercostal space. Decompression should be followed by chest tube placement as soon as possible.

See Chapter 7, Chest Pain.

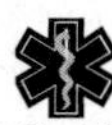

CARDIAC TAMPONADE

Cardiac tamponade is an increase of fluid within the pericardial space that can occur abruptly or over time. Acute effusions are more likely to cause rapid hemodynamic compromise, and if not promptly drained, death may ensue. In the acute setting, tamponade can be difficult to differentiate from tension pneumothorax, which is more common. Immediate ED ultrasound can be diagnostic. Immediate management of tamponade consists of aggressive fluid resuscitation in the prehospital setting followed by pericardiocentesis, operative pericardial window, or ED/operative thoracotomy.

See Chapter 7, Chest Pain.

REFERENCES[www]

Eisenberg MJ, Munoz de Romeral L, Heidenreich PA, et al: The diagnosis of pericardial effusion and cardiac tamponade by 12-lead ECG: a technology assessment, *Chest* 110:318, 1996.

Lange RL, Botticelli JT, Tsagaris TJ, et al: Diagnostic signs in compressive cardiac disorders: constrictive pericarditis, pericardial effusion, and tamponade, *Circulation* 33:763, 1966.

Symmes JC, Berman ND: Early recognition of cardiac tamponade, *Can Med Assoc J* 116:863, 1977.

[www]Additional references are available on the following web site: www.signsandsymptoms.com.

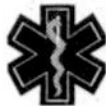

GASTROINTESTINAL BLEEDING

See Chapter 6, Bleeding.

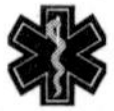

ABDOMINAL AORTIC ANEURYSM AND THORACIC AORTIC DISSECTION

Internal bleeding due to aortic catastrophe can cause immediately life-threatening hypotension.

See Chapter 1, Abdominal Pain, and Chapter 7, Chest Pain.

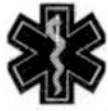

ARRHYTHMIAS

See Chapter 24, Palpitations and Tachycardia, and the emergency algorithm card at the back of the book.

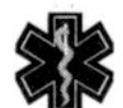

SEPSIS

See Chapter 36, Weakness and Fatigue.

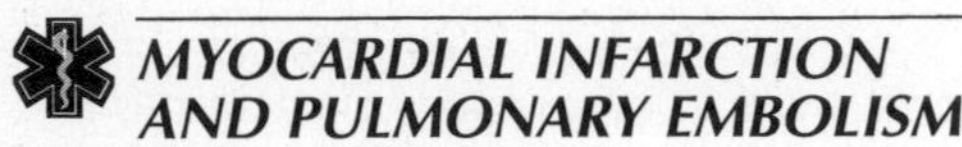

MYOCARDIAL INFARCTION AND PULMONARY EMBOLISM

See Chapter 7, Chest Pain.

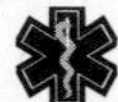

TOXIC INGESTION

See Chapter 32, Toxic Ingestion, Approach to.

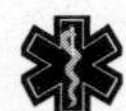

ORTHOSTATIC HYPOTENSION

See Chapter 31, Syncope and Near-Syncope.

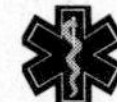

ECTOPIC PREGNANCY

See Chapter 34, Vaginal Bleeding.

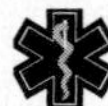

NEUROGENIC/SPINAL SHOCK

Acute spinal cord injury can rarely lead to peripheral vasodilation and hypotension. This is a diagnosis of exclusion.

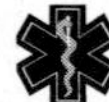

MYXEDEMA COMA

See Chapter 36, Weakness and Fatigue.

CHAPTER 18

The Irritable Child and Vomiting

FRANCES MCCABE and NEAL PEEPLES

Few symptoms in medicine are less specific than crying in an infant. All infants cry and at some point seem irritable to their parents. Indeed, the amount, the intervals, and even the pitch of their cry have been studied. In three population-based studies, "normal infants" cried 1.6 to 2.0 hours a day. While literature on the various causes of inconsolable crying abounds, data on test characteristics of concomitant signs and symptoms are scarce. Inconsolable crying is often attributable to "colic." The occurrence rate of colic varies greatly (3.3% to 25%) depending on the method of the study and the definition of colic used. Much has been written on colic, but unfortunately no reliable method has been developed for diagnosing a child's crying as colic without first excluding a myriad of other potentially serious diagnoses. Only after all emergent diagnoses have been adequately considered and eliminated can a diagnosis of colic be considered. Colic itself is a risk factor for child abuse.

Vomiting frequently accompanies irritability in infants and must be recognized as a potentially ominous sign of a more serious gastrointestinal disease. This chapter reviews a number of serious diagnoses that may all present with the same nonspecific symptoms of irritability, such as crying or vomiting.

REFERENCES

Alvarez M, St James-Roberts I: Infant fussing and crying patterns in the first year in an urban community in Denmark, *Acta Paediatr* 85:463, 1996.

Canivet C, Hagander B, Jakobsson I, Lanke J: Infantile colic—less common than previously estimated? *Acta Paediatr* 85:454, 1996.

Keefe M, Kotzer A, Froese-Fretz A, Curtin M: A longitudinal comparison of irritable and nonirritable infants, *Nurs Res* 45:4, 1996.

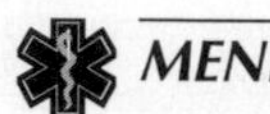 *MENINGITIS*

See Chapter 13, Fever in Children Under 2 Years of Age.

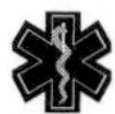 *INTUSSUSCEPTION*

See Chapter 1, Abdominal Pain.

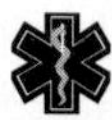 *MALROTATION AND VOLVULUS*

Midgut volvulus (MGV) associated with malrotation most commonly presents in the first month of life but is occasionally seen in infants 1 to 6 months of age. Rarely, MGV develops later in childhood, and patients will give a history of nonspecific intermittent gastrointestinal symptoms for years. Malrotation occurs when the embryonic midgut fails to rotate either partially or completely. Between 30% and 60% of patients with malrotation have additional GI tract abnormalities. MGV can result in obstruction and bowel ischemia if unrecognized. Based on several recent series, mortality is about 5% but has generally decreased in recent years as a result of early surgical intervention.

Symptoms

- Bilious (green) vomiting ++++; most common in patients less than 1 month old. Nonbilious vomiting and irritability and pain are less common.
- Intermittent vomiting
- Poor feeding
- Abdominal bloating

Signs

- Abdominal distention may or may not be present, since obstruction may be proximal.
- Bowel sounds, whether present or absent, are neither sensitive nor specific for malrotation and volvulus.
- Blood in the stool (gross or occult) ++ is an ominous sign that may signal bowel ischemia.

Workup

- Infants who are highly suspected of having MGV or an acute abdominal condition require rapid operative intervention to prevent significant morbidity or mortality; obtaining extensive diagnostic workups on these patients leads to undue and potentially dangerous delays.
- Abdominal x-rays +++; may show evidence of obstruction, loops of small bowel overriding the liver, double-bubble sign of duodenal obstruction, gastric dilatation, and possibly limited gas distal to the obstruction
- Upper gastrointestinal tract series is the study of choice.

Comments and Treatment Considerations

MGV has a high morbidity if the diagnosis is missed or delayed. Patients suspected of MGV should have a nasogastric tube placed for gut decompression and receive fluid resuscitation to make up for fluid and electrolyte losses due to vomiting and bowel edema. The importance of early surgical consultation and repair cannot be overstated.

REFERENCES[www]

Andrassy RJ, Mahour GH: Malrotation in the midgut in infants and children: a 25-year review, *Arch Surg* 116:158, 1981.

Morrison SC: Controversies in abdominal imaging, *Pediatr Clin North Am* 44:555, 1997.

Seashore JH, Touloukian RJ: Midgut volvulus: an ever-present threat, *Arch Pediatr Adolesc Med* 148:43, 1994.

[www]Additional references are available on the following web site: www.signsandsymptoms.com.

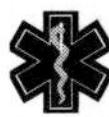

INCARCERATED INGUINAL HERNIA

Inguinal hernias occur in 1% to 4% of children; approximately 10% of these become incarcerated. The male:female ratio is 4:1, but the incarceration rate is higher in girls.

Symptoms

- Irritability
- Vomiting
- History of a scrotal mass that comes and goes

Signs

- Tender scrotal mass
- Abdominal distention
- Fever
- Irritability

Workup

- Thorough physical examination is sufficient to make the diagnosis in most cases.
- Ultrasound may occasionally be useful in differentiating hernia from other scrotal pathology.
- Abdominal x-rays can be used to rule out obstruction.

Comments and Treatment Considerations

Reduction of an incarcerated hernia is necessary. Emergent surgical intervention is required for a nonreducible hernia or if infarcted bowel is present.

REFERENCES

Skoog SJ, Conlin MJ: Pediatric hernias and hydroceles: the urologist's perspective, *Urol Clin North Am* 22:119, 1995.

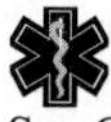

TESTICULAR TORSION

See Chapter 26, Scrotal Pain.

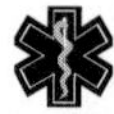

PYLORIC STENOSIS

Pyloric stenosis is the idiopathic hypertrophy of smooth muscle of the pylorus that leads to gastric outlet obstruction in infants. Epidemiology is 1.7 to 2.4/1000 live births (incidence may be declining). Male:female ratio is 4:1. Range of age at presentation is 2 to 26 weeks, with the median age of 6 weeks. It is most common in infants 2 to 4 months of age.

Symptoms

- Vomiting described as nonbilious +++++. Median duration of vomiting before diagnosis is 7 days.

- An infant may appear hungry and feed vigorously between episodes unless, or until, he or she becomes severely dehydrated.

Signs

- Epigastric or right upper quadrant mass +++. The mass is more easily palpable by elevating the child's legs and palpating during a feed just after the stomach has been emptied.
- Volume depletion +++

Workup

- Ultrasound +++++ has nearly replaced upper GI series in the evaluation of pyloric stenosis.
- Upper GI series may be more cost effective than ultrasound because it can demonstrate pathologic conditions other than pyloric stenosis (e.g., reflux) in infants with bilious emesis, but is generally more time consuming and less sensitive and specific than ultrasound for pyloric stenosis.
- Endoscopy is more invasive than ultrasound, and limited data exist on its use in this setting.
- Plain abdominal x-rays are of little value when the diagnosis is suspected.

Comments and Treatment Considerations

Intravenous hydration and electrolyte and dextrose replacement should be administered as guided by clinical volume status and serum electrolytes. Approximately 60% of infants with pyloric stenosis also have a hypochloremic metabolic alkalosis. A recent study suggests atropine administered intravenously may obviate the need for pyloromyotomy in most infants. The correction of metabolic abnormalities is imperative before pyloromyotomy. The lesions can be resected laparoscopically or by traditional open technique.

REFERENCES

Davenport M: Surgically correctable causes of vomiting in infancy, *BMJ* 312:236, 1996.

Hernanz-Schulman M, Sells LL, Ambrosino MM, et al: Hypertrophic pyloric stenosis in the infant without a palpable olive: accuracy of sonographic diagnosis, *Radiology* 193:771, 1994.

Morrison SC : Controversies in abdominal imaging, *Pediatr Clin North Am* 44:555, 1997.

Nagita A, Yamaguchi J, Amemoto K, et al: Management and ultrasonographic appearance of infantile hypertrophic pyloric stenosis with intravenous atropine sulfate, *J Pediatr Gastroenterol Nutr* 23:172, 1996.

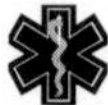

SEPTIC ARTHRITIS AND OSTEOMYELITIS

See Chapter 21, Limping Child/Child Won't Walk.

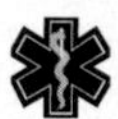

OCCULT INFECTION AND URINARY TRACT INFECTION

Infants with serious occult infections may have few or nonspecific symptoms, such as irritability. Some of the most serious infections, such as meningitis and septic arthritis, are addressed in other chapters. Although not as immediately life or limb threatening, urinary tract infections (UTIs) may be responsible for irritability in infants. UTIs develop in approximately 1% of infants, with premature infants at even higher risk. Because many UTIs are associated with structural urinary tract abnormalities, it is important to diagnose these before permanent renal damage ensues.

Symptoms

- Crying
- Irritability
- Poor feeding

Signs

- Fever ++; occasionally present
- Lethargy
- Vomiting
- Jaundice

Workup

- Urinalysis; dipstick positive for leukocyte esterase or nitrate has only limited sensitivity (+++). Sensitivity of microscopic analysis for leukocytes and bacteria is better (+++) but is still limited.
- Urine culture +++++, obtained by catheterization or suprapubic tap, is the gold standard test and should be obtained even though results will not be available in the ED.
- Urinary tract imaging studies are usually obtained later in the outpatient setting.

REFERENCES

Altieri M, Camarca M, Bock G: Pediatric urinary tract infections, *Emerg Med Reports* 19:1, 1998.

Du J: Colic as the sole symptom of urinary tract infection in infants, *Can Med Assoc J* 115:334, 1976.

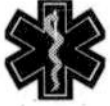

CORNEAL ABRASION

Corneal abrasions are usually thought to be caused by an infant inadvertently scratching his or her own cornea.

Symptoms

- Irritability
- Crying
- Eye pain

Signs

- Inconsolable crying
- Eye redness
- Excessive tearing (tearing begins after age 4 weeks)

Workup

- Topical corneal anesthesia and fluorescein staining with Wood's lamp examination generally establishes the diagnosis of a foreign body or an abrasion. Topical corneal anesthesia should not be prescribed for outpatient use.

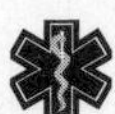

HAIR TOURNIQUET

A hair can become wrapped around a digit or the penis of an infant, causing constriction and potentially resulting in amputation if the hair is not removed.

Symptoms

- Pain in the digit or penis

Signs

- Inconsolable crying
- Erythema and swelling of the digit
- Constricting hair can become enveloped in surrounding edematous tissue, thereby obscuring the correct diagnosis.

Workup

- Thorough physical examination of digits and genitalia.

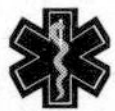

GASTROESOPHAGEAL REFLUX

Gastroesophageal reflux is more common early in infancy and slowly declines in incidence over the first year of life. Nearly all infants have some degree of reflux, but the symptoms vary greatly in severity. Reflux becomes medically important when it causes respiratory symptoms and failure to thrive. The association of reflux with respiratory symptoms (reactive airway disease, stridor, pneumonia, and apnea) is less well substantiated than the GI symptoms. However, occasional resolution of respiratory symptoms with reflux treatment has been demonstrated.

Symptoms

- Irritability
- Regurgitation and nonprojectile vomiting
- Belching, refusal to feed, and rarely, failure to thrive

Signs

- Few clinical signs of reflux
- Abdominal examination is normal.

Workup

- Observation of feeds can be helpful in the evaluation of reflux. Upper GI series may be helpful if more serious diseases are a diagnostic consideration.

Comments and Treatment Considerations

Patients should generally be referred for outpatient evaluation after conditions requiring emergent treatment have been ruled out.

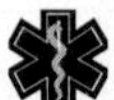

PRENATAL COCAINE EXPOSURE

Neonates exposed to cocaine may develop abnormalities in the dopaminergic system of the CNS.

Symptoms

- Abnormal feeding
- Hypersensitivity to stimuli
- Inability to regulate sleep and wakeful states, with rapid transitions from deep sleep to excessive crying and irritability

Signs

- Hypertonia or hypotonia
- High-pitched cry
- Small head circumference

Workup

- Urine toxicology screen

Comments and Treatment Considerations

Social work or equivalent support and monitoring should be arranged.

REFERENCES[www]

Alpert J, Filler R, Glaser H: Strangulation of an appendage by hair wrapping, *N Engl J Med* 273:866, 1965.

[www]Additional references are available on the following web site: www.signsandsymptoms.com.

Gerardi M: Neonatal emergencies: fever, jaundice, respiratory distress, heart disease, and behavioral complaints, *Pediatr Emerg Med Reports* 1:113, 1996.

Glassman M: Gastroesophageal reflux in children, *Gastroenterol Clin North Am* 24:71, 1995.

Harkness M: Corneal abrasion in infancy as a cause of inconsolable crying, *Pediatr Emerg Care* 5:242, 1989.

Hawley T: The development of cocaine-exposed children, *Curr Probl Pediatr* 24:259, 1994.

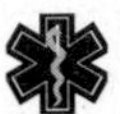

BURNS

It is possible for infants to be accidentally burned or for the caretaker bringing the child for care to be unaware of the mechanism of injury; however, child abuse should always be highly suspected whenever an infant has been burned. The mechanism and pattern of the burn are the greatest clues as to whether the injury was intentional or not. It is also important to realize that infants have thinner skin and, given an equivalent thermal exposure, are more likely to suffer a full-thickness burn than older children. In addition to a detailed history from the caregiver and a physician examination, workup should include a skeletal survey if abuse is suspected in a patient less than 1 year of age.

See Chapter 33, Trauma, Approach to.

REFERENCES

American Burn Association: Hospital and prehospital resources for optimal care of patients with burn injury: guidelines for development and operation of burn centers, *J Burn Care Rehabil* 11:97, 1990.

Banco L, Lapidus G, Zavoski R, Braddock M: Burn injuries among children in an urban emergency department, *Pediatr Emerg Care* 10:98, 1994.

Erdmann C, Feldman K, Rivara F, et al: Tap water burn prevention: the effect of legislation, *Pediatrics* 88:572, 1991.

Jaffe M: Burns. In Fleisher GR, Ludwig T, editors: *Textbook of pediatric emergency medicine*, ed 3, Baltimore, 1993, Williams & Wilkins.

Showers J, Garrison K: Burn abuse: a 4-year study, *J Trauma* 28:1581, 1988.

CHILD ABUSE

Physical child abuse is defined as the nonaccidental injury of a child, ranging from minor bruises and lacerations to severe head trauma and death. It is estimated that 1 million children in the United States are seriously abused by parents or caretakers; approximately 125,000 of these involve physical abuse, i.e., nonaccidental injury, and between 2000 and 5000 deaths annually are attributed to child abuse. Evidence has shown that without intervention 50% of abused children will suffer some escalation of the violence. Although few injuries are pathognomonic for abuse, certain patterns of injury have begun to be associated with nonaccidental injury. Many of these injury patterns are apparent radiographically. Because of the increase in awareness of this important medical issue, with most states mandating reporting of *suspected* abuse, many institutions have developed interdisciplinary teams to investigate and manage suspected cases. Histories that are inadequate or inconsistent with the injury pattern should raise suspicion. Commonly acknowledged risk factors for abuse include premature birth, neonatal hospitalization, or other circumstance that might interfere with normal parent-infant bonding; adolescent parents; children with a congenital abnormality or special needs; and irritability and colic.

Symptoms

- Irritability
- "Clinging"
- Crying
- Poor feeding
- Inability or reluctance to engage with parent or other adult
- Immediate engagement with strangers

Signs

- Bruises +++; combining all age groups, this is the most common sign.
- Welts
- Burns ++; look for small, circular cigarette burns to palms and soles, stocking-glove distribution of immersion burns,

geometric shapes from application of electric appliances, linear marks or bruises from belts or cords, and nonhealed injuries of different ages

- Fractures ++; over half of fractures may be nonaccidental in infants less than 1 year of age. Although not pathognomonic, the following fractures are highly suspicious for abuse: femoral, nonsupracondylar humeral, metaphyseal or "bucket-handle," rib (++, with 90% of these occurring in infants less than age 2), and diaphyseal in conjunction with concurrent skeletal or extraskeletal injury.
- Head injury +++; (majority in those <2 years). Seizures, lethargy, and decreased level of consciousness can be signs of intracranial trauma. Subdural hematoma may be precipitated by violent shaking or blunt trauma.
- Retinal hemorrhages (in most severely shaken infants); concurrent intracranial and skeletal injury has higher specificity for abuse.
- Abdominal injuries (3%, with the majority occurring at age >2 years); signs include bruises on the abdominal wall or manifestations of solid or hollow organ injury.
- Sexual abuse: blood or discharge noted in underwear, bruising on perineum, horizontal diameter of vaginal opening exceeding 4 mm, evidence of a sexually transmitted disease, recurrent UTIs, difficulty walking or sitting
- Signs of *child neglect* include malnutrition and poor hygiene.

Workup

- Consider plot of height, weight, and head circumference
- Radiographic skeletal survey for a child less than 2 years old with evidence of physical abuse or less than 1 year of age with evidence of significant neglect (The survey includes x-ray of the skull, spine, chest, and extremities and should be repeated after 2 weeks.)
- CT of head if intracranial trauma suspected
- Ultrasonography may demonstrate subperiosteal hemorrhages in infants.
- Bone scan is best for diagnosis of rib fractures not evident on x-ray.

- Consider platelet count and coagulation studies in patients with significant bruising to rule out alternative diagnoses.

Comments and Treatment Considerations

Any suspected cases of child abuse or neglect must be reported to child protective services in accordance with local statutes. Visible injuries should be photographed. According to one study, the most common injuries in infants and in children less than 4 years of age were fractures, hemorrhages, and burns. The most frequently injured areas are the skull, brain, feet, genitalia, buttocks, and hips. Infants less than 12 months of age have the highest incidence of head injuries, which cause the greatest morbidity and mortality of all abuse patterns.

REFERENCES[www]

Council On Scientific Affairs: AMA diagnostic and treatment guidelines concerning child abuse and neglect, *JAMA* 254:796, 1985.

Cramer K: Orthopedic aspects of child abuse, *Pediatr Clin North Am* 43:1035, 1996.

Johnson C: Inflicted injury versus accidental injury, *Pediatr Clin North Am* 37:791, 1990.

Merten D, Carpenter B: Radiologic imaging of inflicted injury in the child abuse syndrome, *Pediatr Clin North Am* 37:815, 1990.

Nimkin K, Kleinman P: Imaging of child abuse, *Pediatr Radiol* 44:615, 1997.

Sheridan C, Sherwin T, Mellick L: Child abuse and neglect: recognition and the role of the emergency physician. In *Updates in emergency medicine,* Atlanta, 1995, American Health Consultants, p 21.

Sills R, Pena M, Parsons K: Bones, breaks, and the battered child: is it unintentional or is it abuse? *Emerg Med Reports* 19:68, 1998.

[www]Additional references are available on the following web site: www.signsandsymptoms.com.

CARDIAC DISEASE: STRUCTURAL DEFECTS AND ARRHYTHMIAS

Irritability in infants may be caused by cardiac disease, which can be divided into structural defects and arrhythmias.

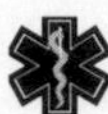

STRUCTURAL DEFECTS

Congestive heart failure (CHF) as a result of left-to-right shunts, and, more rarely, left ventricular dysfunction, may present with an insidious onset of symptoms. The structural lesions most often associated with CHF include ventricular septal defect, atrioventricular canal, large patent ductus arteriosis, myocarditis, cardiomyopathy, and anomalous origin of the coronary arteries.

Symptoms

- Poor feeding
- Crying
- Irritability

Signs

- Sweating with feeding
- Poor weight gain
- Lethargy
- Tachypnea
- Pallor
- Diastolic rumble at the apex, murmur, S3 gallop, and hepatomegaly
- Oliguria
- Poor peripheral perfusion may result from excess sympathetic stimulation and cause peripheral vasoconstriction with cool, pale skin. Poor peripheral perfusion also can cause sluggish capillary refill or weak pulses.
- Rales are often absent.
- Hypotension is a late sign of shock in infants.

Workup

- ECG
- Chest x-ray to look for cardiomegaly or increased pulmonary markings from left-to-right shunting
- Cardiac echocardiography

Comments and Treatment Considerations

In infants with left-to-right shunts the severity of the shunt gradually worsens over the first 2 months of life as pulmonary pressures gradually decrease. This is in contrast to infants with right-to-left shunts—the cyanotic lesions—which may rapidly decompensate in the first few days or weeks of life with closure of the ductus arteriosis.

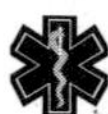

ARRHYTHMIAS

In a British study screening 3300 healthy asymptomatic infants, 1% had arrhythmias detected on ECGs or Holter monitors. Most of these spontaneously resolved by 3 months of age. The most common symptomatic arrhythmia in infants is supraventricular tachycardia (SVT); 80% of cases occur in children less than 12 months of age, and 60% occur in the first 4 months of life. Ventricular tachycardia is much less common in infants and is usually associated with abnormal myocardium, congenital or acquired myopathies, long Q-T syndrome, or postsurgical scarring.

Symptoms

- Crying
- Irritability
- Poor feeding

Signs

- Irritability (possible early sign)
- Feeding intolerance (possible early sign)
- Tachycardia that is sustained can cause poor peripheral perfusion and CHF seen in the structural lesions noted above. Heart rates are in excess of 220, often 250 to 300.

Workup

- ECG (a delta wave indicative of a bypass tract may be visible in infants with SVT ++).
- Electrolytes, K+, Ca++, and Mg++ should also be checked if the patient has a reason for electrolyte abnormality.
- Chest x-ray to look for cardiomegaly
- Cardiac echo, as SVT may be associated with a structural cardiac defect ++ (often done as an outpatient procedure)
- Holter monitor (often done as an outpatient procedure)

Comments and Treatment Considerations

Because of their relatively great cardiovascular reserve, newborns can tolerate high heart rates, even exceeding 300, for long periods. Their symptoms can be very subtle for hours before any significant sign of heart failure is evident. The nonspecific nature of the symptoms of SVT in infants makes early diagnosis difficult. SVT with aberrant conduction is uncommon in children, and, as with adults, wide complex tachycardia should be initially treated as ventricular tachycardia.

REFERENCES[www]

Overholt E, Rheuban K, Gugesell H, et al: Usefulness of adenosine for arrhythmias in infants and children, *Am J Cardiol* 61:336, 1988.

Schamberger M: Cardiac emergencies in children, *Pediatr Ann* 25:339, 1996.

Southall D, Johnson A, Shinebourne E, et al: Frequency and outcome of disorders of cardiac rhythm and conduction in a population of newborn infants, *Pediatrics* 68:58, 1981.

Van Hare G, Stanger P: Ventricular tachycardia and accelerated rhythm presenting in the first month of life, *Am J Cardiol* 67:42, 1991.

[www]Additional references are available on the following web site: www.signsandsymptoms.com.

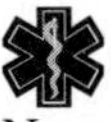

NECROTIZING ENTEROCOLITIS

Necrotizing enterocolitis (NEC) is the most common and lethal surgical abdominal emergency in the newborn. The cause of NEC is unclear. Risk factors include prematurity (++++), hypoxic ischemic insults, aggressive enteral feedings, and a history of infection. In the past 20 years improvements in neonatal intensive care have allowed increased survival in premature infants, and the incidence of NEC has increased concurrently. This disease is seen almost exclusively in the neonatal intensive care unit, although as more infants are sent home earlier in life, NEC presentations to the ED may increase. Extremely premature infants (<28 weeks) remain at high risk until they reach the postconceptual age of 35 to 36 weeks.

Symptoms

- Vomiting and poor feeding ++
- Lethargy
- Irritability
- Episodes of apnea

Signs

- Abdominal distention ++++, may evolve over time
- Blood in the stools, gross or occult ++++
- Fever is uncommon.
- Red streaks on the abdomen are occasionally seen in advanced cases.

Workup

- Abdominal x-rays are the primary diagnostic tool for establishing NEC. X-rays may be normal or show mild ileus pattern early in the course. Pneumatosis intestinalis makes the definitive diagnosis of NEC. Free air indicates intestinal perforation.
- Electrolytes, since abnormalities can result from vomiting and bowel edema
- CBC to assess degree of blood loss in stool

Comments and Treatment Considerations

Treatment of NEC is based on severity. Generally, enteral feedings are discontinued. Intravenous antibiotics, nasogastric decompression, and vigorous hydration are generally recommended for patients with a definitive diagnosis of NEC. If NEC is suspected, early involvement of a neonatologist and pediatric surgeon is essential.

REFERENCES

Albanese CT, Rowe MI: Necrotizing enterocolitis, *Pediatr Surg* 4:200, 1995.

Foglia RP: Necrotizing enterocolitis. Neonatal necrotizing enterocolitis: a 12-year review at a county hospital, *Curr Probl Surg* 32:757, 1995.

Neu J: Necrotizing enterocolitis: the search for a unifying pathologic theory leading to prevention, *Pediatr Clin North Am* 43:409, 1996

CHAPTER 19

Jaundice

ERIC SALK

Jaundice in ED patients is generally caused by hepatitis or alcoholic cirrhosis, gallbladder or biliary duct disease (including tumors that block bile duct drainage), primary or metastatic tumor, or, rarely, hemolysis. History and physical examination alone generally suggest the likely cause of jaundice, which may be confirmed by laboratory tests or imaging studies.

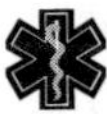

VIRAL HEPATITIS

Hepatitis A, which is transmitted through a fecal-oral route, is a common cause of jaundice in ED patients. In most cases the diagnosis is made on the basis of the patient's history of earlier nonspecific symptoms that have become complicated by jaundice and abdominal pain.

Hepatitis B, C, and D are transmitted parenterally. Hepatitis B, the most virulent, accounts for a large percentage of adult cases. A chronic carrier state develops in up to 10% of patients. Hepatitis C is responsible for 80% to 90% of posttransfusion cases of hepatitis, and approximately one third become chronic. Hepatitis D (delta) requires concomitant hepatitis B infection.

Other viruses (e.g., cytomegalovirus and Epstein-Barr virus), bacteria, rickettsia, and protozoa can also cause liver inflammation.

Symptoms

- Asymptomatic incubation phase of varying length in viral hepatitis (hepatitis A, 2 to 6 weeks; hepatitis B, 2 to 6 months; hepatitis C, 2 to 22 weeks)

- Viral symptoms in prodromal phase, with fever ++++, nausea +++, vomiting +++, malaise, fatigue, anorexia, headache, and chills
- Icteric phase characterized first by dark urine then light (clay-colored) stools, scleral icterus, and jaundice (as serum bilirubin exceeds 3 to 4 mg/dl)
- Pruritic rash, arthralgias, and arthritis, especially with hepatitis B
- Altered mental status and seizures suggest hepatic encephalopathy in fulminant disease.
- Disturbance of taste

Signs

- Jaundice +++
- Tender hepatomegaly +++
- Lymphadenopathy ++
- Splenomegaly +
- Scleral or sublingual icterus
- Low-grade fever
- Skin excoriations caused by itching
- Asterixis, hyperreflexia, and clonus occur with hepatic encephalopathy.

Workup

- Liver function tests: transaminase (AST and ALT) levels greater than 10 times normal strongly suggest acute viral or toxic injury, although some viruses and parasites may cause less significant elevation. Elevations of two to three times normal, with AST higher than ALT, suggest alcoholic injury, although levels may be normal as cirrhosis becomes severe. With significant elevations of alkaline phosphatase, conjugated bilirubin, or GGTP, consider biliary tract obstruction.
- Urinalysis may demonstrate bilirubin in the urine.
- Serum bilirubin is commonly elevated and divided evenly between conjugated and unconjugated varieties.
- Prothrombin time, serum protein, albumin, and glucose are tests of hepatic synthetic function. Hypoglycemia is a late finding of hepatic necrosis.

- Hepatitis serologies should be drawn if hepatitis is suspected. Appropriate initial tests in acute hepatitis include anti-HAV IgM and Hbs Ag. Anti-HBs, anti-HBc and anti-HVC may also be considered.

Comments and Treatment Considerations

Careful travel, exposure, and medication history must be taken. Treatment is largely supportive and directed at controlling symptoms. Avoid use of phenothiazines as antiemetics because they may produce cholestasis. Patients unable to tolerate oral fluids or those with signs or symptoms suggesting fulminant liver failure require admission.

In cases of possible exposure to a hepatitis virus, postexposure prophylaxis should be administered when indicated (Table 19-1) (see also Hepatic Encephalopathy in Chapter 22, Mental Status Change and Coma).

Table 19-1 Postexposure Hepatitis Prophylaxis

Hepatitis A

Nature of Exposure	Recommended Treatment
Close personal contact	ISG 0.02 ml/kg IM
Day care center	
Employee	ISG 0.02 ml/kg IM
Attendee	ISG 0.02 ml/kg IM
School contacts	None
Hospital contacts	None
Workplace contacts	None
Foodborne source	
Within 2 weeks of exposure	ISG 0.02 ml/kg IM
After 2 weeks of exposure	None
After common source outbreaks have begun to occur	None

Table 19-1 Postexposure Hepatitis Prophylaxis—cont'd

Hepatitis B

Nature of exposure	Source	Exposed individual: Unvaccinated	Exposed individual: Vaccinated
Percutaneous/ mucosal	HBsAG+	1. HBIG* 2. HB vaccine†	1. Test HBsAb; if −, then a. HBIG b. HB vaccine
	Known source High-risk HBsAg+	1. HB vaccine 2. Test source; if +, then HBIG	1. Test HBsAb; if − and source HBsAg+ a. HBIG b. HB vaccine
	Low-risk HBsAg+	1. HB vaccine	1. None
	Unknown source	1. HB vaccine	1. None
Intimate sexual	HBsAg+	1. HBIG 2. HB vaccine‡	1. None
Household/ workplace	HBsAg+	1. None	1. None
Perinatal	HBsAg+	1. HBIG§ 2. HB vaccine	NA

Hepatitis C

Unknown benefit from prophylaxis; ISG, 0.06 ml/kg IM should be considered for parenteral exposures from patients with evidence of viral hepatitis and negative serologies.

Hepatitis delta

Same as for hepatitis B

Modified from Centers for Disease Control and Prevention: *Morb Mortal Wkly Rep* 39(RR-2), 1990. In Rosen P, Barkin R, Hockberger RS, et al, editors: *Emergency medicine: concepts and clinical practice,* vol 2, ed 4, St Louis, 1997, Mosby.

**HBIG,* hepatitis B immune globulin, dose 0.6 ml/kg IM.

†HB vaccine, hepatitis B vaccine. (Adequate vaccination requires three injections, so all patients should be referred for follow-up.)

‡Vaccine required only if repeated sexual contacts are likely to occur over an extended period of time and the source becomes a chronic carrier.

§ Dose of HBIG 0.5 ml/kg.

REFERENCES[www]

Alter MJ: Hepatitis surveillance, 1982-1983, *MMWR CDC Surveill Summ* 34:1, 1985.

Alter MJ, Mast EE: The epidemiology of viral hepatitis in the United States, *Gastroenterol Clin North Am* 23:437, 1994.

Balistreri WJ: Viral hepatitis, *Pediatr Clin North Am* 35:637, 1988.

Dienst JA, Tallinn D: Acute viral hepatitis: simplifying a complex clinical syndrome, *Emerg Med Reports* 14:153, 1993.

Go GW, Barr LJ, Schreger DL: Management guidelines for health care workers exposed to blood and body fluids, *Ann Emerg Med* 20:1341, 1991.

[www]Additional references are available on the following web site: www.signsandsymptoms.com.

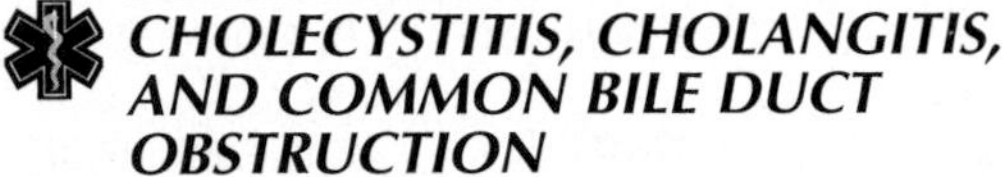

CHOLECYSTITIS, CHOLANGITIS, AND COMMON BILE DUCT OBSTRUCTION

See Chapter 1, Abdominal Pain.

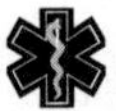

HEMOLYSIS

Hemolysis is an uncommon cause of jaundice. The rate of RBC destruction determines the degree to which jaundice is seen. In most cases, hemolysis occurs in patients with known hemoglobinopathies or RBC diseases (such as sickle cell disease [SCD]) and a concurrent oxidative stress such as hypoxia, infection, acidosis, or oxidative drug usage. Mechanical and infectious hemolysis include microangiopathic hemolytic anemia (MAHA), repetitive trauma to feet or hands, heart valve irregularities, hypersplenism, burns, malaria, and *Mycoplasma* and parvovirus infection. Uremia and hypophosphatemia are metabolic causes. Hemolysis is idiopathic in approximately 50% of cases in which an autoimmune reaction apparently is responsible for RBC destruction.

Symptoms

- Progressive fatigue, weakness, lightheadedness
- Syncope, near-syncope if concomitant vascular disease
- Dyspnea on exertion
- Palpitations
- Abdominal pain, back pain, and black urine can occur in severe intravascular hemolysis.
- Bleeding if associated DIC
- Hemoglobinuria on voiding after sleep (paroxysmal nocturnal hemoglobinuria)

Signs

- An acute drop in hemoglobin from any cause of hemolysis can produce shock, tachypnea, tachycardia, mental status changes, and CHF.
- Pallor
- Jaundice
- Splenomegaly occurs in most forms of immune-mediated hemolysis (not in SCD); children with SCD may exhibit splenomegaly and shock.

Workup

- Hematocrit indicates degree of hemolysis
- Reticulocyte count should be elevated with hemolysis; lack of elevation is a concern for aplastic crisis in SCD. One third of cases of autoimmune and immune hemolysis have reticulocytopenia.
- Direct Coombs in suspected immune and autoimmune cases +++++
- Liver function tests may be useful in diagnosing liver or biliary causes of jaundice.
- Peripheral blood smears can provide evidence that hemolysis is occurring.
- LDH is usually elevated.
- Evaluation for underlying systemic disorder as clinically indicated
- Haptoglobin is often reduced.

Comments and Treatment Considerations

Sepsis occurs more rapidly with SCD; thus a fever necessitates a search for infection and treatment with antibiotics when indicated. Transfusion for anemia due to hemolysis (in consultation with a hematologist) may be required.

REFERENCES[www]

Schrier SL: Anemia: hemolysis. In Dale DC, Federman DD, editors: *Scientific American medicine*, New York, 1995, Scientific American.

Steingart R: Management of patients with sickle cell disease, *Med Clin North Am* 76:669, 1992.

Tabbara IA: Hemolytic anemia: diagnosis and management, *Med Clin North Am* 76:649, 1992.

[www]Additional references are available on the following web site: www.signsandsymptoms.com.

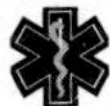

ACETAMINOPHEN OVERDOSE

See Chapter 32, Toxic Ingestion, Approach to.

CHAPTER 20

Joint Pain

SAM ONG

Nontraumatic joint pain may be monoarticular, polyarticular, or migratory. Joint swelling and pain characterize septic arthritis, which is a true medical emergency. Nongonococcal septic arthritis is generally, although not always, monoarticular and most commonly involves the knee, but may involve any joint including the hip. Gonococcal arthritis is the most common cause of bacterial arthritis in sexually active adults and is generally migratory and asymmetric. It often has an associated typical rash.

Distinguishing septic arthritis from other generally monarticular "inflammatory arthritides" (e.g., crystal induced) can be exceedingly difficult on clinical grounds alone. A history of gout or pseudogout and typical location of swelling (e.g., first metacarpophalangeal joint in foot in gout) can be helpful. In most cases, arthrocentesis is *required* to rule out a septic cause of swelling because of the serious implications of a missed infection. Both septic and crystal-induced arthritis generally lead to an increase in synovial fluid WBC >20,000. Visualization of crystals under polarized light establishes the diagnosis of crystal disease, although rarely an infection coexists. Gram staining that shows organisms is relatively insensitive but specific (i.e., if present, establishes the diagnosis; if absent, does not rule out septic joint). Full recovery can be expected if treatment is initiated within the first few days of symptoms. It is also important to remember that osteomyelitis accompanies septic arthritis in about half of the cases seen in neonates and young infants because of vessels that cross the physis before formation of the epiphyseal plate (at 6 months to 1 year). Occasionally, spirochetal infections (e.g., Lyme disease, syphilis) and rarely systemic diseases can also cause monoarticular arthritis. A detailed history, physical examination, and history of possible tick exposure direct the investigation of these conditions.

Polyarticular arthritis can be caused by a number of systemic illnesses, including rheumatoid arthritis, rheumatic fever, Reiter syndrome (nongonococcal urethritis, asymmetric polyarthritis, and conjunctivitis), Lyme disease, serum sickness, SLE, and viral arthritis. Nonarticular signs and symptoms are the key to suspecting these diagnoses in most cases.

Other conditions such as slipped capital femoral epiphysis, Legg-Calvé-Perthes disease, or osteomyelitis may mimic arthritis and should be considered when appropriate.

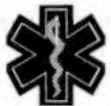

SEPTIC ARTHRITIS OF THE HIP

See Chapter 21, Limping Child/Child Won't Walk.

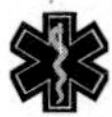

SEPTIC ARTHRITIS (NONGONOCOCCAL)

The knee is by far the most commonly affected joint (~ 50%) followed in order by the hip, ankle, wrist, elbow, and shoulder. The small joints of the hand and foot are infrequently affected in the absence of trauma. The majority of adults have some underlying joint abnormality, most commonly rheumatoid arthritis or osteoarthritis. Children frequently have no underlying disease. A history of trauma, intravenous drug use, or diseases that affect the immune system such as malignancy, diabetes, sickle cell disease, and chronic liver or kidney failure are red flags.

Symptoms

- Swelling
- Joint pain
- Decreased mobility
- Fever ++

Signs

- Erythema, warmth, and joint effusion are usually present but are neither sensitive nor specific for the nature of the arthritis.

- Fever ++
- Monoarticular ++++
- Polyarticular ++
- Most specific sign is limitation of active and passive movement of the joint, but its absence cannot be used to reliably exclude septic arthritis, particularly in very mobile joints such as the shoulder.

Workup

- Arthrocentesis is required.
- WBC >20,000 ++++
- %PMN >75 ++++
- Most aspirates with WBC >50,000 and %PMN >85% will be septic.
- Inoculate blood culture bottles, since recent studies have found fastidious organisms.
- Glucose and protein: neither sensitive nor specific, but if glucose is markedly reduced (<2.8 mmol), increased specificity for septic cause
- Gram stain and culture of joint fluid +++
- Polarizing microscopy to look for crystals; synovial fluid culture
- Blood cultures +++ are warranted because they may be positive when synovial fluid cultures are not. Some data also suggest that blood cultures have prognostic value; when positive, the outcome is worse.
- WBC and ESR are not discriminatory.
- Consider Lyme serology
- Plain radiographs are useful for diagnosing bony disease (e.g., slipped femoral capital epiphysis, Legg-Calvé-Perthes disease, or osteomyelitis) but are not useful for diagnosing septic effusion.
- Ultrasound of the hip is sensitive for effusions and, if negative, essentially excludes the diagnosis of septic arthritis for that joint. Hip effusions should be aspirated under ultrasound guidance by a physician skilled in the procedure.

Comments and Treatment Considerations

Treatment of septic arthritis consists of intravenous antibiotics, ED orthopedic consultation, and hospital admission. When the history, physical examination, and joint fluid analysis suggest the diagnosis, the patient should be admitted to the hospital and treated presumptively for septic arthritis pending the results of cultures. Choice of antibiotics depends on age, comorbidities, and presence of articular foreign body. Antibiotics should cover *Staphylococcus aureus* and *Streptococcus* spp. in addition to other organisms as indicated.

REFERENCES

Del Beccaro MA, Champoux AN, Bockers T, Mendelman PM: Septic arthritis versus transient synovitis of the hip: the value of screening laboratory tests, *Ann Emerg Med* 21:1418, 1992.

Kaandorp CJ, Krijnen P, Bernelot Moens HJ, et al: The outcome of bacterial arthritis: a prospective, community-based study, *Arthritis Rheum* 40:884, 1997.

Shmerling RH, Delbanco TL, Tosteson ANA, Trentham DE: Synovial fluid tests: what should be ordered? *JAMA* 264:1009, 1990.

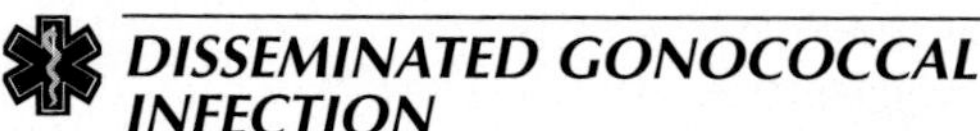

DISSEMINATED GONOCOCCAL INFECTION

Disseminated gonococcal infection is commonly manifested by arthritis, tenosynovitis, and characteristic rash (arthritis-dermatitis syndrome). Other, less common complications include abscesses, pyomyositis, osteomyelitis, pericarditis, and perihepatitis (Fitz-Hugh-Curtis syndrome). Gonococcal arthritis, unlike other causes of bacterial arthritis, has a very good prognosis; full recovery of the joint is the norm. The groups at highest risk include women who are pregnant, postpartum, or near menstruation (1 week) and promiscuous homosexual men.

Symptoms

- Polyarthralgia +++, which is frequently migratory and occasionally progresses to septic arthritis. The wrist, ankle, or knee is commonly involved.
- Periarticular pain ++++ is slightly more common than monarthritis.
- Rash ++++
- Fever and chills +++

Signs

- Rash ++++ ; painful red papules on digits and distal extremities. May have gray necrotic center +++. The lesions are usually few in number ("countable" and often <10). More than 100 suggests the possibility of infection with *Neisseria meningitidis.*
- Tenosynovitis is most commonly seen in the wrist and fingers, whereas arthritis is usually found in the knee, ankle, hip or elbow.

Workup

- Arthrocentesis
- WBC usually >20,000 (i.e., inflammatory) ++++
- Gram stain and culture have limited sensitivity +++.
- Genitourinary tract cultures are highest yield ++++.
- Pharynx and rectum cultures are occasionally diagnostic. Cultures are frequently positive in the absence of localizing symptoms.
- Blood cultures +++

Comments and Treatment Considerations

Small studies have shown polymerase chain reaction to be positive in all culture-proven gonococcal infections along with some that were culture negative. Hospitalization for intravenous antibiotics (e.g., ceftriaxone) is generally required, although outpatient parenteral therapy with close supervision may be appropriate in some cases.

REFERENCES

O'Brien JP, Goldenberg DL, Rice PA: Disseminated gonococcal infection: a prospective analysis of 49 patients and a review of pathophysiology and mechanisms, *Medicine* 62:395, 1983.

Wise CM, Morris CR, Wailaukas BL, Salzer WL: Gonococcal arthritis in an era of increasing penicillin resistance: presentations and outcomes in 41 recent cases (1985-1991), *Arch Intern Med* 154:2690, 1994.

CHAPTER 21

Limping Child/Child Won't Walk

BEVERLY BAUMAN

Determining the cause of acute limping in a child can be a diagnostic challenge. Whereas many of the possible causes are benign, the differential diagnosis includes conditions that can lead to major morbidity or death if not detected early. As in many pediatric illnesses, determining the reason for limping in a child can be much more difficult because of children's inability to describe and localize symptoms. The presentation and frequency of these disorders change with age.

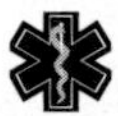

SEPTIC ARTHRITIS

Bacterial infection in a joint is a medical emergency because delay in its diagnosis and treatment can lead to permanent disability from destruction of the joint cartilage. The bacterial etiology and clinical presentation change with age. Although septic arthritis can occur in any joint, the most commonly affected joints in the pediatric age group are the hip (38%) and knee (32%). Toxic synovitis is an inflammatory disease that may cause hip or knee pain and low-grade fever. Aspiration of the hip may be required to distinguish this entity, which is treated with nonsteroidal antiinflammatory agents and follow-up, from a septic joint that requires aggressive management. Specific information relevant to pediatrics is noted here; see Septic Joints in Chapter 20, Joint Pain, for more information.

Symptoms

- Refusal to bear weight or use the affected joint
- "Pseudoparalysis" or prevention of joint movement in infants

Signs

- Infected joint is held in a position that helps to decrease intracapsular pressure and subsequent pain. A septic hip is held in flexion, external rotation, and abduction. The knee is held in mild flexion, and the ankle is held in mild plantar flexion.
- Active or passive movement of the infected joint causes severe pain.
- Warmth of the skin overlying the joint
- Erythema of the skin overlying the joint
- Palpable effusion
- Fever >38° C has limited sensitivity +++.

Workup

See Chapter 20, Joint Pain.

- Ultrasound of the hip; if positive, joint should be aspirated by a physician skilled in the procedure.
- Blood cultures ++; may guide later therapy
- X-rays may demonstrate subtle changes of increased joint space widening from an effusion, soft tissue swelling, or obliteration of normal fat lines around the joint. Their greatest use is to rule out fracture. Osteomyelitis can occur in association with septic joints in children and may be demonstrated on x-rays, which, however, are not sensitive for this condition.
- Urethral, pelvic, or pharyngeal cultures for *Neisseria gonorrhoeae* should be obtained if sexually transmitted diseases could be present at those sites.

Comments and Treatment Considerations

Treatment consists of rapid joint drainage and antibiotic administration. Hematogenous spread is the most common mode of joint infection in children. A thorough physical examination to investigate other sites of infection is mandatory. Overall, *Staphylococcus aureus* is the most common organism. In neonates, *S. aureus,* group A and group B *Streptococci* predominate. *Neisseria gonorrhoeae* should be suspected in sexually active adolescents. Adolescent intravenous drug abusers are at risk for gram-negative organisms. The incidence of *Haemophilus influenzae* septic arthritis has fallen dramatically with the routine administration of HIB vaccine. History of immunization compliance is important to ascertain.

Bacteremia can also lead to meningitis, so the history and physical examination should also be conducted with that possibility in mind.

Orthopedic consultation is indicated for all highly suspected and confirmed cases of septic arthritis.

REFERENCES

Del Beccaro MA, Champoux AN, Bockers T, Mendelman PM: Septic arthritis versus transient synovitis of the hip: the value of screening laboratory tests, *Ann Emerg Med* 21:1418, 1992.

Sonnen GM, Henry NK: Pediatric bone and joint infections: diagnosis and antimicrobial management, *Pediatr Clin North Am* 43:933, 1996.

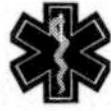

SLIPPED CAPITAL FEMORAL EPIPHYSIS

Slipped capital femoral epiphysis (SCFE) is a displacement of the normal relationship between the femoral head and femoral neck through the growth plate. It is the most common hip disorder in adolescents. It is more common in overweight boys and has a peak age of onset of 12 years. A minority of SCFE is preceded by a traumatic event.

Symptoms

- Pain (hip, knee, thigh, or groin pain) often exacerbated by movement of the hip or ambulation. Hip pain may be referred to the medial knee. Therefore any limping child with knee pain needs an assessment of the hip as well.
- Altered gait
- Pain and limp can be acute or chronic. Small amounts of slippage can occur over a period of months, and an acute slip may be superimposed on chronic slippage after relatively minor trauma (the so-called "acute-on-chronic" slip).

Signs

- The hip is held in relative flexion and external rotation.
- Passive hip flexion may accentuate the external rotation deformity.

- Internal rotation and abduction may be limited.
- Atrophy of the thigh if symptoms have been long-standing
- Shortening of the affected lower extremity depends on the degree of slippage.

Workup

X-ray (anteroposterior view of the pelvis and frog-leg lateral views of both hips) may show subtle findings or gross displacement of the femoral epiphysis on the proximal femoral metaphysis depending on the degree of slippage. Early slips may just show slight irregularity and widening of the epiphysis. On the AP view, a line is drawn from the lateral edge of the femoral neck cephalad toward the joint on the same side. The portion of the epiphysis lateral to this line should be symmetric on both hips. If it is not, SCFE should be suspected. On the frog-leg view, more advanced slips look like a scoop of ice cream slipping off the cone. The slip is not infrequently bilateral (++), so careful examination and radiographic evaluation of the contralateral hip also indicated.

Comments and Treatment Considerations

When the diagnosis has been made, the patient must be admitted and placed at strict bed-rest with no weight bearing to prevent further slippage of the femoral epiphysis. An orthopedic surgeon needs to be consulted. The condition usually requires in situ pinning. SFCE is associated with hypothyroidism and other endocrine disorders.

REFERENCES

Crawford AH: Current concepts review: slipped capital femoral epiphysis, *J Bone Joint Surg* 70A:1422, 1988.

Koop S, Quanbeck D: Three common causes of childhood hip pain, *Pediatr Clin North Am* 43:1053, 1996.

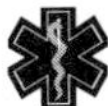

OSTEOMYELITIS

Osteomyelitis should be considered in patients who have bony tenderness and whose history, physical examination, and x-ray findings are suggestive, or if the evaluation does not provide another diagnosis. Trauma may be a precipitating factor of osteomyelitis, but young children are prone to frequent minor trauma in the lower extremities from their normal activities. Osteomyelitis is 2.5 times more common in males than in females.

See Chapter 4, Back Pain, Lower.

Symptoms

- Bone pain
- Fever
- Smaller children and infants may have vague symptoms of irritability and poor feeding or may appear toxic or septic.

Signs

- Bone tenderness +++ in toddlers and young children. The older the patient, the easier to detect the exact site of tenderness on examination.
- Limp or refusal to walk +++
- Fever +++
- Overlying erythema
- Joint motion can be limited from the local muscle spasm caused by inflammation.

Workup

- Bone scan ++++; the method of choice for detecting early pediatric osteomyelitis
- Erythrocyte sedimentation rate ++++
- Blood cultures may help direct therapy +++.
- WBC has low sensitivity ++.
- X-rays are negative early in the disease process but may detect another cause for a limp (e.g., fracture or neoplasm). Before bony changes of osteomyelitis are evident, a plain film may detect soft tissue swelling, blurring of the adjacent fat planes, and periosteal reaction.
- Joint aspiration is indicated for a suspect joint, since this may coexist with osteomyelitis.
- Aspiration of fluid beneath the periosteum for culture may be considered by a consulting orthopedist.

Comments and Treatment Considerations

Over half of pediatric osteomyelitis cases involve bones of the lower extremity. Overall, the most common cause of osteomyelitis is *S. aureus*. In neonates, group B *Streptococcus* and enteric gram-negative organisms are also found. In infants and toddlers who have not been adequately immunized, *H. influenzae* should be considered. *Salmonella* is a common cause of osteomyelitis in patients with sickle cell anemia. *Pseudomonas aeruginosa* is often associated with puncture wounds of the foot, especially those sustained while wearing tennis shoes.

The most common source of bone infection is from hematogenous spread, and the bone metaphysis is the most common site of seeding. Extension from a local skin or muscle infection can also occur. Consider tuberculosis or a fungal cause in appropriate patients.

REFERENCES

Faden H, Grossi M: Acute osteomyelitis in children: reassessment of etiologic agents and their characteristics, *Am J Dis Child* 145:65, 1991.

Myers MT, Thompson GH: Imaging the child with a limp, *Pediatr Clin North Am* 44:637, 1997.

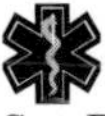

SPINAL EPIDURAL ABSCESS

See Epidural Abscess in Chapter 4, Back Pain, Lower.

REFERENCES

Rubin G, Michowiz SD, Ashkenasi A, et al: Spinal epidural abscess in the pediatric age group: case report and review of the literature, *Pediatr Infect Dis J* 12:1007, 1993.

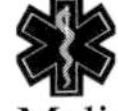

MALIGNANCIES

Malignant bone and soft tissue tumors are uncommon causes of limping in children. However, early diagnosis is critical and can be lifesaving. Leukemia is the most frequent childhood malignancy. The skeleton is often the first body system to display overt manifestations of the acute form of the disease. Osteogenic sarcoma, Ewing sarcoma, leukemia, spinal cord tumors, soft tissue sarcomas, and metastatic tumors of the extremities may cause limb pain or limping.

Symptoms

- Knee pain is a common complaint in adolescents, but the two most common sites for bone tumors are the distal femur and proximal tibia. Knee pain that occurs at rest or at night should be a cause for concern.
- Musculoskeletal pain +++ in cases of acute leukemia; described as intermittent, localized, sharp, severe, and sudden in onset
- Lethargy, fever

Signs

- Focal tenderness at the site of a bony tumor may be elicited by direct palpation.
- Thorough general physical examination may show hepatosplenomegaly, lymphadenopathy, pallor, purpura, or bleeding, which can be signs of leukemia or of other malignancies. Palpation of the muscles in the lower extremity may reveal a soft tissue mass as evidence of a rhabdomyosarcoma or other soft tissue tumor. Hyperreflexia or weakness of the lower extremities can point to a tumor in the spinal area.

Workup

- Plain films of the site of localized pain. Referred pain should be kept in mind and further distal radiographic studies considered if initial ones are negative.
- CBC including leukocyte differential and platelet count

Comments and Treatment Considerations

Appropriate consultation after diagnosis or for further evaluation is required.

REFERENCES

Gallagher DJ, Phillips DF, Heinrich SD: Orthopedic manifestations of acute pediatric leukemia, *Orthop Clin North Am* 27:635, 1996.

Himelstein BH, Dormans JP: Malignant bone tumors of childhood, *Pediatr Clin North Am* 43:967, 1996.

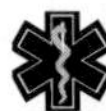

LEGG-CALVÉ-PERTHES DISEASE

Legg-Calvé-Perthes disease is avascular necrosis of the femoral head that occurs most commonly in boys between 5 and 9 years of age and is generally insidious in onset. Hip pain and limp are noted. X-rays may initially be negative; bone scan and MRI are more sensitive. Orthopedic consultation is required.

REFERENCES

Sherk H, Black J: Orthopedic emergencies. In Fleisher GR, Ludwig S, editors: *Textbook of pediatric emergency medicine,* ed 3, Baltimore, 1993, Williams & Wilkins.

Torrey SB: Lower extremity and pelvis. In Barkin RM, editor: *Pediatric emergency medicine: concepts and clinical practice,* ed 2, St Louis, 1996, Mosby.

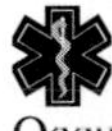

PSOAS ABSCESS AND APPENDICITIS

Occult retroperitoneal, abdominal, or pelvic infections may cause limping in a young child.

See Chapter 1, Abdominal Pain.

Symptoms

- Psoas abscess may present with hip, groin, abdomen, lower back, buttock, or upper thigh pain associated with fever and limping.

Signs

- Hip held in flexion, abduction, and external rotation (like arthritis of the hip)

- Hip extension and internal rotation (stretches the iliopsoas muscle) may cause increased pain.
- Rectal examination may occasionally reveal a mass and tenderness on the affected side.
- Scoliosis to the side of the abscess
- Gait disturbance manifested by a cautious, slow gait and flexion of the trunk may be observed with appendicitis.

Workup

- Abdominal ultrasound may demonstrate a psoas abscess and also may reveal evidence of appendicitis or other pathologic conditions of the pelvis. The value of ultrasound in evaluating for appendicitis is operator-dependent.
- CT scan with intravenous and oral and rectal contrast is an alternative to ultrasound.

Comments and Treatment Considerations

Appendicitis is the most common surgical emergency of childhood. Surgical consultation is needed when appendicitis and psoas abscess are suspected because the treatment is surgical. In cases with an equivocal history, physical examination, and laboratory findings, the patient should be admitted to the hospital for observation and repeat abdominal examinations.

REFERENCES[www]

Gamal R, Moore TC: Appendicitis in children aged 13 years and younger, *Am J Surg* 159:589, 1990.

Schwaitzberg SD, Pokorny WJ, Thurston RS, et al: Psoas abscess in children, *J Pediatr Surg* 20:339, 1985.

Singer J: Neonatal psoas pyomyositis simulating pyarthrosis of the hip, *Pediatr Emerg Care* 9:87, 1993.

[www]Additional references are available on the following web site: www.signsandsymptoms.com.

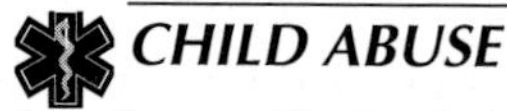

CHILD ABUSE

See Chapter 18, The Irritable Child and Vomiting.

REFERENCES

Clark MC: The limping child: meeting the challenges of an accurate assessment and diagnosis, *Emerg Med Reports* 2:123, 1997.

Meyers MT, Thompson GH: Imaging the child with a limp, *Pediatr Clin North Am* 44:637, 1997.

Renshaw TS: The child who has a limp, *Pediatr Rev* 16:458, 1995.

CHAPTER 22

Mental Status Change and Coma

JULIAN G. LIS

Altered mental status (AMS) represents a spectrum of disability, from mild confusion to deep coma. It is a common occurrence, with approximately 1% of patients arriving at emergency departments comatose and many more with an altered sensorium. The differential diagnosis is large (Table 22-1) and includes numerous life-threatening conditions. An organized approach begins with a rapid initial standard evaluation and stabilization plan that is applicable to most patients. The aim of the initial evaluation is to identify and treat potential immediate threats to life such as ventilatory failure or hypoxia, cardiac dysrhythmia and hypotension, as well as conditions that are easily treated, such as hypoglycemia.

As the patient is stabilized, possible causes for the change in mental status are considered. Potential general causes include primary CNS processes (e.g., infection, bleeding, seizure, and infarction), conditions that reduce CNS perfusion (e.g., hypotension from any cause), decreased oxygen content in the blood (hypoxia or alteration in hemoglobin binding to oxygen), ventilatory failure (hypercapnia), sepsis, toxic or metabolic abnormalities, and other rare conditions. In the setting of possible bacterial meningitis or sepsis, antibiotics should not be unreasonably delayed for any test (including CT or LP). In general, blood and urine cultures should be obtained and antibiotics administered early in the ED evaluation. Only after an exhaustive medical evaluation, which is rarely possible to complete in the ED, can an abnormal mental status be ascribed to psychiatric disease.

INITIAL EVALUATION AND STABILIZATION

A systematic approach is necessary to diagnose and appropriately manage the gamut of causes of AMS. As with all true emergency patients, *evaluation and treatment begin with the ABCs* before a complete history and physical examination are performed. The initial approach is essentially the same for all AMS patients, with physical assessment, diagnostic studies, treatment, and consideration of the differential diagnosis occurring simultaneously.

1. Assess and stabilize the ABCs
2. Establish intravenous access
3. Check pulse oximetry
4. Initiate cardiac monitoring
5. Perform rapid bedside capillary glucose
   a. *Hypoglycemia*: In the context of AMS, administer glucose for a measured glucose <60.
   b. *Hyperglycemia*: Consider DKA and hyperglycemic hyperosmolar nonketotic syndrome (HHNK)
6. Check vital signs
   a. Blood pressure
      (1) Hypotension: see Chapter 17, Hypotension
      (2) Blood pressure: >180/120, consider sympathomimetic abuse, thyroid storm, hypertensive encephalopathy, or primary CNS vascular event (stroke)
      (3) Heart rate: if >150 or <45 and signs of poor perfusion are present, the arrhythmia may be the primary cause of the AMS.
   b. Temperature
      (1) If elevated or depressed, consider sepsis. Temperature may also be normal in patients with sepsis.
      (2) >104° F: consider thyroid storm, neuroleptic malignant syndrome (NMS), malignant hyperthermia, heat stroke, and infection
      (3) <95.0° F: consider myxedema coma, hypothermia
   c. Respiratory rate
      (1) Tachypnea: consider hypoxia, altered hemoglobin oxygen binding, acidosis, sepsis

Table 22-1 Differential Diagnosis of Altered Mental Status

(See specific diagnoses throughout text)

Respiratory	Vascular	Infection	Neurologic
Hypercarbia			
Hypoxia	Hypotension Stroke Hypertensive encephalopathy Thrombotic thrombocytopenic purpura (TTP) CNS vasculitis	Sepsis Meningitis Encephalitis Other intracranial infections (abscess, subdural empyema) Other non-CNS infections	Head trauma Intracranial hemorrhages Intracranial tumors Hydrocephalus Cerebral edema Seizures, including nonconvulsive status epilepticus, temporal lobe epilepsy, and postictal state

(2) Bradypnea: consider opiate abuse; beware of agonal respirations with impending respiratory collapse

7. Assess level of consciousness. If the patient is comatose, test the gag and corneal reflexes.
8. Administer thiamine 100 mg IV. Thiamine is given to alcoholics and others at risk for vitamin deficiency to prevent possible precipitation of Wernicke's encephalopathy by glucose-containing intravenous fluids. This probably is not a truly emergent action but is generally done before glucose administration.

Table 22-1 Differential Diagnosis of Altered Mental Status —cont'd

Toxins	Environmental	Endocrine and Metabolic	Psychiatric
See Chapter 32, Toxic Ingestion, Approach to	Heat stroke Hypothermia	Adrenal insufficiency Hypoglycemia DKA HHNK Thyroid storm Myxedema coma Hypercalcemia Hyponatremia Hypernatremia Hepatic encephalopathy Uremia Wernicke-Korsakoff's syndrome	Psychosis Mania Catatonia Hysteria Malingering

9. Check pupils. Pinpoint pupils and bradypnea or apnea strongly suggest overdose of opiate (rarely other causes, such as pontine hemorrhage) and often dramatically respond to naloxone. A unilateral, dilated, nonreactive pupil indicates probable brainstem herniation from increased intracranial pressure. Emergent management includes intubation, hyperventilation, immediate neurosurgical consultation, and mannitol administration as bridge to OR. An emergent cranial CT scan is indicated.
10. Consider occult trauma. Examine the head and neck. Consider cervical spine immobilization and x-rays.
11. Perform a brief, focused neurologic examination. Emergent cranial CT scanning is a top priority if trauma is evident or focal neurologic deficits are present.

After the immediate life-threatening conditions have been addressed, a more complete history and physical examination can be performed. The circumstances surrounding the onset of the AMS, as well as the patient's past medical history (including medications and any psychiatric history) are often the most helpful factors in determining the cause of AMS. Obtaining a history often entails using all potential sources of information regarding the patient (e.g., calling the nursing home from which the patient was transferred and speaking directly to the paramedics who were on scene).

Common drug overdose toxidromes should be considered when examining patients with AMS (see Chapter 32, Toxic Ingestion, Approach to).

Specific patient populations require additional considerations. For children, consider Reye's syndrome and intussusception. For the elderly, consider polypharmacy and drug interactions, sepsis and other non-CNS infections, dementia, and fluid and electrolyte disorders. For pregnant women, consider HELLP syndrome and eclampsia. For immunocompromised patients, consider opportunistic intracranial infections, intracranial tumors, and hypercalcemia in certain cancer patients. Agitation with AMS suggests a number of possible conditions (e.g., delirium tremens, thyroid storm, adrenergic drug overdose, serotonin syndrome, anticholinergic overdose, NMS, and heat stroke).

DIAGNOSTIC TESTING

Diagnostic studies can be divided into tests reasonably performed routinely whenever the etiology of AMS is uncertain and those performed only as the specifics of the patient's presentation indicate.

Routine Studies

- Urinalysis: especially in the elderly, in whom urosepsis is a frequent cause of AMS
- ECG: In cognitively marginal elderly individuals, an acute myocardial infarction may manifest as AMS. ECG may also be useful in suspected overdoses of cyclic antidepressants (see Chapter 27, Seizure, Adult), type Ia antiarrhyth-

mics (QT prolongation), and digoxin (arrhythmias and heart block).

- Chest x-rays: pneumonia may cause AMS in the frail elderly, who may present without cough, fever, hypoxia, or definitive physical findings. Concomitant sepsis or meningitis must be considered.
- Calcium: hypercalcemia, especially in known malignancy and in the elderly
- Electrolytes, BUN, creatinine, and glucose: hyponatremia, hypernatremia, hyperkalemia (in adrenal insufficiency), anion gap, BUN and creatinine for renal failure, serum glucose to confirm the rapid bedside glucose
- CBC: Although of questionable utility, the WBC is routinely used to detect occult infection, especially in the afebrile elderly.

Specific Studies

- Lumbar puncture (LP): emergent for patients with AMS and evidence of either meningitis or fever without source. Whenever bacterial meningitis is a concern and the LP will be delayed, antibiotics should be given before LP.
- Head CT: All AMS patients should have a cranial CT scan to exclude structural lesions unless a definitive cause for AMS has already been established by the initial evaluation.
- Blood cultures: when considering sepsis. Most useful in the elderly, children <36 months, immunocompromised patients, and when fever accompanies AMS.
- Certain laboratory tests are useful when toxic ingestions are under consideration, including serum osmolality (e.g., for methanol or ethylene glycol), co-oximetry (e.g., for CO or methemoglobin), and possibly qualitative or quantitative toxin screens (see Chapter 32, Toxic Ingestion, Approach to).
- Ethanol level: Although ethanol is a common cause of AMS in every ED, obtaining an alcohol level is not necessary for every AMS patient. While supporting a diagnosis of ethanol intoxication, a high level does not preclude an occult subdural hematoma or other coexistent pathologic condition. A level of "0" in a patient who was presumed drunk should encourage a more aggressive pursuit of alternative causes for

the AMS. Alcohol level also can be used to calculate the osmolal gap (see Chapter 32, Toxic Ingestion, Approach to).

- Liver function tests (AST, ALT, total/direct bilirubin, ammonia level, PT): in children to rule out Reye's syndrome and in patients of any age with suggestive symptoms or physical findings to confirm previously undiagnosed liver disease. Hepatic encephalopathy, however, especially in known chronic liver disease, is largely a clinical diagnosis, and test results rarely change management.
- TSH and Free T4: results not available in the ED, but supports diagnosis of thyrotoxicosis or myxedema coma.
- Serum cortisol: results not available in the ED, but supports diagnosis of adrenal crisis.

There are a number of causes of AMS for which no rapidly available specific test exists and can be diagnosed only on clinical grounds in the ED. (see the box below). Many of these conditions have specific treatments and carry a high mortality if untreated.

Occasionally the cause of AMS remains unknown despite a thorough evaluation. In these cases the patient should generally be cultured and given antibiotics, hospitalized (usually to a monitored bed), and observed. Further diagnostic evaluation and treatment should be individualized.

CAUSES OF ALTERED MENTAL STATUS THAT MUST BE DIAGNOSED ON CLINICAL GROUNDS

- Adrenal crisis
- Delirium tremens
- Heat stroke
- Hypertensive encephalopathy
- Myxedema coma
- Postictal state
- Psychogenic (always a diagnosis of exclusion)
- Sepsis
- Thyroid storm
- Toxicologic causes (e.g., anticholinergic toxicity, cholinergic crisis, and serotonin syndrome)
- Wernicke's encephalopathy

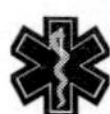

HYPOGLYCEMIA

Hypoglycemia is most often encountered in diabetic patients who fail to balance caloric intake with the amount of insulin or hypoglycemic agent taken. Less commonly, hypoglycemia occurs in fasting alcoholics (owing to the inhibition of gluconeogenesis by alcohol), patients with hepatic dysfunction, and in otherwise healthy elderly adults after a prolonged fast. Hypoglycemia also occurs in infants with poor caloric intake (inadequate glycogen stores) and children who ingest alcohol (owing to inhibition of gluconeogenesis and poor glycogen stores).

Many other medications stimulate insulin secretion or inhibit gluconeogenesis (e.g., pentamidine, propranolol, quinine, and salicylates, among others) and can cause hypoglycemia in overdose. Rarely, an insulinoma is the cause of hypoglycemia.

Symptoms

Signs and symptoms can be categorized into hyperadrenergic (owing to release of counter-regulatory hormones, such as epinephrine, secreted in response to a falling serum glucose) and neuroglucopenic (cerebral dysfunction due to insufficient glucose). Hyperadrenergic manifestations may be absent in long-standing diabetes due to diabetic autonomic neuropathy.

- *Neuroglucopenic:* progress from subtly diminished ability to concentrate to impaired judgment and memory, confusion, drowsiness, and disorientation
- *Hyperadrenergic:* sweating, tremor, sensation of warmth, generalized weakness, hunger, palpitations, and dizziness

Signs

- AMS: confusion ++++, bizarre behavior suggestive of a psychiatric disturbance ++, stupor ++, coma ++
- Seizures ++
- Focal neurologic deficit +; for example, a sudden hemiparesis suggestive of a stroke

Workup

- In the setting of appropriate symptoms, a rapid finger-stick glucose <55 mg/dl establishes the diagnosis. If the diagnosis remains in doubt, dextrose should be given and the low glucose concentration confirmed by the laboratory.

- Renal function (BUN and creatinine) should be checked in diabetics if the cause of the episode is unclear.
- Liver function tests should be considered if hepatic gluconeogenic function is a concern.

Comments and Treatment Considerations

Symptoms and glucose concentrations correlate imperfectly. Some patients are symptomatic with glucose >60, whereas others appear asymptomatic with glucose <40.

Treatment in adults consists of an immediate intravenous bolus of 50 ml (one ampule) of dextrose 50% (D50). In children, 2 to 4 ml/kg of D25 is given intravenously. Neonates should receive D10 intravenously. Glucagon (1 mg subcutaneously or intramuscularly) may be given if venous access is delayed. Glucose determination should be repeated in 30 minutes, and additional dextrose may be administered as necessary. Patients should be fed as soon as they are able to eat safely. One ampule of D50 has only 25 g of carbohydrate, the equivalent of one glass of orange juice.

A period of ED observation with rechecks of serum glucose after feeding is necessary for all patients with an episode of hypoglycemia. Rebound hypoglycemia is common with long-acting insulins and oral hypoglycemics. Hospital admission for observation should be considered if a patient has recurrent or intractable hypoglycemic episodes.

In approximately two thirds of episodes the cause of hypoglycemia can be found, with inadequate caloric intake being the most common cause in diabetics. Increased activity or delayed meals are also frequent causes.

Prevention of subsequent episodes is crucial; this may require decreasing the insulin dose.

REFERENCES

Hepburn DA, Deary IJ: Symptoms of acute insulin-induced hypoglycemia in humans with and without IDDM, *Diabetes Care* 14:949, 1991.

Malouf RM, Brust JC: Hypoglycemia: causes, neurological manifestations, and outcome, *Ann Neurol* 17:421, 1985.

Service FJ: Hypoglycemia, *Med Clin North Am* 79:1, 1995.

ENCEPHALITIS

Encephalitis is an inflammatory disorder of the brain. Common etiologies in immune competent individuals include herpes simplex virus (HSV), arboviruses, and a postviral syndrome mediated by the autoimmune system (30%). In immunocompromised patients, cytomegalovirus (CMV), toxoplasmosis, and fungal infections can cause encephalitis.

HSV causes 2000 cases of encephalitis annually in the United States, with no specific age-related, geographic, or seasonal preference. Mortality is 70% in untreated individuals, and patients with advanced disease almost always become permanently disabled. Herpes encephalitis can cause bizarre behavior that may be misdiagnosed as a psychiatric disorder.

Although the signs and symptoms discussed here pertain specifically to HSV encephalitis, most features are shared by the encephalitides caused by other entities.

Symptoms

- AMS +++++: personality changes ++++, drowsiness ++++
- Onset may be insidious or abrupt
- Headache +++
- History of an antecedent prodromal influenza-like illness +++
- Seizures +++: focal (85%), generalized (15%)

Signs

- Fever +++++
- Focal neurologic signs ++++, hemiparesis +++
- Of those conscious, difficulty speaking or complete aphasia +++
- Meningismus +++
- Evidence of increased intracranial pressure (papilledema or elevated opening pressure on LP) +++

Workup

- CT scan +++; approximately 80% specific for lesions typical of HSV at the time of presentation, increases to ++++ and approximately 90% specific after 6 days of symptoms.

- MRI provides earlier detection and better visualization of lesions than CT.
- CSF analysis initially can be normal and becomes progressively abnormal as illness progresses.
  - WBC: range 0 to 545 WBC/mm^3
  - RBC: elevated +++, range 12 to 4000 RBC/mm^3
  - Protein: elevated in ++++; range, 0.34 to 2.8 g/L
  - Glucose: normal ++++
  - Pressure is usually elevated.
  - PCR analysis of cerebrospinal fluid (CSF-PCR) for herpes simplex virus DNA ++++; approaches 100% specificity
- EEG ++++, but only 33% specific. Diffuse slowing or unilateral (or bilateral) periodic discharges in the temporal lobes. Slow-wave complexes at regular intervals of two or three per second are classic.

Comments and Treatment Considerations

Acyclovir (10 mg/kg IV q8h) has decreased 6-month mortality from 70% to 19% and should be administered. Early diagnosis is essential, and in most cases presumptive treatment with acyclovir until CSF-PCR results return is indicated whenever the diagnosis is entertained.

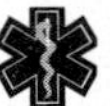

DIABETIC KETOACIDOSIS

Diabetic ketoacidosis (DKA) is a syndrome defined by a constellation of clinical findings and laboratory abnormalities (typically blood glucose >250, pH <7.30, serum HCO_3^- <15 to 20 mmol/L, and ketonemia >1:4 dilution). Between 60% and 80% of DKA occurs in known diabetics; the remaining 20% to 40% occurs with the onset of diabetes. Relative or absolute insulin deficiency is the cause of DKA.

As a result of insulin deficiency, peripheral glucose uptake is impaired and hepatic gluconeogenesis increases, resulting in hyperglycemia. As the glucose concentration rises, the renal threshold for glucose is exceeded; glucosuria ensues, creating an osmotic diuresis, which in turn leads to volume depletion. A serum glucose greater than 400 in a patient with normal renal function implies a significant total body water deficit. Increasing serum osmolarity causes progressive obtundation. Fat cells, without the action of insulin, release fatty acids into the blood, which are converted by the liver into ketoacids. Acidosis accounts for the symptoms of tachypnea, Kussmaul respirations, nausea, vomiting, and abdominal pain.

Symptoms

Symptoms vary with severity of the DKA episode.

- Polydipsia and polyuria
- Weight loss
- Fatigue ++++
- Muscle cramps +++
- Abdominal pain, nausea, and vomiting +++
- AMS ++: confusion and lethargy to coma ++

Signs

- Vital signs: tachypnea ++++, tachycardia ++++, hypotension ++, hypothermia
- Evidence of volume depletion: dry oral mucosa, dry skin ++++
- AMS (50% to 60%): drowsiness to coma
- Kussmaul respirations ++++
- Odor of acetone on breath +++
- Abdominal tenderness without rebound +++ or less commonly with rebound and guarding +

Workup

- Serum glucose to confirm bedside glucose
- Electrolytes: HCO_3^- to determine the severity of the acidosis. The potassium concentration is critically important. Rehydration and insulin therapy with correction of the acidosis acutely decrease the serum potassium concentration, which must be monitored closely. Serum sodium may be low initially owing to the dilutional effect of the movement of water from the intracellular to the extracellular space due to the osmotic effect of serum hyperglycemia.
- BUN, creatinine: to assess renal function

- Serum ketones
- ECG: for evidence of hyperkalemia (peaked T waves), hypokalemia (U waves), presence of acute myocardial infarction
- Consider CBC, blood and urine cultures, and chest x-rays as appropriate.
- ABG: if the patient appears severely ill, to assess the severity of the acidosis (may not be needed if quick electrolytes are rapidly available) and ventilatory status

Comments and Treatment Considerations

The most important treatment in the ED management of DKA is volume replacement (generally at least 2 L of normal saline in adults who are not at risk for CHF). Unless the ECG shows evidence of hyperkalemia, insulin therapy is not needed immediately and should generally be held until the potassium level is known, since insulin can cause life-threatening hypokalemia.

In addition to intravenous fluids, insulin therapy is required in order to stop ketogenesis and subsequent acidosis. Bicarbonate is generally not indicated. Regular insulin (0.1 units/kg/hr in adults and children) may be given by intravenous infusion with or without a bolus dose (0.1 units/kg of regular insulin). The blood sugar may drop before ketogenesis is reversed (generally monitored by normalization of the anion gap). Therefore glucose should be added to intravenous fluids when the blood sugar begins to approach "normal" levels (usually glucose is added to IVF when level is 200 to 250 mg/dl). Intravenous potassium replacement is usually also necessary even when initial serum K is "normal," since total body potassium is decreased and insulin further decreases extracellular levels. Glucose and potassium levels should be monitored closely (every hour) during initial treatment.

A search for the precipitating cause of the episode of DKA is necessary. Common precipitating factors include insufficient insulin (including noncompliance and new onset), infection +++, alcohol or drug abuse ++, pancreatitis or other abdominal disorders +, myocardial infarction +, and patients older than 50 years of age ++.

REFERENCES

Kitabchi AE, Wall BM: Diabetic ketoacidosis, *Med Clin North Am* 79:9, 1995.

Snorgaard O, Eskildsen PC: Diabetic ketoacidosis in Denmark: epidemiology, incidence rates, precipitating factors, and mortality rates, *J Intern Med* 226:223, 1989.

Umpierrez GE, Kelly JP: Hyperglycemic crises in urban blacks, *Arch Intern Med* 157:669, 1997.

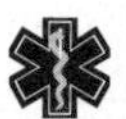

HYPEROSMOLAR HYPERGLYCEMIC NONKETOTIC SYNDROME

Hyperosmolar hyperglycemic nonketotic syndrome (HHNK) is a condition that usually occurs in older type 2 diabetics in whom severely elevated serum glucose results in an osmotic diuresis, electrolyte abnormalities, profound dehydration, and frequently AMS. HHNK is defined as a serum glucose >600 mg/dl, serum osmolarity >320 to 330 mOsm/L, arterial pH >7.30, and negative or trace serum ketones. HHNK has an incidence roughly equivalent to DKA, and the two syndromes have significant overlap. HHNK differs from DKA in the more severely elevated glucose levels reached and the absence of ketoacidosis. Approximately half of patients with HHNK do not have a history of known diabetes. Many patients have precipitant medical or surgical conditions such as infection, MI, or stroke.

Symptoms

- Weakness ++++
- Polyuria ++++
- Polydipsia +++
- Anorexia +++
- Nausea and vomiting +++
- Dizziness ++
- Confusion

Signs

- Volume depletion +++++: dry oral mucosa, dry skin with poor turgor, orthostatic hypotension, and tachycardia (moderate to severe +++; mild ++)

- AMS: alert ++, lethargic +++, comatose +++. Mental status correlates with serum osmolarity; coma is rare below 350 mOsm/L.
- Seizures ++
- Altered mental status

Workup

- Glucose: 800 to 1000 mg/dl
- Electrolytes, BUN, creatinine, and serum osmolarity. Severe hyperglycemia results in a pseudo-hyponatremia; the sodium concentration must be corrected by adding 1.6 mEq/L for every 100 mg/dl elevation of glucose over the normal value of 100 mg/dl.
- Serum ketones to differentiate from DKA
- Search for a precipitating cause: chest x-rays, urinalysis and urine culture, and blood cultures for infection
- ECG to investigate acute MI
- Head CT or MRI to look for a concomitant stroke

Comments and Treatment Considerations

Hydration, initially with intravenous normal saline, is the cornerstone of therapy. Insulin is routinely administered but is less crucial than with DKA and lower doses are required. Otherwise treatment is similar to DKA, that is, fluids, insulin, replacement of electrolytes, and specific treatments for precipitant illnesses. Hyperglycemia and hyperosmolarity should be corrected gradually to prevent hypokalemia and cerebral edema due to rapid shifting of fluid into the intracellular space.

Mortality has ranged from 10% to 17% in recent series and is predominantly related to the severity of the precipitating illness. A higher serum osmolarity and higher serum sodium also correlate with a poor outcome.

REFERENCES

Lorber D: Nonketotic hypertonicity in diabetes mellitus, *Med Clin North Am* 79:39, 1995.

Pinies JA, Cairo G, Gaztambide S, Vazquez JA: Course and prognosis of 132 patients with diabetic nonketotic hyperosmolar state, *Diabete Metab* 20:43, 1994.

Wachtel TJ, Tetu-Mouradjian LM: Hyperosmolarity and acidosis in diabetes mellitus: a three-year experience in Rhode Island, *J Gen Intern Med* 6:495, 1991.

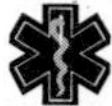

HYPERCALCEMIA

Malignancy is the most common cause of severe hypercalcemia resulting in AMS. Malignancies most likely to cause hypercalcemia are breast cancer (30% to 40%), multiple myeloma (20% to 40%), squamous cell carcinomas of the lung (12% to 35%), the head, neck, or esophagus (19%), non-Hodgkin's lymphoma (3% to 13%), leukemias (2% to 11%), renal cell carcinoma (8%), cervical carcinoma (7%), and colon cancer (5%). Of these, the only malignancies that commonly present *initially* with signs of hypercalcemia are adult T-cell lymphoma (45%) and multiple myeloma. Although hyperparathyroidism is a more common cause of hypercalcemia, most patients with that disorder have less severe hypercalcemia and are asymptomatic. Hypercalcemic crisis is usually defined as a serum calcium concentration >14 mg/dl with acute signs and symptoms.

Symptoms

Although symptoms are determined by both the absolute serum calcium concentration and the rate of rise, certain generalizations apply (Table 22-2).

- Polyuria and polydipsia ++++ due to inhibition of ADH
- Nausea and vomiting

Table 22-2 Correlation of Calcium Concentration with Symptoms of Hypercalcemia

Calcium Concentration	Symptoms
<12 mg/dl	Often asymptomatic; polyuria and polydipsia may be present
12-14 mg/dl	Moderate weakness and fatigue
14-16 mg/dl	Extreme weakness, lethargy, and confusion

Signs

- Evidence of extreme dehydration: dry mucous membranes, tachycardia, and orthostasis
- Increased vascular tone may lead to normal blood pressures despite severe dehydration.
- Coma, if present, usually occurs at concentrations >15 mg/dl.

Workup

- Total or ionized serum calcium concentrations. Total serum calcium must be corrected for low albumin states (such as cancer), as ionized levels may be normal. These corrections can be avoided by measuring ionized serum calcium directly (normal range, 4.2 to 4.8 mg/dl).
- Check electrolytes for evidence of hypokalemia, hypomagnesemia, and hypernatremia
- ECG: shortening of the QT interval; bradyarrhythmias, heart block, and asystole can occur.

Comments and Treatment Considerations

Initial treatment consists of hydration with normal saline, since correction of volume depletion increases calcium excretion. Furosemide may also be used. Other pharmacologic therapy is not usually begun in the ED.

Serum phosphate will be low but should not be replaced because of the danger of precipitating calcium phosphate crystals in the blood and tissues.

REFERENCES

Edelson GW, Kleerekoper M: Hypercalcemic crisis, *Med Clin North Am* 79:79, 1995.

Fisken RA, Heath DA: Hypercalcaemia in hospital patients, *Lancet* 1:202, 1981.

Ralston SH, Gallacher SJ: Cancer-associated hypercalcemia: morbidity and mortality. Clinical experience in 126 treated patients, *Ann Intern Med* 112:499, 1990.

DELIRIUM TREMENS AND ALCOHOL WITHDRAWAL

Delirium tremens (DTs) occurs in chronic alcoholics who are withdrawing from alcohol. Alcohol withdrawal causes a spectrum of clinical manifestations from mild tremulousness to seizures, hallucinations (may be auditory or visual and are often dramatic, e.g., bugs crawling on patient, or persecutory), and delirium. Aggressive treatment with benzodiazepines is required when early symptoms and signs are present to prevent progression of alcohol withdrawal syndrome. DTs can lead to death.

Symptoms

Depend on stage of withdrawal

- Early: Shaking, anxious, nausea, vomiting
- Late: Seizures, altered mental status

Signs

Depend on stage of withdrawal

- Early: tremor, increasing levels of autonomic activity as condition progresses (tachycardia, hypertension, hyperreflexia)
- Late: diaphoresis, seizures, hallucinations, delirium

Workup

- Clinical diagnosis
- Rule out other conditions such as infection or CNS trauma that frequently coexist (e.g., urinalysis, chest x-rays, CT, LP as indicated)
- Electrolytes, glucose, magnesium (frequently low)
- CBC

Comments and Treatment Considerations

The mainstay of treatment is benzodiazepine administration. Large doses of IV benzodiazepines are often required. Thiamine 100 mg IV should also probably be given because of the possibility of inducing Wernicke's encephalopathy with delivery of glucose-containing solutions. Patients are generally given magnesium because they are frequently hypomagnesemic. Patients with DTs require hospital admission, often to the ICU. Patients with mild withdrawal controlled with benzodiazepine administration in the ED may be discharged. Caution needs to be exercised in prescribing benzodiazepines for outpatient alcoholic patients, because the combination of alcohol and benzodiazepines can lead to lethal respiratory depression.

REFERENCES[www]

Nolop KB, Natow A: Unprecedented sedative requirements during delirium tremens, *Crit Care Med* 13:246, 1985.

Thompson WL: Management of alcohol withdrawal syndromes, *Arch Intern Med* 138:278, 1978.

Turner RC, Lichstein PR, Peden JG Jr, et al: Alcohol withdrawal syndromes: a review of pathophysiology, clinical presentation, and treatment, *J Gen Intern Med* 4:432, 1989.

[www]Additional references are available on the following web site: www.signsandsymptoms.com.

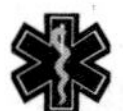

HYPERNATREMIA

Hypernatremia is defined as a serum sodium concentration >145 mmol/L. Hypernatremia is unlikely to be the cause of AMS until the sodium concentration is >155 mEq/L.

Hypernatremia generally occurs in infants, the debilitated, and the elderly; that is, generally in those who do not control their own dietary intake. Even a slight increase in serum sodium levels (3 mEq/L) above baseline triggers an intense thirst response in patients with normal physical abilities, mentation, and an intact thirst mechanism. This triggers water intake and a correction of the serum sodium before significant hypernatremia ensues.

Hypernatremia is usually precipitated by an illness that increases water loss, or, less commonly, by excessive sodium intake. Diarrhea accounts for the majority of cases in young children (40% to 90%). Other precipitants in pediatric patients include pneumonia (10%), urinary tract infections, various CNS diseases, and inadequately diluted infant formulas. Complications include intracranial hemorrhages and arterial thrombosis. Permanent brain damage affects 10% to 15% of survivors.

Half of elderly patients with hypernatremia live in nursing homes. Hypernatremia is frequently precipitated by infection (pneumonia, 39%; urinary tract infections or urosepsis, 28%; bacteremia, 17%). In adults, co-morbidities result in a higher mortality (40% to 60%) and incidence of permanent neurologic sequelae (38%).

Undiagnosed diabetes insipidus (DI) is a rare cause of hypernatremia in the ED but should be considered in patients who have recently undergone intracranial surgery. Persistently high urine output with concomitant volume depletion is a clue to this diagnosis.

Symptoms

- AMS +++++, with severe hypernatremia causing lethargy to coma. Infants may be irritable and have a high-pitched cry.
- Infants are more likely to have seizures +++ to ++++, depending on severity of hypernatremia and rapidity of rise, than adults ++
- Anorexia (infants: decreased feeding), nausea, and vomiting
- Oliguria ++++
- Symptoms stemming from the precipitating illness may predominate; diarrhea (90%) in infants, infection in any age group.

Signs

- AMS: lethargy to coma
- The features of volume depletion (weak pulses, and poor capillary perfusion) may be absent until late in the course.
- A doughy consistency of the skin is common.

Workup

- A workup for sepsis (chest x-rays, blood and urine cultures, and often an LP) is indicated.
- Electrolytes, BUN, creatinine, and glucose: the serum

sodium concentration establishes the diagnosis of hypernatremia. The serum sodium concentration must be corrected if severe hyperglycemia is present (see HHNKS section).

- A cranial CT scan may be indicated to rule out an intracranial hemorrhage, especially in children.
- Urine specific gravity is inappropriately low with DI.

Comments and Treatment Considerations

Initial treatment of hypernatremia due to dehydration is saline 0.9% IV until the intravascular volume is restored as indicated by normalization of pulse, BP, and urine output. Correction can then continue with 0.45% saline. Correction of serum Na^+ should be gradual to prevent cerebral edema.

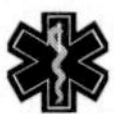

HEPATIC ENCEPHALOPATHY

Hepatic encephalopathy is an uncommon cause of AMS that results from severe hepatic dysfunction. Patients' mental status varies from mildly depressed to coma in severe cases. Asterixis and sequelae of chronic liver disease may be found during physical examination, and plasma ammonia levels may be increased. Other conditions associated with liver failure, such as GI bleeding, must be considered. Treatment includes lactulose, and most patients are hospitalized as an evaluation for the precipitating cause is initiated.

REFERENCES

Fraser C, Arieff AI: Hepatic encephalopathy, *N Engl J Med* 313:865, 1985.

Gammal SH, Jones EA: Hepatic encephalopathy, *Med Clin North Am* 73:793, 1989.

Guss DA: Disorders of the liver, bilary tract, and pancreas. In Rosen P, Barkin RM, Hockberger RS, et al, editors: *Emergency medicine: concepts and clinical practice,* ed 4, St Louis, 1997, Mosby.

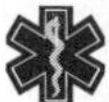

MYXEDEMA COMA

Myxedema coma is the most severe expression of decompensated hypothyroidism. The true incidence is unknown; however, only 200 cases were reported between 1953 and 1986. It is more common in the elderly (70% >60 years of age) and women (80%) and presents almost invariably during winter months (95%). Only approximately a third of patients have a history of hypothyroidism. The diagnosis is often delayed because of the coexistence of a precipitating factor (infection, stroke, hypothermia, sedative-hypnotic use, recent surgery, trauma, or other severe illness), which is presumed to be the cause of the patient's AMS. The diagnosis is then entertained only when initial management fails. Previous mortality was 80%; it is now 15% to 20% principally because of the availability of intravenous levothyroxine.

Symptoms

- AMS: lethargy, confusion, or psychosis; often a gradual deterioration over weeks
- Symptoms of hypothyroidism: fatigue, weakness, cold intolerance, muscle cramps, constipation, weight gain

Signs

- Coma +++
- Seizures: ++ in patients with coma
- Hypothermia (T < 35.5° C) ++++ in comatose patients
- Vital signs reflect the state of overall decreased metabolism: bradycardia ++++, SBP <100 +++, hypoventilation (with hypoxemia and hypercarbia).
- Signs of long-standing hypothyroidism: periorbital edema, macroglossia, hoarse voice, dry and cool skin, nonpitting edema of the lower extremities, fine hair texture with diminished eyebrows, and delayed relaxation of deep tendon reflexes
- Many of the signs of myxedema are indicative of a lowered basal metabolic rate and a lack of stimulation of beta-adrenergic receptors.

- Abdominal distention is common from either ileus or constipation; megacolon and fecal impaction can occur.
- Heart sounds are frequently distant due to pericardial effusion +++. Congestive heart failure is also frequent.
- Fever may develop and heart rate can be "normal" if sepsis is also present.

Workup

- Diagnosis is clinical in the ED setting.
- Serum TSH and free T_4 index are sent to the laboratory to confirm the clinical diagnosis. If available, a free T_3 and free T_4 by dialysis may be more clinically useful. A serum cortisol level is useful to exclude coexisting adrenal insufficiency.
- Other tests may assist in ruling out other conditions. Results are inconsistent in myxedema.
  - Electrolytes: hyponatremia +++, hypochloremia +++, hypoglycemia +
  - CK levels: frequently mildly elevated to 500 to 1000 U/L (MM fraction)
  - CBC: macrocytic anemia; WBC rarely exceeds 10,000/mm^3 even with infection, although bandemia may be present.
  - ECG: low voltage, sinus bradycardia, prolonged PR and QT intervals, and inverted or flattened T waves without ST segment changes
  - LP: increased opening pressure and increased protein
  - Chest x-rays: cardiomegaly
  - Abdominal x-rays: constipation, ileus, or megacolon
  - ABG: hypoxia (Po_2 <75 mm Hg), hypercarbia, and respiratory acidosis

Comments and Treatment Considerations

Treatment must be initiated on the basis of clinical suspicion. Debate is ongoing concerning the optimal formulation and dose of thyroid hormone replacement in myxedema coma. Most experts recommend treatment with intravenous levothyroxine (T_4).

Possible coexisting adrenal insufficiency should be treated empirically with hydrocortisone (100 mg IV q8h). Alternatively, dexamethasone phosphate (4 mg IV q6-8h) allows for an ACTH stimulation test after initial cortisol measurement, although this may not be necessary in all patients.

REFERENCES

Forester CF: Coma in myxedema: report of a case and review of the world literature, *Arch Intern Med* 111:734, 1963.

Nicoloff JT, LoPresti JS: Myxedema coma: a form of decompensated hypothyroidism, *Endocrinol Metab Clin North Am* 22:279, 1993.

Olsen CG: Myxedema coma in the elderly, *J Am Board Fam Pract* 8:376, 1995.

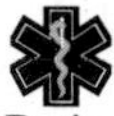

NONCONVULSIVE STATUS EPILEPTICUS

Patients who have AMS, even to thc point of being comatose, may in fact be in nonconvulsive status epilepticus (NCSE). Nonconvulsive seizures occur in nonmotor areas of the brain (usually the temporal, frontal, or parietal regions), can be simple or complex (relating to whether consciousness is affected), and focal (partial) or generalized. Nonconvulsive status epilepticus is defined as continuous or intermittent seizure activity for more than 30 minutes as evidenced by impaired mental status, without motor convulsions.

Symptoms

Patients in NCSE are often unaware of their seizures and do not voice any complaint. Family members who become concerned about the patient's behavior typically bring him or her to medical attention.

Signs

- Automatisms, such as repetitive lip smacking, picking at clothes, smiling, head nodding, laughing inappropriately, and verbal perseveration are common.

- Level of consciousness often fluctuates. Patients may appear awake but withdrawn and confused. Alternatively, they may be drowsy and slow to respond or even comatose.
- NCSE may progress to convulsive seizure activity, resulting in focal signs such as clonic jerking of the eyelids or an extremity or tonic deviation of the head.

Workup

An EEG is ultimately needed to diagnose the seizure activity.

Comments and Treatment Considerations

NCSE is frequently misdiagnosed as psychiatric illness (40%), a metabolic encephalopathy, or a prolonged postictal phase. The diagnosis of NCSE should be considered in patients who (1) have AMS and fail to awaken after a seizure and all other medical workup is negative; (2) have AMS and exhibit automatisms or minor myoclonic jerking of the arms or facial region; or (3) have a new-onset "psychiatric" illness, especially if consciousness or symptoms wax and wane.

Patients in NCSE often respond dramatically to diazepam, with improvement of their mental status within 4 to 5 minutes in many cases.

REFERENCES

Jagoda A: Nonconvulsive seizures, *Emerg Med Clin North Am* 12:963, 1994.

Kaplan PW: Nonconvulsive status epilepticus in the emergency room, *Epilepsia* 37:643, 1995.

Scholtes FB, Renier WO: Non-convulsive status epilepticus: causes, treatment, and outcome in 65 patients, *J Neurol Neurosurg Psychiatry* 61:93, 1996.

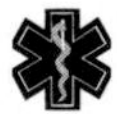

REYE'S SYNDROME

Reye's syndrome is an acute, noninflammatory encephalopathy that usually occurs in children and is associated with fatty degeneration of the liver. Case fatality rates range from 26% to 42%, and any delay in recognition, aggressive management, or disposition is strongly associated with a poor outcome.

Symptoms

- History of a prodromal illness in 75% to 95%, either influenza B or varicella infection ++++ ; followed by severe, repetitive vomiting 3 to 6 days later during apparent convalescence ++++ ; then altered behavior, usually irritability and lethargy
- History of therapeutic dosages of salicylate during the antecedent infection ++++; 75% to 95% sensitivity, limited specificity
- Approximately 75% of cases occur in winter months.
- Between 75% to 80% of cases occur in children 5 to 15 years old, the rest in children under 5. These cases may be more difficult to detect because the differential diagnosis for vomiting and lethargy is large; adult cases are rare but can occur, following the same history, clinical course, and laboratory values as pediatric cases.
- Afebrile by the time of presentation

Signs

- Disease progresses in stages; 70% to 80% present in precomatose stages (I-II).
  - Stage I—lethargy only
  - Stage II—combative or stuporous; inappropriate verbalizing; sluggish pupillary reaction; conjugate deviation on doll's eyes maneuver; may have nonpurposeful response to pain; seizures
  - Stage III—same as stage II except comatose with decorticate posture and response to pain
  - Stage IV—same as stage III except decerebrate posture and response to pain, inconsistent or absent oculocephalic reflex
  - Stage V—same as stage IV except flaccid with no response to pain, no pupillary response, no oculocephalic reflex
- Tachypnea ++++
- Lack of jaundice or nuchal rigidity ++++

- Hepatomegaly +++
- Dehydration ++
- Arrhythmias and myocarditis can occur rarely in advanced stages.

Workup

- Hypoglycemia occurs in 40% of all children and more commonly affects younger children; adults are rarely hypoglycemic.
- ALT and AST levels are 3 to 30 times normal but significantly lower than in fulminant hepatitis.
- PT abnormal in 90% ++++; low specificity
- CSF cell counts and bilirubin levels are normal ++++.
- Ammonia levels initially may be normal ++; levels greater than 300 mcg% are associated with increased mortality; comatose patients have levels 3 to 20 times normal ++++.
- Salicylate levels help differentiate liver failure from toxicity; Reye's syndrome occurs in the absence of toxicity.
- CT of the head should be done before LP in patients with neurologic symptoms; absence of papilledema does not reliably rule out increased intracranial pressure in children.

Comments and Treatment Considerations

All patients with Reye's syndrome must be admitted to the hospital. Those with stage II or higher disease require admission to an ICU with ICP monitoring capability; stage III or higher generally require intubation.

REFERENCES[www]

Dezateux CA, Dinwiddie R, Helms P, Matthew DJ: Recognition and early management of Reye's syndrome, *Arch Dis Child* 61:647, 1986.

Hurwitz ES: Reye's syndrome, *Epidemiol Rev* 11:249, 1989.

Louis PT: Reye syndrome. In Oski PA, DeAngelis CD, Feigin RD, et al, editors: *Principles and practice of pediatrics,* ed 2, Philadelphia, 1994, JB Lippincott.

[www]Additional references are available on the following web site: www.signsandsymptoms.com.

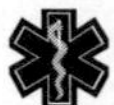

HYPOMAGNESEMIA

Those at high risk for hypomagnesemia include chronic alcoholics, patients with cirrhosis or who are taking diuretics, malnourished patients, patients requiring tube feeding or total parenteral nutrition, and patients with renal failure. The clinical syndrome of hypomagnesemia is similar to hypocalcemia.

Symptoms

- Anorexia
- Nausea and vomiting
- Fatigue
- Irritability
- Generalized weakness

Signs

- Tremor
- Muscular twitching and tetany
- Chvostek's sign
- Trousseau's sign
- Hyporeflexia
- Altered mentation: delirium, hallucinations
- Hypotension and hypothermia (occasional)
- Seizures (usually generalized)

Workup

- If a patient has signs or symptoms of hypomagnesemia or is in a high-risk group, serum magnesium, calcium, and electrolytes should be measured. However, serum magnesium levels do not reflect the total body tissue depletion of magnesium. Severe symptoms, such as seizures, are associated with serum magnesium levels below 1.5.
- ECG: a prolonged PR interval, prolonged QT interval, ST segment depression, and T wave abnormalities are characteristic of hypomagnesemia. Arrhythmias may be seen.

Comments and Treatment Considerations

Magnesium depletion is almost always associated with hypocalcemia and hypokalemia. Acid-base abnormalities are also common. In clinical practice, patients who are at high risk for hypomagnesemia typically also have many other risk factors for seizures (e.g., alcohol abuse or withdrawal, other electrolyte abnormalities, and so forth). Seizures associated with hypomagnesemia are likely multifactorial. Experimentally induced hypomagnesemia in humans has failed to induce seizures.

REFERENCES[www]

Shils ME: Experimental human magnesium depletion, *Medicine* 48:61, 1969.

Suter C, Klingman WO: Neurologic manifestations of magnesium depletion states, *Neurology* 5:691, 1955.

Turnball TL, Vanden Hoek TL, Howes DS, Eisner RF; Utility of laboratory studies in the emergency department patient with a new-onset seizure, *Ann Emerg Med* 19:373, 1990.

[www]Additional references are available on the following web site: www.signsandsymptoms.com.

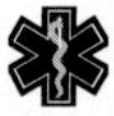

CYANIDE POISONING

Cyanide poisoning is very rare, but frequently fatal, and is a potentially treatable cause of AMS. Routes of exposure include oral ingestion (often suicidal), cutaneous exposure (usually industrial), and inhalational (e.g., smoke from a fire).

Cyanide inhibits oxygen metabolism at the cellular level. The clinical appearance of these patients is therefore similar to those who are hypoxic, except that the blood of patients with cyanide poisoning is well oxygenated; therefore cyanosis does not appear until the onset of respiratory failure. Patients have a severe metabolic acidosis as a result of anaerobic cellular metabolism. An odor of almonds also may be detected.

Symptoms

- Rate of symptom development depends on form, concentration, and route of ingestion: inhalation (seconds to minutes), oral ingestion of cyanide salts (several minutes to 1 hour), organic cyanides (up to 12 hours).

- AMS: initial stimulation followed by a rapid loss of consciousness
- Nausea and vomiting
- Palpitations

Signs

- AMS: agitation, confusion, coma
- Seizures
- Arrhythmias, asystole
- Profound hypotension

Workup

- Clinical diagnosis on the basis of a history of exposure and concordant physical findings
- ABG and electrolytes; profound anion gap metabolic acidosis supports the diagnosis.
- O_2 saturation and Po_2 are normal.
- Other laboratory results are often too delayed to be helpful in the most serious cases of cyanide poisonings.
- CO level

Comments and Treatment Considerations

100% oxygen should be administered. The Lilly Cyanide Antidote Kit (contains amyl nitrate inhaler; sodium nitrite—adult: 10 ml of 3% solution IV, children: 0.2 ml/kg not to exceed 10 mg; and sodium thiosulfate—adults: 50 ml of 25% solution, children: 1.65 ml/kg) is the only antidote combination available in the United States and should be administered to all patients with serious symptoms of cyanide poisoning. Nitrates are thought to affect the production of methemoglobin, which subsequently binds to cyanide. This can be very dangerous in patients with carboxyhemoglobin from CO poisoning because oxygen delivery will be further compromised. Sodium thiosulfate is given after the more rapidly acting nitrate preparations and enhances endogenous detoxification mechanisms. Sodium thiosulfate alone (without nitrates) may be the treatment of choice for cases involving smoke inhalation in which CO poisoning may also have occurred.

REFERENCES[www]

Baud FH, Barriot P, Torris V, et al: Elevated blood cyanide concentrations in victims of smoke inhalation, *N Engl J Med* 325:1761, 1991.

Clark CJ, Campbell D, Reid WH: Blood carboxyhaemoglobin and cyanide levels in fire survivors, *Lancet* 1:1332, 1981.

Hall AH, Rumack GH: Clinical toxicology of cyanide, *Ann Emerg Med* 15:1067, 1986.

[www]Additional references are available on the following web site: www.signsandsymptoms.com.

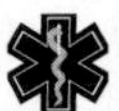

METHEMOGLOBINEMIA

Many drugs and substances, including nitrates, benzocaine, and dapsone, can induce methemoglobinemia. Because of an alteration in the properties of hemoglobin and its subsequent ability to bind oxygen, the oxygen-carrying capacity of the blood is reduced. Similar in mechanism to CO poisoning, patients have central cyanosis but "normal" blood gases. Dissolved oxygen in the blood (Pao_2) is unaffected by the process. Direct measurement of oxygen saturation by co-oximetry and methemoglobin levels confirm the diagnosis. Treatment is with methylene blue. See Chapter 32, Toxic Ingestion, Approach to.

REFERENCES[www]

Curry S: Methemoglobinemia, *Ann Emerg M*ed 11:4, 1982.

Harwood-Nuss AL, Kunisaki T: *Cyanosis in emergency medicine: a comprehensive study guide,* New York, 1996, McGraw-Hill.

Horne MK III, Waterman MR, Garriot JC, et al: Methemoglobinemia from sniffing butyl nitrate, *Ann Intern Med* 91:417, 1982.

[www]Additional references are available on the following web site: www.signsandsymptoms.com

CHAPTER 23

Neck Pain and Stiffness

THOMAS GRAHAM

Patients with neck pain or stiffness as a result of trauma should be considered to have a cervical spine fracture or ligamentous injury until proven otherwise. In the absence of trauma, meningitis and encephalitis must be considered, since bacterial meningitis can progress from an initially mild-appearing illness to death within hours. Subarachnoid hemorrhage may lead to neck pain as blood irritates the meninges.

Local spinal processes (e.g., epidural abscess, cervical disc disease, and osteomyelitis) should also be considered as potential causes of posterior neck or extremity pain. Anterior and internal structures in the neck can cause neck and throat discomfort.

Dystonic reactions are common after short- or long-term neuroleptic use and often are manifested by marked neck stiffness. This causes tremendous discomfort and requires urgent treatment. Tetanus often causes trismus and may cause neck and back stiffness.

Patients with significant head or cervical spine trauma, in particular those with neck pain, cervical spine tenderness, alteration in mentation, or distracting injuries, must be immobilized with a hard cervical collar (taped in place) and be placed on a backboard until a fracture is excluded. Patients who are able to turn their head or move their body off the board have not been adequately immobilized. Immobilized patients must be monitored to prevent aspiration and asphyxiation.

CERVICAL SPINE FRACTURE AND LIGAMENTOUS INJURY

Symptoms

- Neck pain occurring at rest or during range of motion ++++. Patients may not complain of neck pain if they are intoxicated or have an altered level of alertness or have distracting injuries (e.g., other fractures, intraabdominal bleeding, or extensive lacerations). Neck pain is present in nearly 100% of patients in the absence of these complicating circumstances.
- Weakness, numbness, paresthesias, or pain in a radicular pattern suggests possible concurrent spinal cord or nerve root injury.
- Dysesthesias, paresthesias, or even paresis of the upper extremities may indicate a central spinal cord injury (central cord syndrome) and may occur despite the absence of significant neck pain or abnormal neurologic findings in the lower extremity.

Signs

- Midline neck tenderness ++++
- Neck pain with active range of motion (should not be attempted before radiologic clearance in patients who are not fully alert and oriented or in those who are intoxicated or have a distracting injury)
- Soft tissue swelling is usually not appreciated.
- Weakness or sensory deficit ++ may occur with spinal cord involvement.

Workup

Rule out bony injury

- Three-view x-ray series of cervical spine (Figs. 23-1 to 23-3). A cervical spine series is incomplete until it contains a lateral film(s) showing C1 through and including the entire upper border of T1, an anteroposterior (AP) view, an AP projection, and an open-mouth odontoid view demonstrating the dens and the lateral masses of C1. These films must be of adequate quality to analyze the prevertebral soft tissue, as well as the cervical vertebrae and their alignment. When one fracture is seen, often another, less obvious fracture is present. Examples of cervical spine fractures are shown in Figures 23-4 to 23-7).

- Transaxillary (swimmer's) view of cervical spine: It may be necessary to apply gentle traction to both arms during the lateral film to visualize the lower cervical spine adequately in patients wearing cervical collars or in those who are muscular or obese. If this does not lead to visualization of the lower vertebrae, one of the patient's arms may be raised above the head (transaxillary view). No traction or arm movement

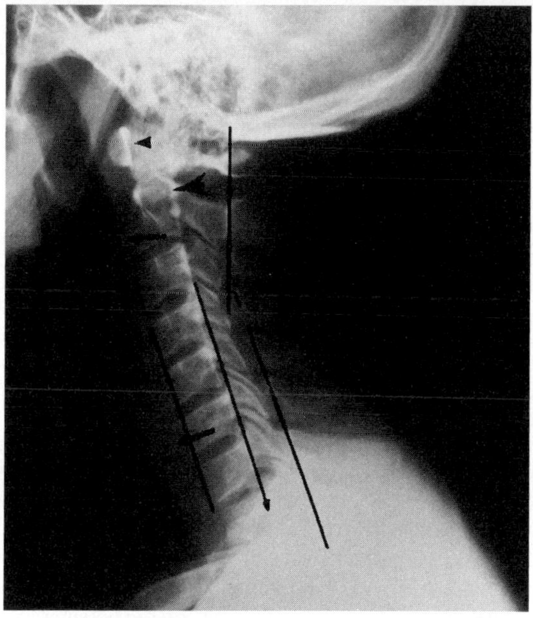

Fig. 23-1 Lateral view of normal cervical spine. Predental space *(arrowhead)*. Harris' ring *(barbed arrow)*. Prevertebral soft tissues *(arrows)*. Posterior cervical line, anterior and posterior body lines, spinolaminar lines *(long arrows)*. (Courtesy Michael Zucker, MD, Los Angeles.)

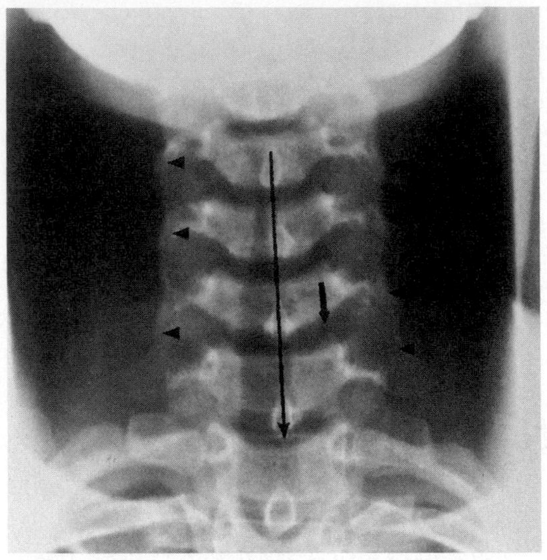

Fig. 23-2 Anteroposterior view of normal cervical spine. Lateral masses *(arrowheads)*. Spinous processes are aligned *(line)*. (Courtesy Michael Zucker, MD, Los Angeles.)

should be ordered, however, in the setting of neurologic abnormalities.

- CT scan is indicated to: (1) evaluate a fracture or suspicious finding seen on plain films; (2) search for a fracture when plain films are normal but clinical suspicion for fracture is high (neurologic signs or symptoms or persistent pain); (3) evaluate areas of the cervical spine not adequately visualized on plain x-rays.
- Oblique views may assist in diagnosing facet dislocation (Figs. 23-8 and 23-9).

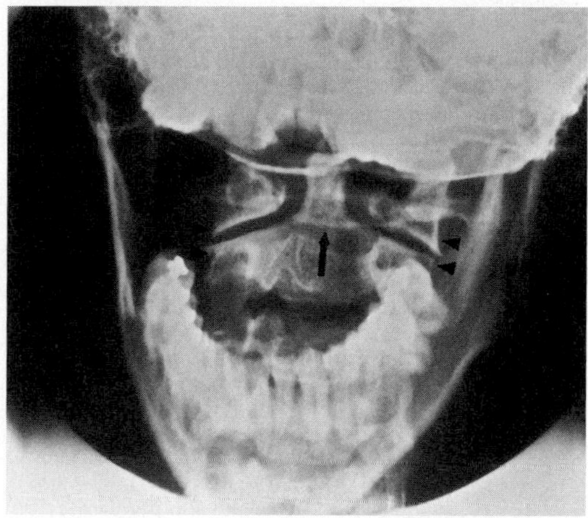

Fig. 23-3 Open-mouth odontoid view of normal cervical spine. Lateral masses C1-2 are aligned *(arrowheads)*. Dens is unremarkable *(arrow)*. (Courtesy Michael Zucker, MD, Los Angeles.)

Rule out ligamentous injury

- Flexion-extension views of cervical spine. Consider flexion-extension x-rays (after obtaining a three-view cervical spine series that is normal) in patients with persistent neck pain, a normal sensorium and no distracting injury to evaluate for ligamentous stability. Patients initiate active flexion and extension (never assisted by others) and should not flex nor extend past a point where pain is felt. Flexion-extension x-rays may not definitively rule out ligamentous injury.
- MRI is less sensitive than CT for the evaluation of fractures; however, it is superior to flexion-extension films in demonstrating ligamentous injury, spinal cord injury, and intervertebral disc herniation.

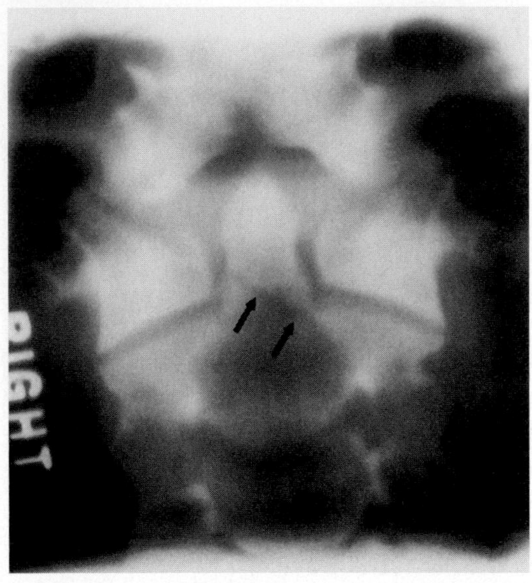

Fig. 23-4 Anteroposterior tomogram of dens fracture, type II. Oblique fracture at base of dens *(arrows).* (Courtesy Michael Zucker, MD, Los Angeles.)

Comments and Treatment Considerations

Cervical spine precautions must be observed until a fracture or ligamentous injury has been reliably excluded. If neck pain persists in neurologically normal patients after a negative cervical spine evaluation, patients should be discharged with a hard collar (e.g., Philadelphia collar) in place. These patients require orthopedic or neurosurgical follow-up.

Controversy exists over whether cervical spine fractures can reliably be excluded by clinical examination alone. Case reports of "occult" cervical spine injuries occurring in asymptomatic patients have been published, although whether the injuries were truly occult is debatable. Proposed guidelines for

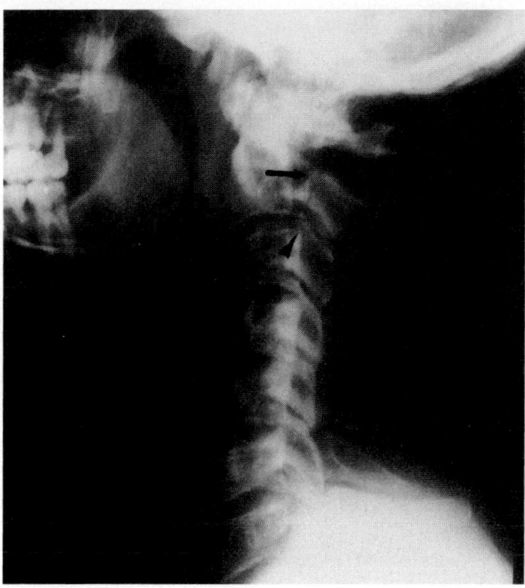

Fig. 23-5 Lateral view of pars fracture of C2 (hangman's fracture) *(arrow)*. Mild subluxation *(arrowhead)*. (Courtesy Michael Zucker, MD, Los Angeles.)

ruling out cervical spines in awake, alert, nonintoxicated patients without midline neck pain or bony cervical spine tenderness are currently being evaluated.

Cervical spine fractures in children are uncommon. However, because of the higher incidence of subluxation and spinal cord injury without radiographic abnormality (SCIWORA) in children, careful neurologic assessment and aggressive imaging must be performed for all pediatric trauma patients who have a mechanism for or clinical evidence of neck injury. MRI should be considered after normal plain films or CT if suspicion for injury remains.

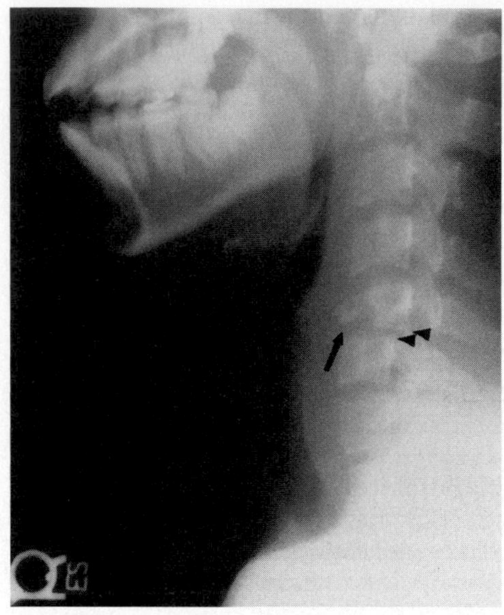

Fig. 23-6 Lateral view of hyperflexion tear drop fracture-dislocation of C5 *(arrow)*. Posterior subluxation of C5 and C6 *(arrowheads)*. (Courtesy Michael Zucker, MD, Los Angeles.)

The majority of cervical spine fractures occur at level C2 and C5-6. In the elderly, odontoid fractures predominate. However, any spinal column fracture, whether cervical or thoracolumbar, should heighten suspicion for other (often noncontiguous) spinal column fractures.

REFERENCES[www]

Hadley M, Zabramski J, Browner C, et al: Pediatric spinal trauma, *J Neurosurg* 68:18, 1988.

Hoffman J, Schriger D, Mower W, et al: Low-risk criteria for cervical-spine radiography in blunt trauma: a prospective study, *Ann Emerg Med* 21:1454, 1992.

[www]Additional references are available on the following web site: www.signsandsymptoms.com.

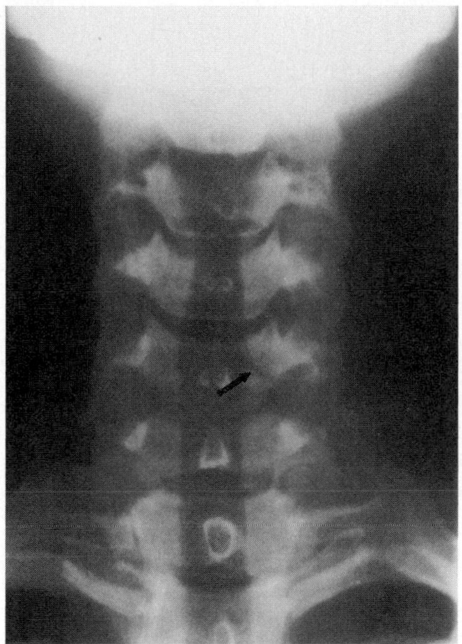

Fig. 23-7 Anteroposterior view of burst fracture of C6. Oblique fracture line *(arrow)*. (Courtesy Michael Zucker, MD, Los Angeles.)

Jacobs L, Schwartz R: Prospective analysis of acute cervical spine injury: a methodology to predict injury, *Ann Emerg Med* 15:44, 1986.

el-Khoury G, Kathol MH, Daniel W: Imaging of acute injuries of the cervical spine: value of plain radiography, CT, and MR imaging, *Am J Roentgenol* 164:43, 1995.

Ringenberg B, Fisher A, Urdaneta L, et al: Rational ordering of cervical spine radiographs following trauma, *Ann Emerg Med* 17:792, 1988.

Shaffer M, Doris P: Limitation of the cross table lateral view in detecting cervical spine injuries: a retrospective analysis, *Ann Emerg Med* 10:508, 1981.

Woodring J, Lee C: Limitations of cervical radiography in the evaluation of acute cervical trauma, *J Trauma* 34:32, 1993.

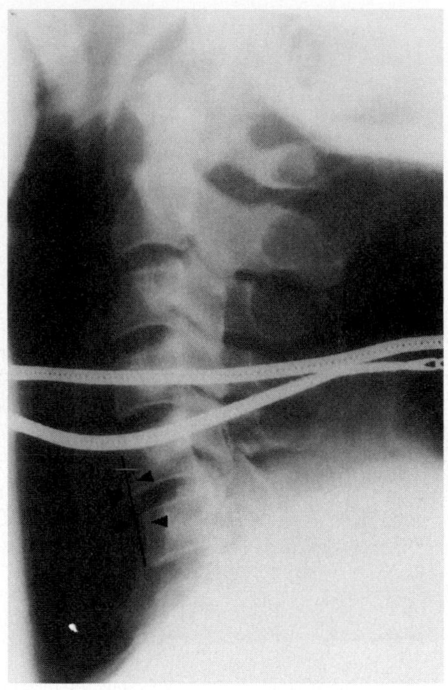

Fig. 23-8 Lateral view of unilateral interfacetal dislocation of C5-6. Subtle anterior subluxation of C5 on C6 *(arrowheads* and *line)*. (Courtesy Michael Zucker, MD, Los Angeles.)

MENINGITIS AND SUBARACHNOID HEMORRHAGE

Neck pain and stiffness due to inflammation of the meninges (meningismus) may indicate a true medical emergency requiring timely diagnosis and treatment.

See Chapter 15, Headache.

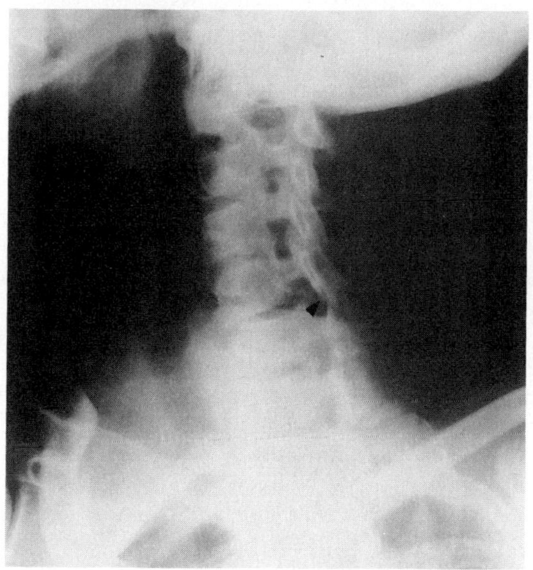

Fig. 23-9 Oblique view of unilateral interfacetal dislocation of C5-6. Facets are reversed *(arrowhead).* (Courtesy Michael Zucker, MD, Los Angeles.)

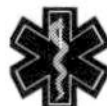

CERVICAL SPINE DISC HERNIATION

Symptoms

- Neck pain that may radiate to the scalp, shoulder, or down an extremity in a radicular pattern

Signs

- Weakness or sensory deficit of the upper extremities

- Fasciculations, loss of deep tendon reflexes, and atrophy of muscles in the affected nerve distribution have also been described.

Workup

- Cervical spine x-rays are usually negative in the investigation of possible disc herniation but may be helpful in ruling out other causes of neck pain.
- Flexion-extension x-rays can be used to evaluate for ligamentous instability if routine x-rays are normal.
- Oblique x-rays can indicate bony impingement of cervical nerve roots causing symptoms.
- MRI is the study of choice, although more costly and less readily available.

Comments and Treatment Considerations

Chronic disc disease may present as a slow progression of symptoms. Disc levels most commonly involved are C5-6 and C6-7. Conservative treatment with analgesics and a soft cervical collar are reasonable. Neurosurgical consultation should be obtained for significant neurologic symptoms or signs.

REFERENCES

Dillon W, Booth R, Cuckler J, et al: Cervical radiculopathy: a review, *Spine* 11:986, 1986.

Saal JS, Saal JA, Yurth EF: Nonoperative management of herniated cervical intervertebral disc with radiculopathy, *Spine* 21:1877, 1996.

Schimandle JH, Heller JG : Nonoperative treatment of degenerative cervical disk disease, *J South Orthop Assoc* 5:207, 1996.

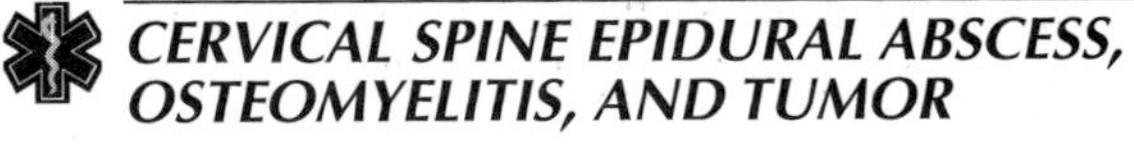

CERVICAL SPINE EPIDURAL ABSCESS, OSTEOMYELITIS, AND TUMOR

Neck pain and midline cervical spine tenderness not associated with trauma may indicate a serious pathologic condition.

See Chapter 4, Back Pain, Lower.

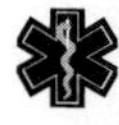

EPIGLOTTITIS, PERITONSILLAR/ RETROPHARYNGEAL/PARAPHARYNGEAL ABSCESSES, LUDWIG'S ANGINA

Anterior neck pain may suggest conditions that can lead to airway compromise.

See Chapter 30, Sore Throat.

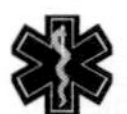

THYROIDITIS

See Chapter 24, Palpitation and Tachycardia.

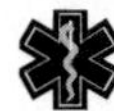

DYSTONIC REACTION

Neuroleptic agents, antiemetics (e.g., prochlorperazine [Compazine] or metoclopramide [Reglan]), and occasionally other agents can cause extrapyramidal side effects. Dystonia, akathisia, and akinesis may occur with phenothiazine use and are generally responsive to treatment; tardive dyskinesia occurs after longer-term neuroleptic therapy and is usually not reversible. Patients with dystonia are most likely to seek treatment in the ED because symptoms are acute in onset and severe. Dystonia may develop hours or days after drug exposure.

The diagnosis of dystonia should be entertained in patients currently taking a suspected medication (or those who have recently taken a single dose) and report a characteristic onset of muscle spasms of the neck or face. Patients should be specifically questioned about exposure to drugs that commonly cause dystonia. The presentation is often dramatic and, when suspected, is easily treated.

Symptoms

- Severe neck discomfort and stiffness
- Difficulty with speech

Signs

- Acute torticollis
- Elevation of the shoulder
- Upward deviation of the eyes (oculogyric crisis)
- Protrusion of tongue
- Arching of back (opisthotonos)

Workup

- Diagnosis is established by the findings of the drug history and physical examination.
- Laboratory tests are of no value for diagnosing dystonic reaction.

Comments and Treatment Considerations

Treatment with an anticholinergic agent such as diphenhydramine (adults: 50 mg IV preferred/IM; children: 1 to 2 mg/kg IV preferred/IM) or benztropine mesylate (adults: 1 to 2 mg IM; children [over 3 years only]: 0.02 to 0.05 mg/kg IM) is diagnostic and therapeutic when the typically rapid relief of symptoms occurs. Patients should be instructed to continue diphenhydramine or benztropine therapy for 3 or 4 days.

REFERENCES[www]

Corre KA, Niemann JT, Bessen HA: Extended therapy for acute dystonic reactions, *Ann Emerg Med* 13:194, 1984.

Lee A: Treatment of drug-induced dystonic reactions, *J Am Coll Emerg Physicians* 8:453, 1979.

McCormick MA, Manoguerra AS: Dystonic reactions. In Harwood-Nuss A, Linden CH, Luten RC, et al, editors: *The clinical practice of emergency medicine,* ed 2, Philadelphia, 1996, JB Lippincott..

Rodgers C: Extrapyramidal side effects of antiemetics presenting as psychiatric illness, *Gen Hosp Psych* 14:192, 1992.

[www]Additional references are available on the following web site: www.signsandsymptoms.com.

TETANUS

Characterized by severe generalized muscle rigidity and spasms, tetanus is an acute illness caused by the exotoxin tetanospasmin, which is secreted by the bacterium *Clostridium tetani. C. tetani,* an anaerobic gram-positive rod with vegetative and sporulated forms, is present in soil and feces worldwide. Tetanospasmin, a potent neurotoxin, diffuses into the nervous system, where it causes disinhibition of the autonomic and motor nervous systems. Although the incubation period can be as short as 1 day or as long as 1 month, symptoms usually develop over 2 to 5 days approximately 1 to 2 weeks after the initial injury. A shorter incubation period portends a more severe course. Although rare in the United States, tetanus causes an estimated 800,000 deaths per year worldwide, principally as a result of neonatal tetanus.

Tetanus should be considered particularly in older patients (women may not have been vaccinated because of lack of military service), those with recent wounds (contaminated, operative, or burns), and in intravenous drug users. In some cases, no history of skin break is noted.

Symptoms

- Jaw pain or tightness
- Neck or back pain or stiffness
- Dysphagia
- Extremity pain, especially in the wounded extremity
- Cranial nerve palsies +

Unless treated, symptoms progress from pain and stiffness to rigidity and violent convulsive spasms.

Signs

- Trismus
- Tetanic spasms, especially in the face (risus sardonicus) and back muscles (opisthotonus)
- Hypersympathetic autonomic disturbances: tachycardia, labile blood pressure, hyperpyrexia, dysrhythmias

Workup

- No diagnostic tests exist for tetanus. The diagnosis is made on clinical grounds.
- The site of infection should be sought.
- Diagnostic studies including a chest x-ray, ECG, CBC, electrolytes, calcium, BUN, creatinine, creatine kinase, and uri-

nalysis are usually performed in anticipation of intensive supportive care.

- An ABG is warranted if ventilatory failure is a concern.

Comments and Treatment Considerations

A reliable history of active immunization within the past 10 years makes the diagnosis very unlikely.

The early stages of tetanus may mimic dystonia or hypocalcemic tetany, whereas a more severe episode must be differentiated from strychnine poisoning. In contradistinction to tetanus, the jaw muscles are often spared in strychnine poisoning and rigidity is typically absent between spasms.

Treatment of tetanus consists of five components:

1. Aggressive supportive care including, in severe cases, intubation and paralysis to ensure adequate ventilation
2. Human tetanus immune globulin (TIG) to neutralize circulating and wound tetanospasmin
3. Treatment of muscle spasm with benzodiazepines in milder cases and with paralysis in severe cases
4. Antibiotics (penicillin 24 mu/day in divided doses; metronidazole 500 mg IV q6h may be preferable)
5. Wound debridement

All patients with suspected tetanus should be admitted to an ICU. The typical duration of illness is 4 to 6 weeks. Patients who have recovered from tetanus require active immunization because the disease does not confer immunity.

REFERENCES

Ahmadsyah I, Salim A: Treatment of tetanus: an open study to compare the efficacy of procaine penicillin and metronidazole, *Br Med J* 291:648, 1985.

Bleck TP: Tetanus: pathophysiology, management, and prophylaxis, *Dis Mon* 37:545, 1991.

Groleau G: Tetanus, *Emerg Med Clin North Am* 10:351, 1992.

Kefer MP: Tetanus, *Am J Emerg Med* 10:445, 1992.

CHAPTER 24

Palpitations and Tachycardia

MEL E. HERBERT and MARY L. LANCTOT

Palpitations are a common and frequently perplexing presenting complaint in emergency medicine. Patients ultimately may have a life-threatening disease, a benign rhythm disturbance, or simply "anxiety." Definitive diagnosis on initial presentation to the ED is uncommon. The ED physician must distinguish high-risk patients needing treatment or hospitalization from low-risk patients who can be evaluated in an outpatient setting. The sensation of a beating heart is normal in many situations. The normal contraction and movement of the heart is generally not felt at rest. A normal sinus tachycardia may be noted during exercise, high-stress situations, or after drug ingestion.

CAUSES

1. Arrhythmias (ultimately diagnosed in 45% of unselected patients): Almost any arrhythmia can cause palpitations; however, most arrhythmias are clinically silent. Sinus pause or extrasystole may be felt as a pounding in the chest. Paradoxically, patients with serious heart disease frequently have the most arrhythmias and the least sensation of palpitation.
2. High-output states: Patients with high-output states such as anemia, fever, hypoglycemia, or thyrotoxicosis may feel the compensatory sinus tachycardia associated with the underlying condition.
3. Drug ingestion: Many legal and illegal drugs can cause palpitations.
4. Caffeine: Coffee, various teas, and even sodas high in caffeine
5. Illicit drugs: Cocaine, amphetamines

6. Prescribed drugs: Epinephrine, aminophylline, and thyroid replacements
7. Anxiety (ultimately diagnosed in 30% of unselected cases): A common cause of palpitations but a risky diagnosis to make in the ED, since only after serious diseases have been excluded should this diagnosis be made.

SYMPTOMS

Although it remains good practice to determine the onset, timing, rate, and rhythm of the palpitations, the usefulness of many of these features is in doubt (Table 24-1).

1. Palpitations associated with the following suggest potentially serious cardiac disease and generally require hospital admission:
   a. Syncope or near-syncope. This suggests a hypoperfusion state caused by an arrhythmia, which usually is an indication for admission and monitoring, although results of inpatient workup are frequently negative.
   b. History of underlying ischemic heart disease. A history of prior myocardial infarction (MI) or congestive heart failure (CHF) is a serious risk factor for ventricular arrhythmias. All patients with this history and with palpitations should be admitted to the hospital to rule out ventricular tachycardia.
   c. Chest pain. A history of ischemic-sounding chest pain in association with palpitations is cause for concern. Tachycardia can be thought of as a cardiac stress test. Symptoms of cardiac ischemia suggest the patient has failed the stress test.
   d. Shortness of breath. This suggests possible transient pulmonary congestion of heart failure. Congestive heart failure in association with palpitations may suggest a serious arrhythmia or underlying heart disease.
2. Palpitations associated with the following suggest a potentially serious cardiac condition but may not require hospital admission:
   a. Sustained palpitations. Patients who have palpitations that last more than 5 minutes frequently have a cardiac cause of their symptoms.

Table 24-1 Patient History and Possible Arrhythmic Events

Historical Feature	Consider
Isolated skips or jumps	Dropped beats or extrasystole
Paroxysms of rapid palpitations that appear irregular	Atrial fibrillation Atrial flutter with variable block MAT
Paroxysms of rapid palpitations that appear regular	SVT or VT
On standing or change in posture	Postural hypotension
In women, associated with sweats, flushes, and so forth	Menopause

b. Irregular palpitations. Palpitations clearly described as irregular are strongly predictive of an underlying cardiac cause. Rapid irregular palpitations are usually episodes of atrial fibrillation.

SIGNS

- The physical examination is rarely helpful in patients with palpitations, as they have generally resolved. If palpitations occur during the examination, a rhythm strip should be obtained. A normal physical examination does not rule out a serious cause for the palpitation.
- Underlying signs of cardiac disease should be sought (e.g., cardiomegaly, signs of heart failure, and murmurs).
- Conditions that could cause a high-output state should be investigated (e.g., goiter from thyroid disease, anemia from GI bleed, and so forth).

WORKUP

1. ECG in currently symptomatic patients allows a diagnosis to be made in most cases. If present, an arrhythmia should be treated appropriately. If no arrhythmia is noted, this information can be used to reassure the patient, or as evidence for

an alternative, frequently psychiatric, diagnosis. Patients should be questioned about stress and suicidal or homicidal thoughts.

2. ECG in currently asymptomatic patients yields limited information. A completely normal, one-time ECG is consistent with a cardiac cause. However, ECG may show the following:
   a. *Evidence of old MI (pathologic Q waves).* Patients with ECG evidence of an old MI are at higher risk of ventricular arrhythmias.
   b. *Evidence of preexcitation.* The most common form of preexcitation is Wolff-Parkinson-White syndrome (WPW). The usual manifestations are a short PR interval and a delta wave. WPW is associated with a number of arrhythmias that can present as palpitations. (Fig. 24-1).
   c. *Long QT interval.* Prolongation of the QT interval is associated with ventricular arrhythmia and sudden death. Long QT syndrome may be congenital or the result of drug or electrolyte abnormalities. A simplified approach to determining if the QT interval is long is to divide the R-R interval in half. If the T wave lies past the midpoint of the R-R interval, then a long QT interval is present (for QTc calculation, see Appendix or www.signsandsymptoms.com).
   d. *Conduction blocks.* Although conduction blocks are common in patients without symptoms, their presence should suggest the possibility of an intermittent high-grade block that may cause palpitations.
3. Holter and event monitoring: Most ED patients require an event monitor (or Holter monitor), since generally an ECG cannot be obtained during symptoms. These tests are performed in the outpatient setting in low-risk patients. Event monitors are by far the more useful and cost-effective test. Approximately 30% of patients initially given a psychiatric diagnosis for their palpitations will have arrhythmias noted on subsequent investigation.

COMMENTS AND TREATMENT CONSIDERATIONS

Traditionally, all patients with syncope, near-syncope, pulmonary edema, or ischemic-sounding chest pain in association with pal-

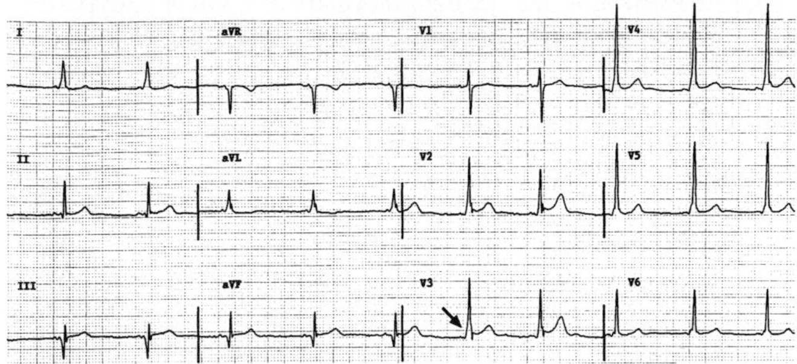

Fig. 24-1 Wolff-Parkinson-White syndrome. Note delta wave.

pitations have been admitted to the hospital. For many of these patients, unfortunately, the yield of inpatient evaluation is low.

Most discharged patients should have event monitoring performed to rule out cardiac arrhythmia as the cause of palpitations.

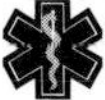

THYROTOXICOSIS AND THYROID STORM

Thyrotoxicosis and the more severe form—thyroid storm—are uncommon but important causes of palpitations. Symptoms and signs of mild thyrotoxicosis are those expected from catecholamine excess. Patients with mild symptoms require no immediate treatment or only symptomatic therapy in the ED. Undiagnosed or undertreated Graves' disease is the most common cause of thyrotoxicosis.

Thyroid storm is a medical emergency that may mimic or complicate other conditions such as sepsis, sympathomimetic intoxication, or drug withdrawal. Findings defining thyroid storm include the following:

- Elevated temperature +++++ (T >38.7° C, but may be as high as 41° C)
- CNS dysfunction ++++ (anxiety, emotional lability, delirium)
- Cardiovascular dysfunction

- Gastrointestinal dysfunction (nausea, vomiting, hyperdefecation or diarrhea, crampy abdominal pain)

Symptoms

- Anxiety
- Tremor
- Weakness
- Heat intolerance
- Weight loss
- Hyperdefecation
- Sweating
- Angina and CHF may be present in the absence of prior known heart disease and indicate either the unmasking of a previously existing condition or severe hyperthyroidism overtaxing a healthy heart.

Signs

- Sinus tachycardia is almost always present in thyrotoxicosis and serves as a marker of the severity of catecholamine excess.
- PACs and PVCs may be present.
- Atrial fibrillation ++
- Enlarged thyroid gland may be palpable or have bruit on physical examination.
- Proptosis and other eye findings indicative of Graves' disease
- Brisk reflexes

Workup

- Primarily a clinical diagnosis in the ED because the results of thyroid function tests (TFTs) are generally not immediately available. The differentiation between hyperthyroidism and thyroid storm is based on clinical judgment. Laboratory values for hyperthyroidism without storm and true storm overlap.
- TFTs are used to confirm the clinical diagnosis. In general, an elevated free T4 and a suppressed (unmeasurably low) TSH establishes the diagnosis.
- Glucose (may be elevated)
- ECG

Comments and Treatment Considerations

In most cases of mild thyrotoxicosis, patients can be referred for outpatient evaluation and treatment without ED therapy. In patients who are symptomatic but not acutely ill, beta-adrenergic blockade with propranolol (slow 1 mg IV bolus, may repeat) alone is generally adequate. Angina should be treated with a beta-blocker. The treatment of CHF with thyroid storm is controversial. Since the underlying precipitant is beta-agonist excess, beta-adrenergic blockade with propranolol or esmolol is the best approach.

Only the sickest patients (i.e., those with thyroid storm) need more specific treatment in the ED. Treatment of thyroid storm consists of five components:

1. Supportive care including cooling measures
2. Inhibition of thyroid hormone synthesis: propylthiouracil (PTU) 100 to 200 mg po tid
3. Inhibition of thyroid hormone release: iodine (e.g., SSKI gtt 4 po tid); wait at least 1 hour after PTU administration.
4. Inhibition of peripheral conversion of T_4 to T_3: dexamethasone 2 mg IV or po q6h. PTU and propranolol have minor effects.
5. Blockade of peripheral thyroid hormone effects: beta-adrenergic blockade with propranolol. As an alternative, an esmolol drip can be considered.

It is also imperative to consider other processes as precipitants of thyroid storm or as the primary cause of the symptoms. These include infection, surgery, trauma, contrast studies, DKA/HHNKS, and emotional stress. Patients require ICU admission and consultation with an endocrinologist.

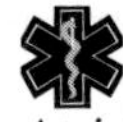

ATRIAL FIBRILLATION

Atrial fibrillation is a common cause of palpitations. Patients are frequently older but may be in their thirties or forties. Atrial fibrillation is one of the more benign causes of palpitations. In general, palpitations presumed to be ventricular in origin are considered far more serious. The search for the cause of the atrial fibrillation is generally more important than the disease itself, since it may be caused by a serious medical condition (e.g., MI, hypertension, pulmonary embolism, hyperthyroidism, alcohol withdrawal or use, hypertension, or valvular disease).

Symptoms

- Palpitations, irregular
- Chest pain, shortness of breath, if decompensated from the arrhythmia
- Syncope (rarely)
- Symptoms of the cause of the atrial fibrillation (see above)

Signs

- Rapid irregular heartbeat
- Peripheral pulse, heart one dissociation (i.e., more heartbeats heard than felt at the radial pulse)
- Signs of CHF, if decompensated
- Slow irregular heartbeat can occur if AV node disease
- No signs (between episodes)
- Signs of the underlying cause

Workup

- ECG is diagnostic and assists in evaluating for ischemia.
- Chest x-ray is used to evaluate for heart failure or evidence of valvular disease (calcified value or atrial hypertrophy).
- Outpatient event monitor may be placed in patients who are otherwise medically stable for discharge and with normal sinus rhythm but for whom there is a concern of paroxysmal atrial fibrillation or other arrhythmia.

Comments and Treatment Considerations

The goal of therapy for ED patients with rapid atrial fibrillation is rate control. In patients without evidence of end-organ compromise (e.g., no CHF or chest pain and stable blood pressure), rate control can be achieved with a number of agents (e.g., diltiazem 5 mg IVP administered q5min to a heart rate of approximately 90 and SBP >100, up to a total dose of 50 mg; diltiazem infusion can follow at 5 to 15 mg/hr; beta-blockers are another alternative.). Most patients should be anticoagulated (and/or evaluated for thrombus) before cardioversion because of the risk of embolization after return to a normal rhythm. Conversion to sinus rhythm is a secondary goal usually best performed as an inpatient service, as patients' symptoms may not correlate with the time of onset of atrial fibrillation and because of rare instances of clot preexistent to the current episode of atrial fibrillation.

Emergent ED cardioversion at 200J (increase as needed) should be reserved for unstable patients and is considered a form of rate control. It frequently is unsuccessful in patients with underlying heart disease.

REFERENCES[www]

Barsky AJ, Clearly PT, Barnett MC, et al: The accuracy of symptom reporting by patients complaining of palpitations, *Am J Med* 97:214, 1994.

Brugada P, Gursoy S, Brugada J, et al: Investigation of palpitations, *Lancet* 341:1254, 1993.

Kinlay S, Leitch JW, Neil A, et al: Cardiac event recorders yield more diagnoses and are more cost-effective than 48-hour Holter monitoring in patients with palpitations: a controlled clinical trial, *Ann Intern Med* 124:16, 1996.

Lochen ML, Snaprud T, Zhang W, et al: Arrhythmias in subjects with and without a history of palpitations: the Tromso study, *Eur Heart J* 15:345, 1994.

Zimetbaum P, Josephson M: Current concepts: evaluation of patients with palpitations, *N Engl J Med* 19:338, 1998.

[www]Additional references are available on the following web site: www.signsandsymptoms.com.

CHAPTER 25

Rash

PAMELA DYNE, JOLIE HALL PFAHLER, and JONATHAN EDLOW

The evaluation and treatment of a patient with a chief complaint of rash can be very intimidating, since, to the uninitiated, all rashes look alike. However, only four principal categories of rashes exist: (1) erythematous and maculopapular, (2) petechial and purpuric, (3) vesiculobullous, and (4) urticarial. From an emergency physician's perspective, a rash is generally only one component of a constellation of signs and symptoms that can be brought together to establish a definitive diagnosis. Although most illnesses with an associated rash are not life threatening, a few emergent conditions must be understood and recognized readily.

TERMINOLOGY

Macule: flat, nonpalpable discoloration <1 cm
Patch: flat, nonpalpable discoloration >1 cm
Papule: solid, raised, palpable lesion < 1 cm
Nodule: rounded, raised, palpable lesion >1 cm
Plaque: flat-topped, raised, palpable lesion <1.5 cm
Maculopapular: flat or raised red, pink, or tan discoloration of varying sizes and textures
Vesicle: well-circumscribed, fluid-filled, raised lesion < 1 cm
Bullae: well-circumscribed, fluid-filled, raised lesion >1 cm
Pustule: well-circumscribed, pus-filled, raised lesion
Wheal: pink, raised, usually pruritic, transient lesion
Purpura: blue-to-purple lesion, secondary to hemorrhage into the skin, usually nonblanching
Petechia: round, pinpoint, flat purplish spot caused by intradermal or subdermal hemorrhage

ERYTHEMATOUS AND MACULOPAPULAR RASHES

ERYTHEMA MULTIFORME AND STEVENS-JOHNSON SYNDROME

Erythema multiforme (EM) and Stevens-Johnson (SJ) syndrome constitute two ends of a spectrum of the same disease. EM is the mild form; SJ is the more severe, potentially fatal form. In patients who have Stevens-Johnson syndrome, the skin eruption generally involves the mucous membranes. Patients appear clinically ill and may suffer from multisystem dysfunction. EM/SJ is usually the result of a hypersensitivity (allergic) reaction either to a medication or infection (*Mycoplasma pneumoniae* and herpes simplex most frequently), although a cause is not identified in half of the cases.

Symptoms

- SJ usually begins with a prodrome: upper respiratory tract infection, fever, headache, malaise.
- Rash

Signs

- *EM:* rash usually begins as erythematous macules and papules, found symmetrically on the hands and feet. The rash spreads and evolves into the classic target-appearing lesions (dark center with a lighter outside ring) (Fig. 25-1).
- *SJ:* erythematous blisters are also seen on the mucous membranes of the eyes, mouth, and genitalia. The lesions may progress to bullae and then slough. The patient's lips may have a characteristic thick hemorrhagic crust.

Workup

The diagnosis is made clinically.

Comments and Treatment Considerations

In EM, topical corticosteroids can be used but should not be applied to eroded areas. The use of systemic steroids is controversial. A 3- to 5-day course probably provides some benefit with a limited risk of complications. Analgesics and antipruritics or antihistamines should be provided and follow-up with a dermatologist arranged.

Patients with SJ should generally be admitted to the hospital because their condition can rapidly deteriorate. Nutrition, analgesia, and other supportive care should be provided and fluid and electrolyte balance maintained. An ophthalmologist should be consulted for eye care. Sitz bath and whirlpool are used for wound care. Patients with severe symptoms may be best served in a burn center. Topical and systemic antibiotics are used for specific infections only.

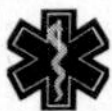

TOXIC EPIDERMAL NECROLYSIS

Toxic epidermal necrolysis (TEN) is a rare, life-threatening syndrome characterized by erythema and exfoliation of the skin. TEN is usually the result of a drug hypersensitivity reaction, although it may rarely be seen as a manifestation of graft-versus-host disease in a transplant recipient.

Symptoms

- 24- to 48-hour prodrome of high fever, headache, intense malaise, myalgias, arthralgias, diarrhea, vomiting, conjunctival irritation, and skin tenderness

Signs

- Lesions are usually a morbilliform ("sandpaper") eruption or diffuse macular erythema. The skin is often tender. The lesions can progress to form vesicles, which then coalesce and slough, leaving large denuded areas (Fig. 25-2).
- Mucous membranes are often involved, with erosions and sloughing occurring as well.
- Fingernails and toenails may slough or develop Beau's lines.

Workup

- Diagnosis is generally made clinically.
- Skin biopsy shows necrosis of the epidermis with detachment from the dermis.

Comments and Treatment Considerations

Treatment is similar to that for severe burns. Patients are admitted to an ICU or burn unit and are provided with aggressive intravenous hydration, nutritional support, infection control, and measures to stop the effects of the offending drug. The use of systemic corticosteroids is controversial. Antibiotic coverage for *Staphylococcus aureus* should be considered because the differential diagnosis includes staphylococcal scalded skin syndrome (see below).

Researchers disagree on whether TEN is related to EM and SJ.

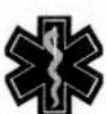

NECROTIZING FASCIITIS

Necrotizing fasciitis ("flesh-eating" bacteria) is an invasive soft tissue bacterial infection of the skin, often developing in patients who have had minor skin trauma (50% to 85%). The disease is also seen in immunocompromised and postoperative patients. If the area of infection involves the perineum, the disease is called Fournier's gangrene.

Symptoms

- Patients usually have severe pain in a localized area. This is the earliest and most consistent symptom.

Signs

- May be very minimal initially (i.e., pain is out of proportion to physical findings)
- Erythema and swelling without demarcated margins initially
- Rapidly evolves to include the development of reddish purple patches and then bullae
- Area becomes necrotic, edematous, and possibly crepitant
- Surrounding surface becomes involved as the infection spreads along the subcutaneous tissue and fascia.
- Fever is common as disease progresses.

Workup

- X-rays of the area involved may demonstrate subcutaneous gas, although they may be negative.

- Blood cultures
- Wound culture is required to determine bacterial etiology (*Streptococcus, Clostridium*, or polymicrobial).
- During surgical exploration, the surgical instrument easily passes through planes of fascia.

Comments and Treatment Considerations

This is a disease for which a high index of suspicion can be life- or limb-saving. Patients present along the continuum of disease, with those in the early stages showing only minimal local symptoms. This aggressive infection rapidly advances to involve contiguous areas, eventually causing generalized sepsis. Early diagnosis is made by a high level of concern for patients complaining of intense pain without significant physical findings.

Regardless of the severity of illness at presentation, this is a surgical emergency. The patient needs immediate wide surgical debridement along with antibiotic treatment. The antibiotic chosen should cover gram-negative and gram-positive organisms and anaerobes. Clindamycin 900 mg IV q8h plus Pen G 24 mu/day IV divided q4-6h and an aminoglycoside is reasonable first-line therapy. A penicillinase-resistant penicillin is added if a skin source is suspected. Patients in shock need to be treated, and supportive care is provided as necessary.

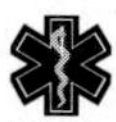

TOXIC SHOCK SYNDROME

Toxic shock syndrome (TSS) is a multisystem illness caused by an exotoxin usually produced by certain strains of *S. aureus*. The site of the S. *aureus* infection is often a tampon (85%), catheter, nasal packing, or other foreign body.

Symptoms

- Fever
- Chills
- Dizziness
- Myalgias

- Headache
- Red, nonpruritic rash that includes the palms and soles

Signs

- Diffuse, nonpruritic, blanching macular (or maculopapular or petechial) erythematous rash
- Patient may appear clinically ill with hypotension and other clinical signs of shock.
- Desquamation of skin (usually hands or feet) may occur by the second to fifth day.

Workup

- Culture: blood, urine, sites of potential foreign bodies (vagina, nares, and so forth)
- Laboratory evaluation for possible multiorgan dysfunction: CBC, platelet count, PT/PTT, electrolytes, liver function tests, urinalysis

Comments and Treatment Considerations

The offending foreign body needs to be sought and subsequently removed. Patients should be admitted to the hospital and the infection treated with beta-lactamase-resistant antistaphylococcal antibiotics. Patients in shock must be treated and given supportive care as needed.

A very similar illness also can be caused by a toxin-producing streptococcal infection.

STAPHYLOCOCCAL SCALDED SKIN SYNDROME

Staphylococcal scalded skin syndrome (SSSS) is an illness caused by an exfoliative exotoxin produced by certain strains of *S. aureus*. The primary infection (of the nose, conjunctiva, or umbilicus) is often clinically inapparent. SSSS usually occurs in children.

Symptoms

- Rash
- Fever

- Malaise
- Irritability

Signs

- Diffuse, tender, red rash, sometimes with a sandpaper texture initially
- Bullae and vesicles may appear over the course of a few days.
- Exfoliation of large sheets of epidermis, with a positive Nikolsky's sign (the skin sloughs easily if the examiner applies lateral pressure to the area) may follow (Fig. 25-3).

Workup

Definitive diagnosis is usually made by skin biopsy.

Comments and Treatment Considerations

Large volume losses may occur in these patients secondary to insensible losses without intact skin. Fluid resuscitation is initiated and electrolyte abnormalities corrected. Attempts should be made to identify the source of the staphylococcal infection. SSSS is treated with beta-lactamase-resistant anti-staphylococcal antibiotics (e.g., nafcillin 100 mg/kg/day divided q4-6h).

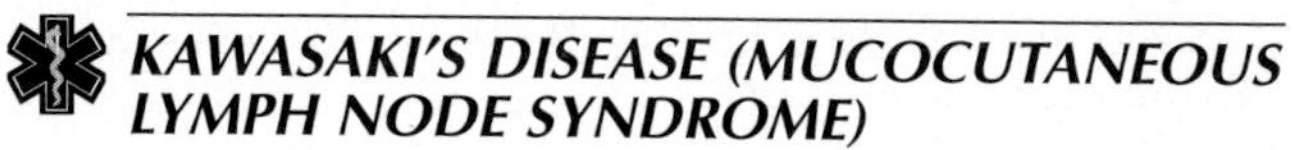

KAWASAKI'S DISEASE (MUCOCUTANEOUS LYMPH NODE SYNDROME)

Kawasaki's disease is an idiopathic disease of children less than 5 years of age. It is characterized by a systemic illness and usually has a cutaneous manifestation. To make the diagnosis, fever must be present for 5 or more days.

Symptoms

- Sore throat
- Headache
- Malaise
- Nausea, vomiting, diarrhea
- Rash

Signs

- The diagnosis is made when any four of the following physical findings are found: cervical lymphadenopathy, dry, fissured lips (Fig. 25-4), strawberry tongue, pharyngitis, peripheral edema or erythema, desquamation of the finger tips.
- The conjunctivae are usually injected but without exudate.
- Rash may be any nonvesicular rash, although usually is maculopapular. It commonly involves the perineum.

Workup

The diagnosis is made clinically based on the presence of the above signs and symptoms. However, these children need to be evaluated for the complications of this disease, namely cardiac abnormalities, which occur in 20% of cases. They require cardiac echocardiography at the time of diagnosis to evaluate for coronary artery aneurysm or pericardial effusions. Consultation with a pediatric cardiologist or a pediatric infectious disease specialist is recommended.

Comments and Treatment Considerations

Many patients need to be admitted for further evaluation and treatment. Intravenous immunoglobulin and oral salicylates, in addition to supportive measures, are suggested by most pediatric cardiologists, since these may decrease cardiac complications.

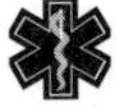

LYME DISEASE

Lyme disease is a multisystem infection caused by the bite of a tick infected with the spirochete *Borrelia burgdorferi*. Systemic dissemination can occur within days to weeks. The symptoms tend to occur in stages, somewhat arbitrarily divided into early localized, early disseminated, and late. Prompt diagnosis is crucial because early treatment is highly effective, whereas late disease is more difficult to eradicate. In addition to the symptoms and signs, the history of *possible* exposure to ticks is extremely important, as there is a history of tick bite in less than

30% of cases. In patients with later manifestations of Lyme disease, there may be a history of earlier manifestations (e.g., in a patient presenting with seventh nerve palsy, history of prior rash should be solicited).

Symptoms

Early localized disease

- Rash: solitary erythema migrans (EM, see below), which may be pruritic, painful, or neither ++++
- Flulike symptoms: fatigue, headache, fever, stiff neck

Early disseminated disease (may occur in various combinations)

- Rash: multiple EM
- Flulike illness with fevers, chills, fatigue
- Neurologic: facial weakness or paralysis, headache and stiff neck, painful or weak limb, dysesthesias
- Cardiac (more common in males): palpitation, dyspnea, syncope, chest pain
- Musculoskeletal: arthralgias, pain over muscles, tendons, and bursae
- Ocular (resulting from conjunctivitis, iritis, or keratitis): red eye, eye pain, blurred vision

Signs (may occur in various combinations)

Early localized disease

- EM: large (median size, 15 cm), red, usually flat, round, or oval eruption at the site of tick bite. Rash morphology can be variable. It is typically located at skin creases or thorax and appears 1 to 33 days after exposure, typically between 7 and 10 days (Fig. 25-5).

Early disseminated disease

- Fever with or without rash
- Cutaneous: multiple EM (secondary lesions are usually smaller and lack the central punctum)
- Neurologic: most commonly facial nerve palsy, which can be bilateral
- Cardiac: irregular pulse, cardiac rub or gallop

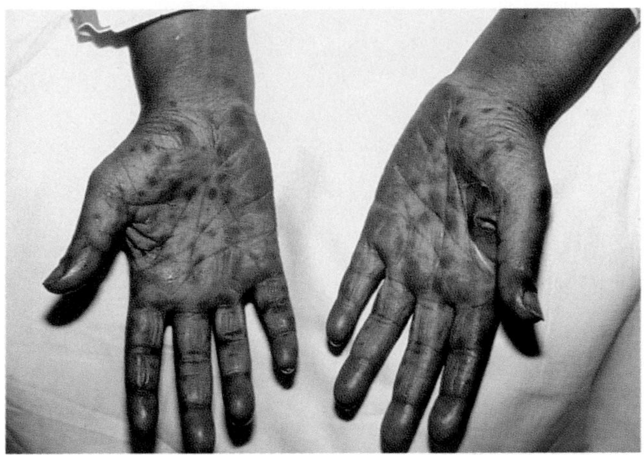

Fig. 25-1 Erythema multiforme. "Target" lesions on the palms. (Courtesy Anthony J. Mancini, MD, Chicago.)

- Ocular: conjunctival injection, corneal fluorescein uptake from keratitis, cells in the anterior chamber; rarely, disc edema and retinal changes from vasculitis or inflammation
- Musculoskeletal: frank synovitis occasionally found in this stage
- GI: rarely, hepatomegaly or splenomegaly

Workup

- In patients with typical EM, diagnosis is clinical. No testing (including serologic testing) is indicated.
- In patients with symptoms of early disseminated and late disease, Lyme serology is usually positive.
- In patients with isolated facial palsy, some practitioners recommend examining the cerebrospinal fluid for a pleocytosis, which, if present, argues for parenteral rather than oral therapy. Definitive data are lacking.
- ECG: in patients with cardiac symptoms or disseminated disease

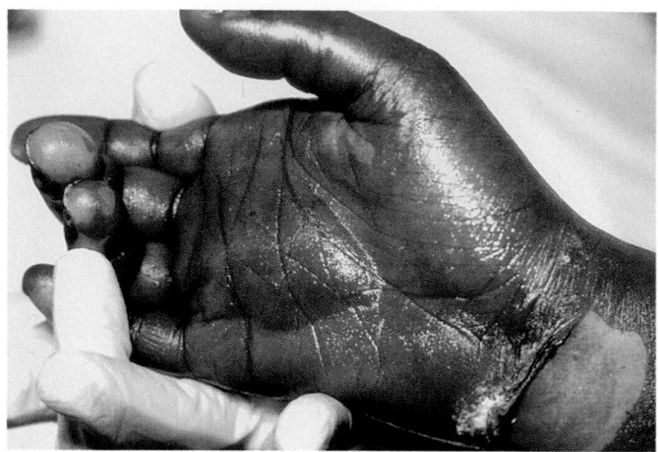

Fig. 25-2 Toxic epidermal necrolysis. Blisters and epidermal sloughing. (Courtesy Anthony J. Mancini, MD, Chicago.)

- Hepatic transaminases: in an atypical case, this may support the diagnosis (at least one LFT is elevated in +++ of cases of Lyme disease) and can also be a clue of ehrlichiosis.

Comments and Treatment Considerations

In patients with prominent flulike illness or atypical manifestations, co-infection with *Babesia microti* and human Ehrlichia pathogens should be considered. Treatment is as follows:

- Early localized disease: 21 days of oral doxycycline (100 mg bid), amoxicillin (500 mg tid), or cefuroxime axetil (500 mg bid). Doxycycline cannot be used in children under 9 years of age or in pregnant or lactating women; in others, it has the advantage of covering co-infected ehrlichiosis.
- Early disseminated disease: Without CSF pleocytosis or second- or third-degree heart block, treatment is same as for solitary EM. If either of the above is present, treat with

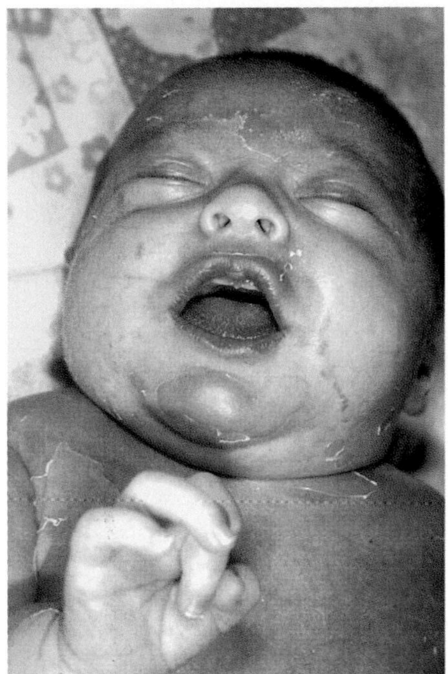

Fig. 25-3 Staphylococcal scalded skin syndrome. Epidermolysis in a 3-week-old infant. (Courtesy Anthony J. Mancini, MD, Chicago.)

ceftriaxone, 2 g/day IV for 2 to 4 weeks, depending on clinical variables and response to treatment (in children, ceftriaxone 75 mg/kg/day IV).

Follow-up by a primary care physician is important to confirm success of the treatment. Late disease, mainly arthritis (most commonly of the knee) and neurologic syndromes (most commonly encephalopathy and peripheral neuropathy), requires prompt referral for diagnosis and treatment.

REFERENCES[www]

Brenner BE, Vitullo M, Simon RR: Necrotizing fasciitis, *Ann Emerg Med* 11:384, 1982.

Edlow JA: The multiple faces of Lyme disease and other common tick-borne conditions, *Emerg Med Reports* 18:103, 1997.

Feder HM Jr, Whitaker DL: Misdiagnosis of erythema migrans, *Am J Med* 99:412, 1995.

Kotrappa KS, Bansal RS, Amin NM: Necrotizing fasciitis, *Am Fam Physician* 53:1691, 1996.

Magnarelli LA: Current status of laboratory testing for Lyme disease, *Am J Med* 98:10, 1995.

Nadelman RB, Wormser GP: Erythema migrans and early Lyme disease, *Am J Med* 98:15, 1995.

Strausbaugh LJ: Toxic shock syndrome: are you recognizing its changing presentations? *Postgrad Med* 94:107, 1993.

[www]Additional references are available on the following web site: www.signsandsymptoms.com.

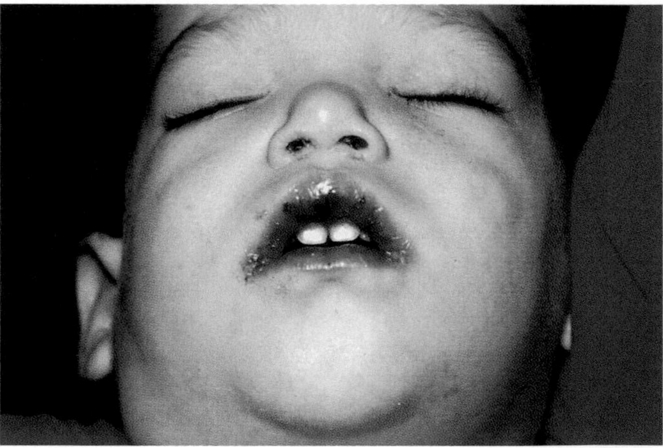

Fig. 25-4 Kawasaki's disease. Dry, fissured lips. (Courtesy Anthony J. Mancini, MD, Chicago.)

PETECHIAL AND PURPURIC RASHES

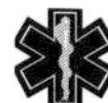

MENINGOCOCCEMIA

Meningococcemia is a disease caused by the gram-negative diplococci *Neisseria meningitidis* and usually is seen in young people (under 20 years old). This infection can cause pharyngitis, meningitis, sepsis, or a combination of CNS and systemic infection. Infection usually begins 3 to 4 days after exposure and can rapidly progress from very mild symptoms to death in a few hours.

Symptoms

- Rash
- Headache
- Fever
- Nausea
- Sore throat
- Vomiting
- Myalgias
- Arthralgias
- Stiff neck
- Confusion

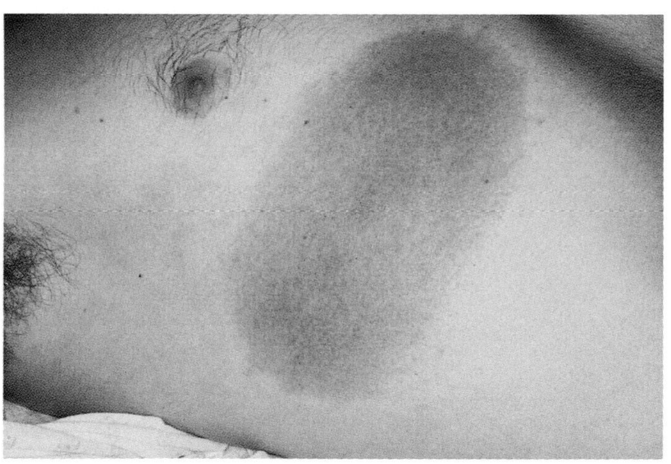

Fig. 25-5 Lyme disease, erythema migrans.

Signs

- Rash classically begins as petechiae (extremities, trunk, palms, soles, head, and mucous membranes).
- Petechiae develop into palpable purpura with gray necrotic centers (Fig. 25-6).
- Rash can also manifest as urticaria, hemorrhagic vesicles, macules, and maculopapules.
- Occasionally presentation as fulminant meningococcal disease characterized by shock, with petechial and ecchymotic areas ++. Purpura fulminans, a severe form of disseminated intravascular coagulation, may develop in these patients. Some affected ecchymotic areas become necrotic and gangrenous and must be amputated.

Workup

- Antibiotics must not be delayed for tests, including lumbar puncture.
- Diagnosis is often made clinically: an ill patient with rapidly progressive symptoms, a petechial rash, fever, headache, and altered mental status.

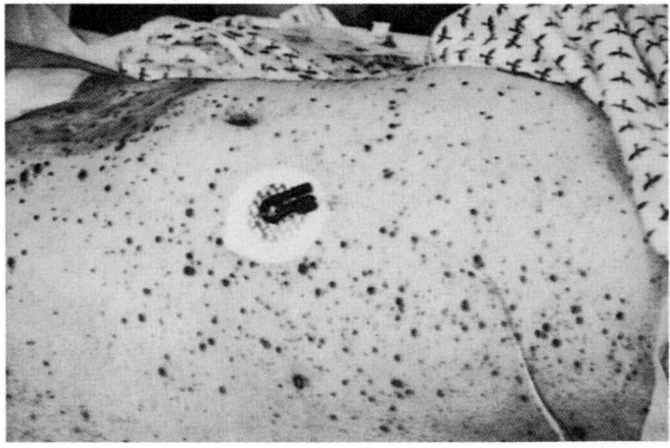

Fig. 25-6 Meningococcemia. Purpura and petechiae. (Courtesy Javier Gonzalez del Rey, MD.)

- Blood cultures
- Lumbar puncture
- Gram stain of the skin lesions

Comments and Treatment Considerations

Immediate treatment with a third-generation cephalosporin (e.g., ceftriaxone, adult: 2 g IV; child: 40 mg/kg IV) after rapidly obtaining blood cultures, if possible. Supportive care and hemodynamic stabilization are provided as needed in an intensive care unit with isolation from other patients. Once the diagnosis is confirmed, penicillin is the drug of choice.

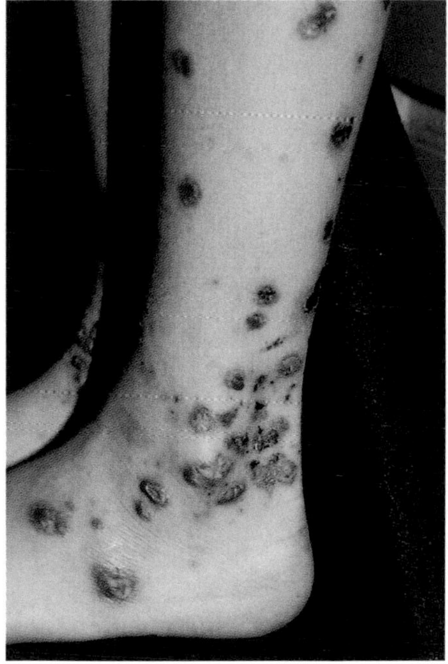

Fig. 25-7 Henoch-Schönlein purpura. Raised, palpable hemorrhagic lesions on a child's leg. (Courtesy Anthony J. Mancini, MD, Chicago.)

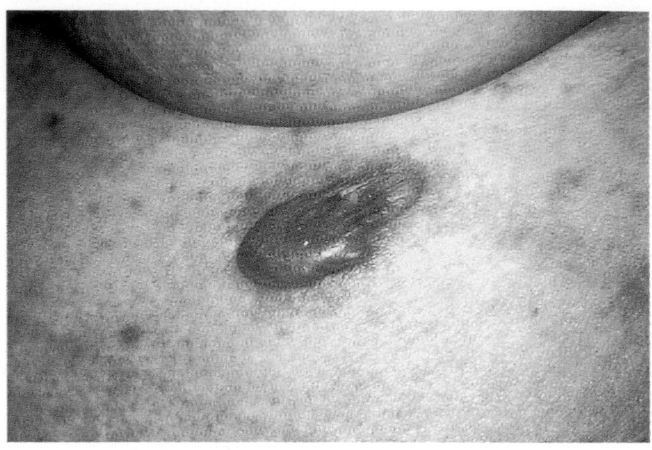

Fig. 25-8 Pemphigus vulgaris. Vesicle. (Courtesy Anthony J. Mancini, MD, Chicago.)

Patients should be placed in respiratory isolation. Since this is a very contagious and severe illness, individuals who have been in close proximity to the patient's oral secretions or have had prolonged exposure to the patient's respiratory secretions should be treated with antibiotics to help prevent subsequent contraction of the illness. The latest CDC recommendation for prophylaxis for those exposed to *N. meningitides* is a single dose of ciprofloxacin 500 mg po (do not give ciprofloxacin to children or pregnant women). An alternative is rifampin 600 mg po q12h for 2 days (children, 10 mg/kg/dose).

See Chapter 15, Headache.

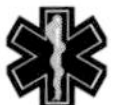

ROCKY MOUNTAIN SPOTTED FEVER

Rocky Mountain spotted fever (RMSF) is a multisystem disease caused by the parasite *Rickettsia rickettsii*. The parasite is usually transmitted through the bite of an infected wood or dog tick. However, 40% of patients do not recall being exposed to a tick at the time of diagnosis. RMSF must be suspected in a patient with possible tick exposure. A clinical triad of fever, headache, and myalgias is commonly present. There is a regional distribution of this disease to the central and southern Atlantic seaboard states and is most common in children.

Symptoms

- Common triad, usually presenting 1 week after tick bite: fever +++++, headache ++++, myalgias ++++
- Rash begins approximately 4 days after these symptoms begin ++++.
- Rash: palms and soles ++++
- Nausea and vomiting +++
- Abdominal pain +++
- Confusion ++
- Diarrhea ++
- Meningismus ++

Signs

- Rash commonly begins on the wrists and ankles and then spreads more centrally to the palms and soles, proximal extremities, trunk, and face.
- Rash consists of blanching macules or maculopapules, which evolve into diffuse petechiae over 2 to 4 days.
- Systemic signs develop if multiorgan (e.g., cardiovascular, renal) involvement.

Workup

- Diagnosis is usually clinical.
- Diagnosis can be confirmed with a rise in antibody titer after 10 days to 2 weeks or by immunofluorescent staining of skin biopsy.

Comments and Treatment Considerations

Doxycycline (100 mg po bid for 7 days or for 2 days after normal temperature; do not use in children and pregnant women) or chloramphenicol (50 mg/kg/day) should be used to treat RMSF. Remove any ticks and provide supportive care as needed. Without appropriate antibiotic treatment, there is a high rate of mortality due to complications, some of which include shock, congestive heart failure, renal insufficiency, meningitis, DIC, and hepatic dysfunction.

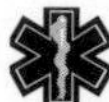

HENOCH-SCHÖNLEIN PURPURA

Henoch-Schönlein purpura (HSP) is an immune-mediated anaphylactoid reaction to bacterial or viral infection (especially beta-hemolytic streptococcus), drugs (penicillin, sulfonamides, and sedatives), and chemical toxins. It is idiopathic and causes vasculitis of the small vessels. It most commonly affects school-aged children.

Symptoms

- Migratory joint pain and swelling
- Colicky abdominal pain
- Rash on the lower extremities or dependent regions

Signs

- Physical findings of this illness are the result of showers of immune complexes throughout the body with resultant microhemorrhages at sites of deposition. The skin, joints, gut, and kidney are affected.
- Rash is purpuric with isolated petechiae at the ankles, lower extremity, and buttocks, along with edematous plaques, vesicles, and central necrosis (Fig. 25-7).

Workup

- Diagnosis is made clinically.
- Evaluation of the patient's renal function, urine, and CBC to evaluate for hematuria and proteinuria is indicated.

Comments and Treatment Considerations

Treatment is generally supportive only, with NSAIDs given as needed for arthralgias. Steroids may be indicated in some cases. Renal insufficiency, hypertension, and GI bleeding are complications.

REFERENCES

Brady WJ, DeBehnke D, Crosby DL: Dermatological emergencies, *Am J Emerg Med* 12:217, 1994.

Silber JL: Rocky Mountain spotted fever, *Clin Dermatol* 14:245, 1996.

VESICULOBULLOUS RASHES

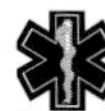

PEMPHIGUS VULGARIS

Pemphigus vulgaris (PV) is a blistering disease caused by the development of autoantibodies against epidermal intercellular material. PV usually affects the middle-aged and elderly. A genetic link may be associated with this disease, but other etiologic factors include drug associations or other autoimmune diseases.

Signs and Symptoms

- Blisters on erythematous skin (Fig. 25-8) and on mucous membranes with positive Nikolsky's sign (lateral stress to the skin causes exfoliation)
- Tremendous epidermal disruption is possible, resulting in large fluid and electrolyte disturbances, causing potentially serious illness.

Workup

- Skin biopsy: immunofluorescent and histopathologic studies

Comments and Treatment Considerations

Treatment initially consists of intravenous corticosteroids and aggressive supportive care. Adjunct immunosuppressive therapy may be added (cyclophosphamide [Cytoxan], azathioprine [Imuran], and similar drugs); antibiotics to cover skin flora may be considered. With current therapies and early diagnosis, the mortality rate is low.

REFERENCES

Becker BA, Gaspari AA: Pemphigus vulgaris and vegetans, *Dermatol Clin* 11:429, 1993.

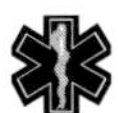

CHICKEN POX

Varicella zoster virus causes both chicken pox and herpes zoster (shingles). Chicken pox presents as a generalized viral infection with a typical skin eruption. The rash is initially maculopapular and becomes vesicular after several days. Chicken pox in adults, especially those who are pregnant or immunocompromised, can cause life-threatening pneumonitis or encephalitis. Intravenous acyclovir and varicella-zoster immunoglobulin (VZIG) have been shown to decrease mortality in immunocompromised patients. Routine use of oral acyclovir for treatment of children with chicken pox in is controversial.

REFERENCES

Fitzpatric TB, Johnson RA, Polano MK, et al: *Color atlas and synopsis of clinical dermatology,* ed 2, New York, 1994, McGraw-Hill.

Polis MA: Viral infections in emergency medicine. In Rosen P, Barkin RM, Hockberger RS, editors: *Emergency medicine: concepts and clinical practice,* ed 4, St Louis, 1998, Mosby.

URTICARIAL RASHES

There are many causes of urticarial rashes. Most of these rashes are the result of mild allergic reactions to skin or GI contacts. They are self-limited or respond to oral antihistamines (e.g., diphenhydramine 25 to 50 mg po q6h). More serious eruptions may require topical or oral steroid treatment. Patients who do not respond to this treatment and who are otherwise clinically well should be referred to a dermatologist for further evaluation.

Occasionally, allergic reactions are more serious and cause life-threatening respiratory or hemodynamic compromise. These patients require intravenous antihistamine, steroids, epinephrine, and possibly advanced airway management.

See Chapter 29, Shortness of Breath.

CHAPTER 26

Scrotal Pain

BRIAN MIURA

A patient who has acute scrotal pain must be evaluated promptly, since testicular torsion, one of the key diagnostic considerations, has a time-dependent testicular salvage rate (90% salvageable if detorsion occurs within 6 hours of pain onset; 20% salvageable if greater than 12 hours). Other diagnoses not to miss include strangulated inguinal hernia, Fournier's gangrene, appendicitis, and abdominal aortic aneurysm.

All patients with scrotal pain warrant an abdominal examination, and all patients with lower abdominal pain require a scrotal examination, since pain can often be referred and poorly localized. Testicular torsion, frequently misdiagnosed as epididymo-orchitis, should be the key diagnosis to entertain in any patient with unilateral testicular pain or tenderness. In patients with scrotal pain but a normal scrotal examination, referred causes of scrotal pain such as appendicitis and abdominal aortic aneurysm must be considered. Renal calculus can also cause scrotal pain, but is diagnosed only after determining that an emergent condition is not present.

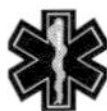

TESTICULAR TORSION VERSUS EPIDIDYMO-ORCHITIS (Table 26-1)

Patients with any of the following clinical features should be considered to have testicular torsion until proven otherwise:

1. Recent history of similar painful episodes resolving spontaneously
2. Sudden onset of testicular pain
3. Absent or diminished ipsilateral cremasteric reflex

Table 26-1 Signs and Symptoms of Testicular Torsion and Epididymo-orchitis

Signs and Symptoms	Testicular Torsion	Epididymo-orchitis
Age	Newborn to 20 years (80%)	Adolescent to adult
Risk factors	Prior orchiopexy	Sexually active, genitourinary anomalies, recent genitourinary instrumentation
Onset of pain	Sudden (90%)	Gradual
History of similar painful episodes	30%	Rare
History of trauma	Possible	Possible
Nausea or vomiting	30%	Rare
Dysuria	Rare	Common
Fever >101° F	Rare	30%
Tenderness, swelling	Testicle/global	Epididymis/global
Cremasteric reflex present	Substantial minority	Many
Testicle position (standing)	Usually high-riding and horizontal lie (50%)	Normal position and vertical lie
Contralateral testicle	Horizontal lie (if "bell clapper deformity")	Normal vertical lie
Pyuria (>10 WBC/hpf)	<10%	50%

4. Horizontal testicular lie of ipsilateral or contralateral testis
5. High-riding ipsilateral testicle
6. Absence of pyuria

In some patients it may not be possible to distinguish by history and physical examination between torsion and epididymo-orchitis.

Workup

- Immediate urologic evaluation is required when testicular torsion is suspected. A delay in urologic evaluation and repair while performing ancillary tests can lead to "castration by neglect."
- Color Doppler ultrasonography ++++ or nuclear scintigraphy ++++ should be performed in patients with an equivocal presentation and in all pediatric patients who are suspected of having epididymo-orchitis while awaiting the arrival of the urologist. Definitive operative treatment should not be delayed for testing. Color Doppler ultrasound is preferred over nuclear scintigraphy because it is noninvasive and provides information more expeditiously.
- Doppler ultrasound stethoscope +++ can be a quick bedside test (listen for arterial flow at the inferior pole of the testicle). Although insensitive, a diminished or absent testicular pulse as compared to the contralateral testicle strongly supports the diagnosis.

Comments and Treatment Considerations

No single clinical feature or diagnostic test can absolutely exclude testicular torsion. The diagnosis may be derived from the entire clinical picture. The diagnosis of epididymo-orchitis should be made hesitantly in a pediatric patient.

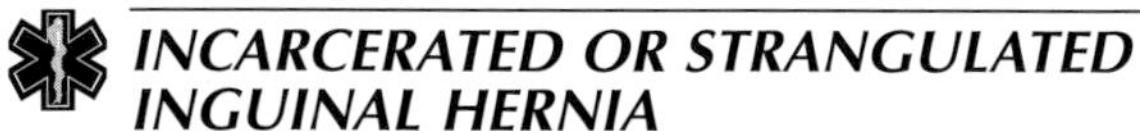

INCARCERATED OR STRANGULATED INGUINAL HERNIA

Incarcerated or strangulated inguinal hernias are typically noted as firm, tender masses in the inguinal canal or superior scrotum. The ipsilateral testicle and scrotum are normal. Nausea, vomiting, and other signs of bowel obstruction may develop. Tachycardia, low-grade fever, and toxic appearance are also common.

See Chapter 1, Abdominal Pain.

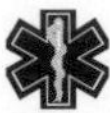

FOURNIER'S GANGRENE

Fournier's gangrene, a rapidly progressive scrotal infection from mixed bacterial flora, commonly occurs in diabetic or other immunocompromised patients between 50 to 70 years of age. Fever, toxic appearance, scrotal edema and erythema, focal necrotic areas, crepitus, and foul odor and discharge are some of the common features. This is a medical-surgical emergency and requires aggressive treatment.

See Chapter 25, Rash.

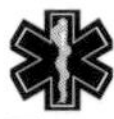

ABDOMINAL AORTIC ANEURYSM

Expanding or leaking abdominal aortic aneurysms (AAA) should be considered in older men with scrotal pain but with unimpressive findings on genital examination. Pain is usually severe and constant and may persist for weeks.

See Chapter 1, Abdominal Pain.

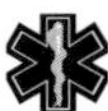

APPENDICITIS

Appendicitis is a referred cause of scrotal pain and should be considered in a patient with a normal genital examination. Patients may have fever, vomiting, anorexia, right lower abdominal tenderness, a positive iliopsoas or obturator sign, and hypoactive bowel sounds. Mild pyuria can be noted secondary to ureteral irritation from an adjacent retrocecal inflamed appendix.

See Chapter 1, Abdominal Pain.

REFERENCES[www]

Flanigan RC, DeKernion JB, Persky L: Acute scrotal pain and swelling in children: a surgical emergency, *Urology* 17:51, 1981.

[www]Additional references are available on the following web site: www.signsandsymptoms.com.

Haynes BE: Doppler ultrasound failure in testicular torsion, *Ann Emerg Med* 13:1103, 1984.

Lindsey D, Stanisic TH: Diagnosis and management of testicular torsion: pitfalls and perils, *Am J Emerg Med* 6:42, 1988.

McGee SR: Referred scrotal pain: case reports and review, *J Gen Intern Med* 8:694, 1993.

Melloul M: The value of radionuclide scrotal imaging in the diagnosis of acute testicular torsion, *Br J Urol* 76:628, 1995.

Patriquin HB, Yazbeck S, Trinh B, et al: Testicular torsion in infants and children: diagnosis with Doppler sonography, *Radiology* 188:781, 1993.

Petrack EM: Testicular torsion versus epididymitis: a diagnostic challenge, *Pediatr Emerg Care* 8:347, 1992.

Steinhardt GF, Boyarsky S, Mackey R: Testicular torsion: pitfalls of color Doppler sonography, *J Urol* 150:461, 1993.

CHAPTER 27

Seizure, Adult

MICHELLE KRUEGER

Seizures are a common complaint among patients seeking ED care. Chronic recurrent seizures with an established cause are usually not a major concern in the ED, since most patients with recurrent seizures require nothing more than (1) observation until the postictal state resolves and the patient's neurologic baseline is reached and (2) measurement of serum concentration (if available) of any anticonvulsants that the patient is known to be taking to help assess if dose adjustment is indicated.

The evaluation of a new-onset seizure is of greater concern because of the many disease processes that can cause seizures, as well as significant morbidity or mortality if not promptly diagnosed. Even in recurrent seizures, however, it is important to realize that new medical conditions can precipitate increased seizure activity. A directed search for an underlying cause is appropriate in patients with a dramatic increase in seizure activity (rather than a single seizure) or with clinical suspicion of another process (fever, persistent or new focal neurologic findings, shortness of breath, and so forth), as well as in those whose mental status and neurologic function fail to normalize within the first few hours.

Initial evaluation must include an assessment of airway, breathing, and circulation. Patients who are seizing on arrival to the ED should have an immediate check of glucose level and possibly administration of intravenous dextrose (consider pretreatment with thiamine 100 mg IV in appropriate patients). If intravenous access is unavailable and the patient is found to be hypoglycemic, glucagon 1 mg subcutaneously or intramuscularly may be administered. Diagnostic tests and subsequent treatment should be directed toward an identifiable cause of seizure that can be specifically treated. Whenever meningitis is a serious consideration, antibiotics should be given (after quickly obtaining blood cultures but before LP if a delay in obtaining CSF is anticipated). Emergent CT neuroimaging is warranted for patients who are at risk for a structural intracranial lesion. Many drugs and toxins can cause seizures, and administration of charcoal and specific antidotes should be considered.

Most nonhypoglycemic seizures cease spontaneously or respond to administration of a benzodiazepine (e.g., lorazepam [Ativan], children: 0.05 to 0.1 mg/kg, maximum of 4 mg; adults: 1 to 2 mg/min, maximum of 10 mg). In cases of status epilepticus, additional treatment is required. Phenytoin (Dilantin) may be given only intravenously (children: 20 mg/kg at 1 mg/kg/min; adults: 20 mg/kg at <50 mg/min). Fosphenytoin (Cerebyx) dosing (15 to 20 mg phenytoin equivalents per kilogram) is similar to phenytoin. It may be given intravenously at a rate of 100 to 150 phenytoin sodium equivalents/min or intramuscularly. If this is ineffective, phenobarbitol (20 mg/kg IV at 60 to 100 mg/min) may be administered. General anesthesia (or barbiturate coma) and subsequent EEG monitoring are necessary if these interventions are ineffective.

REFERENCES[www]

Turnbull TL, Vanden Hoek TL, Howes DS, Eisner RF: Utility of laboratory studies in the emergency department patient with a new-onset seizure, *Ann Emerg Med* 19:373, 1990.

[www]Additional references are available on the following web site: www.signsandsymptoms.com.

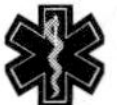

HYPOXIA

Adequacy of ventilation and oxygen saturation should be checked for all patients who are seizing. Hypoxia may be a cause of seizure or be caused by ventilatory insufficiency as a result of the seizure. Initial airway and ventilatory stabilization must take priority over ancillary testing.

See Chapter 29, Shortness of Breath.

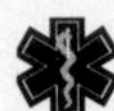

HYPONATREMIA

Hyponatremia is the cause of new-onset seizures in up to 5% of patients. The severity of the clinical manifestations of hyponatremia depends on the absolute reduction in serum sodium and the rapidity with which this reduction has occurred. Hyponatremia can be life threatening and requires laboratory testing for diagnosis. Hyponatremia is unlikely to be the cause of seizures until the sodium concentration is less than 120 mEq/L.

Symptoms

- Lethargy
- Confusion or agitation
- Headaches
- Nausea and vomiting
- Muscle cramps or generalized weakness
- Seizures

Signs

- Altered mentation: agitation, lethargy, and coma
- Seizures are usually generalized and may be refractory or recurrent.

Workup

- Serum sodium level confirms the diagnosis of hyponatremia.
- CT scan may be indicated to rule out a CNS process.

Comments and Treatment Considerations

If hyponatremia is present, a thorough investigation is necessary to identify its cause. Causes of hyponatremia include retention of water (SIADH, CHF, cirrhosis, and so on) and sodium losses (GI tract, skin, renal). Severe hyperglycemia, hypertriglyceridemia, and hyperproteinemia cause a pseudohyponatremia (measured sodium concentrations are low without actual hyponatremia), which does not cause seizure. Hyponatremic seizures are frequently refractory to standard anticonvulsant therapy and require serum sodium supplementation for seizure abatement. Controlled delivery of hypertonic saline is the treatment of choice. Careful attention to the rate in the rise of serum sodium is crucial to prevent central pontine myelinolysis.

REFERENCES[www]

American College of Emergency Physicians: Clinical policy for the initial approach to patients presenting with a chief complaint of seizure who are not in status epilepticus, *Ann Emerg Med* 29:706, 1997.

[www]Additional references are available on the following web site: www.signsandsymptoms.com.

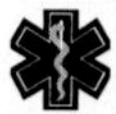

HYPERNATREMIA

Hypernatremia is a rare cause of new-onset seizures. Patients at risk for hypernatremia are generally debilitated individuals who do not control their own dietary intake. Patients with normal mentation and intact thirst mechanisms have an intense thirst response to even a slight increase in the serum sodium level (3 mEq/L) above baseline. This triggers water intake and a correction of the serum sodium. Seizures are usually generalized.

See Chapter 22, Mental Status Change and Coma.

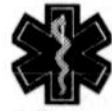

HYPOCALCEMIA

Hypocalcemia is the cause of new-onset seizures in up to 4% of patients. Most of these individuals have other signs of or risk factors for hypocalcemia (pancreatitis, renal failure, and thyroid surgery with hypoparathyroidism). Patients without risk factors or signs of hypocalcemia after seizure activity are very unlikely to have hypocalcemia as the cause of seizure and will not likely benefit from measurements of serum calcium levels.

Symptoms

- Anorexia
- Nausea and vomiting
- Fatigue
- Paresthesias (especially perioral)
- Muscle twitching
- Generalized weakness

Signs

- Tremor
- Muscular twitching
- Chvostek's sign: tapping over the facial nerve causes twitching of the mouth
- Trousseau's sign: carpal spasm induced by inflating the blood pressure cuff between the systolic and diastolic pressures and leaving it inflated for 3 minutes
- Tetany and hyperreflexia
- Altered mentation: delirium and hallucinations
- Seizures are usually generalized and may be recurrent or refractory.

Workup

- Ionized calcium should be measured in patients with seizures who have signs or symptoms of or risk factors for hypocalcemia. Hypocalcemia is defined as ionized calcium <2.0 mEq/L. Serious effects, however, are not usually seen until the level falls below 1.6 mEq/L.
- Electrolytes, magnesium, phosphorous, and creatinine
- ECG: a prolonged QT interval is characteristic of hypocalcemia.

Comments and Treatment Considerations

Patients with hypocalcemic seizures require parenteral calcium replacement with 10 ml of 10% calcium gluconate given slowly (over 10 to 20 minutes) and repeated until hypocalcemia is corrected and the seizures resolve.

REFERENCES[www]

American College of Emergency Physicians: Clinical policy for the initial approach to patients presenting with a chief complaint of seizure who are not in status epilepticus, *Ann Emerg Med* 22:875, 1993.

Aminoff MJ, Simon RP: Status epilepticus: causes, clinical features, and consequences in 98 patients, *Am J Med* 69:657, 1980.

Eisner RF, Turnbull TL, Howes DS, Gold IW: Efficacy of a "standard"

[www]Additional references are available on the following web site: www.signsandsymptoms.com.

seizure workup in the emergency department, *Ann Emerg Med* 15:33, 1986.

Petch CP: Hypoparathyroidism presenting with convulsions 27 years after thyroidectomy, *Lancet* 2:124, 1963.

Powers RD: Serum chemistry abnormalities in adult patients with seizures, *Ann Emerg Med* 14:416, 1985.

Rosenthal RH, Heim ML, Waeckerle JF: First time major motor seizures in an emergency department, *Ann Emerg Med* 9:242, 1980.

Wijdicks EFM, Sharbrough FW: New-onset seizures in critically ill patients, *Neurology* 43:1042, 1993.

Working Group on Status Epilepticus: Treatment of convulsive status epilepticus, *JAMA* 270:854, 1993.

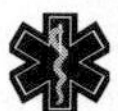

HYPOMAGNESEMIA

Hypomagnesemia accounts for <1% of new-onset seizures and is usually seen in patients who have many other risk factors for seizures. It is likely that seizures associated with hypomagnesemia are multifactorial. Experimentally induced hypomagnesemia in humans has failed to induce seizures.

See Chapter 22, Mental Status Change and Coma.

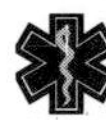

UREMIA

Seizures are usually a late manifestation of renal failure. Seizures can also be associated with the dialysis dysequilibrium syndrome (headache, nausea, muscle cramps, agitation, delirium, and convulsions), which usually occurs near the end of or just after a rapid dialysis or ultrafiltration procedure. Seizures generally respond well to conventional therapy. Many anticonvulsant drug dosages have to be adjusted in renal failure.

See Chapter 22, Mental Status Change and Coma.

REFERENCES[www]

Wijdicks EFM, Sharbrough FW: New-onset seizures in critically ill patients, *Neurology* 43:1042, 1993.

[www]Additional references are available on the following web site: www.signsandsymptoms.com.

HYPOGLYCEMIA

Hypoglycemic seizures generally occur in patients with a history of treatment for diabetes and do not resolve until the hypoglycemia is corrected. These patients present in status epilepticus until therapy is initiated. Patients with cirrhosis, alcoholism, sepsis, and malnutrition are also predisposed to hypoglycemia. In up to 10% of patients with hypoglycemia, seizure is the principal manifestation of hypoglycemia.

A finger-stick glucose is a rapid, safe, inexpensive screening test that should be performed for all patients with altered mental status or seizures. The treatment of hypoglycemic seizures consists of dextrose (consider thiamine 100 mg IV beforehand in appropriate patients), not standard anticonvulsants. If IV access is not available, glucagon 1 mg IM/SC may be given to transiently increase serum glucose levels. Careful serial examinations and a thorough search for the cause of the hypoglycemia are required.

See Chapter 22, Mental Status Change and Coma.

REFERENCES[www]

American College of Emergency Physicians: Clinical policy for the initial approach to patients presenting with a chief complaint of seizure who are not in status epilepticus, *Ann Emerg Med* 29:706, 1997.

Aminoff MJ, Simon RP: Status epilepticus: causes, clinical features, and consequences in 98 patients, *Am J Med* 69:657, 1980.

Baraff LJ, Schriger DL, Starkman S: Compliance with a standard for the emergency department management of epileptics who present after an uncomplicated convulsion, *Ann Emerg Med* 19:367, 1990.

Browning RG, Olson DW, Steven HA, Mateer JR: 50% dextrose: antidote or toxin? *Ann Emerg Med* 19:683, 1990.

Cahill GF, Soeldner JS: A non-editorial on non-hypoglycemia, *N Engl J Med* 291:905, 1974.

Carter WP Jr: Hypothermia: a sign of hypoglycemia, *J Am Coll Emerg Room Physicians* 5:594, 1976.

Inglefinger FJ: Debates on diabetes, *N Engl J Med* 296:1228, 1977.

Jones JL, Ray VG, Gough JE, et al: Determination of prehospital blood glucose: a prospective, controlled study, *J Emerg Med* 10:679, 1992.

[www]Additional references are available on the following web site: www.signsandsymptoms.com.

Merimee TJ, Tyson JE: Hypoglycemia in man: pathologic and physiologic variants, *Diabetes* 26:161, 1977.

Powers RD: Serum chemistry abnormalities in adult patients with seizures, *Ann Emerg Med* 14:416, 1985.

Rosenthal RH, Heim ML, Waeckerle JF: First time major motor seizures in an emergency department, *Ann Emerg Med* 9:242, 1980.

Wijdicks EFM, Sharbrough FW: New-onset seizures in critically ill patients, *Neurology* 43:1042, 1993.

Working Group on Status Epilepticus: Treatment of convulsive status epilepticus, *JAMA* 270:854, 1993.

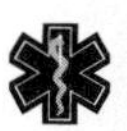

HYPERGLYCEMIA, DIABETIC KETOACIDOSIS, AND HYPEROSMOLAR HYPERGLYCEMIC NONKETOTIC SYNDROME (HHNKS)

Mild hyperglycemia (glucose <200 mg/dl) may occur after generalized seizures. Seizures attributable to hyperglycemia, however, usually occur in the setting of severe hyperglycemia and multiple metabolic abnormalities. The mechanism is thought to involve hyperosmolality. Hyperglycemia accounts for up to 4% of new-onset seizures. The majority of patients with seizures attributable to hyperglycemia have a history of diabetes; however, up to two thirds of patients with HHNKS do not have a history of diabetes.

The seizures associated with complicated hyperglycemia frequently do not respond to anticonvulsant therapy, and correction of the metabolic abnormalities including a reduction in serum glucose is required to terminate the seizures. The underlying cause (infection, myocardial infarction, stroke, or noncompliance) of the complicated hyperglycemia must be thoroughly investigated.

See Chapter 22, Mental Status Change and Coma.

REFERENCES

American College of Emergency Physicians: Clinical policy for the initial approach to patients presenting with a chief complaint of seizure who are not in status epilepticus *Ann Emerg Med* 22:875, 1993.

Aminoff MJ, Simon RP: Status epilepticus: causes, clinical features, and consequences in 98 patients, *Am J Med* 69:657, 1980.

Aquino A, Gabor AJ: Movement-induced seizures in non-ketotic hyperglycemia, *Neurology* 30:600, 1980.

Maccario M, Messis CP, Vastola EF: Focal seizures as a manifestation of hyperglycemia without ketoacidosis, *Neurology* 15:195, 1965.

Rosenthal RH, Heim ML, Waeckerle JF: First time major motor seizures in an emergency department, *Ann Emerg Med* 9:242, 1980.

Vastola EF, Maccario M, Homan R: Activation of epileptogenic foci by hyperosmolarity, *Neurology* 17:520, 1967.

Wijdicks EFM, Sharbrough FW: New-onset seizures in critically ill patients, *Neurology* 43:1042, 1993.

Working Group on Status Epilepticus: Treatment of convulsive status epilepticus, *JAMA* 270:854, 1993.

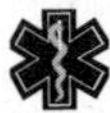

HYPOTHYROIDISM

Hypothyroidism is a rare cause of seizures in adults, and the seizures that have been reported occur in the presence of myxedema coma. Patients usually have a history of hypothyroidism and other manifestations of myxedema coma, although seizures may be the initial presentation in up to 25% of patients. The mortality from myxedema coma is greater than 50%.

See Chapter 22, Mental Status Change and Coma.

REFERENCES[www]

Catz B, Russell S: Myxedema, shock, and coma: seven survival cases, *Arch Intern Med* 108:407, 1961.

[www]Additional references are available on the following web site: www.signsandsymptoms.com.

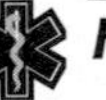

HYPERTHYROIDISM

Seizures attributable to hyperthyroidism are rare, are associated with thyrotoxicosis, and are limited to case reports in the literature.

REFERENCES[www]

Urbanic RC, Mazzaferri EL: Thyrotoxic crisis and myxedema coma, *Heart Lung* 7:435, 1978.

Waldstein SS, Slodki SJ, Kaganiec GI, et al: A clinical study of thyroid storm, *Ann Intern Med* 52:626, 1960.

[www]Additional references are available on the following web site: www.signsandsymptoms.com.

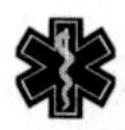

INTRACEREBRAL HEMORRHAGE, EPIDURAL HEMATOMAS, AND SUBDURAL HEMATOMAS

Intracranial hemorrhages account for about 2% of new-onset seizures, and subdural hematomas are the most common type of hemorrhage associated with seizures. The seizures may be focal or generalized, and status epilepticus is not uncommon. Seizures occur in up to 15% of patients with lobar parenchymal brain hemorrhages (secondary to tumors, arteriovenous malformations, hypertension, angiomas, and so forth), and 70% of these patients will have recurrent seizures. Patients with a significant head injury should receive prophylactic anticonvulsant therapy because seizures may worsen the outcome of the head injury.

See Chapter 15, Headache.

REFERENCES[www]

American College of Emergency Physicians: Clinical policy for the initial approach to patients presenting with a chief complaint of seizure who are not in status epilepticus, *Ann Emerg Med* 29:706, 1997.

American College of Emergency Physicians, American Academy of Neurology, American Association of Neurologic Surgeons, and the American Society of Neuroradiology: Practice parameter: neuroimaging in the emergency patient presenting with seizure (summary statement), *Ann Emerg Med* 27:114, 1996.

Aminoff MJ, Simon RP: Status epilepticus: causes, clinical features, and consequences in 98 patients, *Am J Med* 69:657, 1980.

[www]Additional references are available on the following web site: www.signsandsymptoms.com.

Horton JM: The immediate care of head injuries, *Anaesthesia* 30:212, 1975.

Javid M: Head injuries, *N Engl J Med* 291:890, 1974.

Lobato RD, Rivas JJ, Gomez PA, et al: Head-injured patients who talk and deteriorate into coma, *J Neurosurg* 75:256, 1991.

Ramirez-Lassepas M, Cipolle RJ, Morillo LR, Gumnit RJ: Value of computed tomographic scan in the evaluation of adult patients after their first seizure, *Ann Neurol* 15:536, 1984.

Ransohoff J, Fleischer A: Head injuries, *JAMA* 234:861, 1975.

Reinus WR, Wippold FJ, Erickson KK: Seizure patient selection for emergency computed tomography, *Ann Emerg Med* 22:1298, 1993.

Ropper AH, Davis KR: Lobar cerebral hemorrhages: acute clinical syndromes in 26 cases, *Ann Neurol* 8:141, 1980.

Stone JL, Rifai MH, Sugar O, et al: Subdural hematomas. I. Acute subdural hematoma: progress in definition, clinical pathology, and therapy, *Surg Neurol* 19:216, 1983.

Talalla A, Morin MA: Acute traumatic subdural hematoma: a review of 100 consecutive cases, *J Trauma* 11:771, 1971.

Weisberg LA: CT in intracranial hemorrhage, *Arch Neurol* 36:422, 1979.

Wijdicks EFM, Sharbrough FW: New-onset seizures in critically ill patients, *Neurology* 43:1042, 1993.

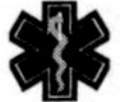

SUBARACHNOID HEMORRHAGE

Seizures occur in a significant minority of patients with subarachnoid hemorrhages, and approximately 60% occur near the time of hemorrhage. Up to 5% of adults with a new-onset seizure have a subarachnoid hemorrhage as the underlying cause.

See Chapter 15, Headache.

REFERENCES[www]

Eisner RF, Turnball TL, Howes DS, Gold IW: Efficacy of a "standard" seizure work-up in the emergency department, *Ann Emerg Med* 15:33, 1986.

Fontanarosa PB: Recognition of subarachnoid hemorrhage, *Ann Emerg Med* 18:1199, 1989.

[www]Additional references are available on the following web site: www.signsandsymptoms.com.

Mayberg MR, Batjer HH, Dacey R, et al: Guidelines for the management of aneurysmal subarachnoid hemorrhage, *Circulation* 90:2592, 1994.
Reinus WR, Wippold FJ, Erickson KK: Seizure patient selection for emergency computed tomography, *Ann Emerg Med* 22:1298, 1993.
van der Wee N, Rinkel GJ, Hasan D, et al: Detection of subarachnoid hemorrhage on early CT: is lumbar puncture still needed after a negative CT scan? *J Neurol Neurosurg Psychiatry* 58:357, 1995.

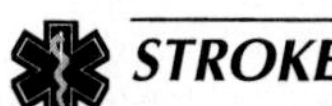

STROKE

Stroke is a common cause of a new-onset seizure in patients over the age of 50; up to 20% of new-onset seizures in adults may be caused by stroke. Conversely, seizure is the presenting symptom of a stroke in less than 7% of patients. Recurrent seizures occur in as many as one third of patients after a stroke.

See Chapter 36, Weakness and Fatigue.

REFERENCES[www]

American College of Emergency Physicians: Clinical policy for the initial approach to patients presenting with a chief complaint of seizure who are not in status epilepticus, *Ann Emerg Med* 29:706, 1997.
American College of Emergency Physicians, American Academy of Neurology, American Association of Neurologic Surgeons, and the American Society of Neuroradiology: Practice parameter: neuroimaging in the emergency patient presenting with seizure (summary statement), *Ann Emerg Med* 27:114, 1996.
Aminoff MJ, Simon RP: Status epilepticus: causes, clinical features, and consequences in 98 patients, *Am J Med* 69:657, 1980.
Berlin L: Significance of grand mal seizures developing in patients over 35 years of age, *JAMA* 152:794, 1953.
Cocito L, Favale E, Reni L: Epileptic seizures in cerebral arterial occlusive disease, *Stroke* 13:189, 1982.
Ettinger AB, Shinnar S: New-onset seizures in an elderly hospitalized population, *Neurology* 43:489, 1993.
Greenberg MK, Barsan WG, Starkman S: Neuroimaging in the emergency patient presenting with seizure, *Neurology* 47:26, 1996.

[www]Additional references are available on the following web site: www.signsandsymptoms.com.

Gupta SR, Naheedy MH, Elias D, Rubino FA: Postinfarction seizures: a clinical study, *Stroke* 19:1477, 1988.

Livingston S: Etiologic factors in adult convulsions, *N Engl J Med* 254:1211, 1956.

Luhdorf K, Jensen LK, Plesner AM: Etiology of seizures in the elderly, *Epilepsia* 27:458, 1986.

Reinus WR, Wippold FJ, Erickson KK: Seizure patient selection for emergency computed tomography, *Ann Emerg Med* 22:1298, 1993.

Rosenthal RH, Heim ML, Waeckerle JF: First time major motor seizures in an emergency department, *Ann Emerg Med* 9:242, 1980.

Wijdicks EFM, Sharbrough FW: New-onset seizures in critically ill patients, *Neurology* 43:1042, 1993.

Working Group on Status Epilepticus: Treatment of convulsive status epilepticus, *JAMA* 270:854, 1993.

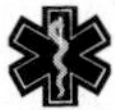

MENINGITIS AND ENCEPHALITIS

Central nervous system infections account for up to 4% of new-onset seizures and between 3% to 14% of cases of status epilepticus. Following generalized seizures or status epilepticus, patients commonly have a mild transient elevation in CSF white blood cell count. Nevertheless, patients with a mild CSF pleocytosis should be treated as if they have a CNS infection if there is any doubt.

See Chapter 15, Headache, and Chapter 22, Mental Status Change and Coma.

REFERENCES[www]

American College of Emergency Physicians: Clinical policy for the initial approach to patients presenting with a chief complaint of seizure who are not in status epilepticus, *Ann Emerg Med* 29:706, 1997.

American College of Emergency Physicians, American Academy of Neurology, American Association of Neurologic Surgeons, and the American Society of Neuroradiology: Practice parameter: neuroimaging in the emergency patient presenting with seizure (summary statement), *Ann Emerg Med* 27:114, 1996.

[www]Additional references are available on the following web site: www.signsandsymptoms.com.

Aminoff MJ, Simon RP: Status epilepticus: causes, clinical features, and consequences in 98 patients, *Am J Med* 69:657, 1980.

Barry E, Hauser WA: Antecedents, precipitants, and prognosis of patients with status epilepticus, *Epilepsia* 24:519, 1983.

Garvey G: Current concepts of bacterial infections of the central nervous system, *J Neurosurg* 59:735, 1983.

Hauser WA: Status epilepticus: epidemiologic considerations, *Neurology* 40(suppl 2):9, 1990.

Janz D: Conditions and causes of status epilepticus, *Epilepsia* 2:170, 1961.

Lothman E: The biochemical basis and pathophysiology of status epilepticus, *Neurology* 40(suppl 2):13, 1990.

Rosenthal RH, Heim ML, Waeckerle JF: First time major motor seizures in an emergency department, *Ann Emerg Med* 9:242, 1980.

Schmidley JW, Simon RP: Postictal pleocytosis, *Ann Neurol* 9:81, 1981.

Simon RP: Physiologic consequences of status epilepticus, *Epilepsia* 26(suppl 1):58, 1985.

Wijdicks EFM, Sharbrough FW: New-onset seizures in critically ill patients, *Neurology* 43:1042, 1993.

Working Group on Status Epilepticus: Treatment of convulsive status epilepticus, *JAMA* 270:854, 1993.

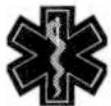

BACTERIAL BRAIN ABSCESSES

In most studies, brain abscesses account for less than 2% of new-onset seizures, although up to 50% of patients with brain abscesses have seizures during the course of their illness. Brain abscesses are frequently misdiagnosed on initial presentation because physical signs may be limited. The majority of patients are not correctly diagnosed within 10 days of symptom onset.

See Chapter 15, Headache.

REFERENCES[www]

American College of Emergency Physicians: Clinical policy for the initial approach to patients presenting with a chief complaint of seizure who are not in status epilepticus, *Ann Emerg Med* 29:706, 1997.

[www]Additional references are available on the following web site: www.signsandsymptoms.com.

American College of Emergency Physicians, American Academy of Neurology, American Association of Neurologic Surgeons, and the American Society of Neuroradiology: Practice parameter: neuroimaging in the emergency patient presenting with seizure (summary statement), *Ann Emerg Med* 27:114, 1996.

Reinus WR, Wippold FJ, Erickson KK: Seizure patient selection for emergency computed tomography, *Ann Emerg Med* 22:1298, 1993.

Rosenblum ML, Mampalam TJ, Pons VG: Controversies in the management of brain abscesses, *Clin Neurosurg* 33:603, 1986.

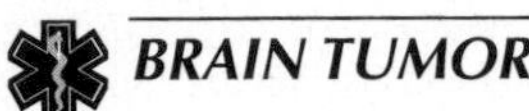

BRAIN TUMOR

See Chapter 15, Headache.

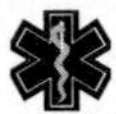

CYCLIC ANTIDEPRESSANT TOXICITY

Cyclic antidepressants (CAs) account for approximately 25% of drug-induced seizures, and 20% to 30% patients with significant CA overdose have seizures. Although CA-induced seizures can occur without cardiac toxicity, most CAs are major cardiotoxins, and patients with seizures frequently manifest serious cardiovascular toxicity as well. Risk of mortality is significant.

See Chapter 32, Toxic Ingestion, Approach to.

REFERENCES[www]

Boehnert MT, Lovejoy FH Jr: Value of the QRS duration versus the serum drug level in predicting seizures and ventricular arrhythmias after an acute overdose of tricyclic antidepressants, *N Engl J Med* 313:474, 1985.

Litovitz RL, Troutman WG: Amoxapine overdose: seizures and fatalities, *JAMA* 250:1069, 1983.

Niemann JT, Bessen HA, Rothstein RJ, Laks MM: Electrocardiographic criteria for tricyclic antidepressant cardiotoxicity, *Am J Cardiol* 57:1154, 1986.

Olson KR, Kearney TE, Dyer JE, et al: Seizures associated with poisoning and drug overdose, *Am J Emerg Med* 11:565, 1993.

[www]Additional references are available on the following web site: www.signsandsymptoms.com.

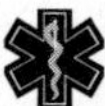

ISONIAZID TOXICITY

Isoniazid (INH) toxicity should be considered in any patient who has intractable seizures (typically associated with severe metabolic acidosis) and is unresponsive to standard antiepileptics. This is particularly true in patients from high-risk groups who are likely to have ready access to INH (e.g., AIDS patients, recent immigrants, Native Americans, homeless patients, and those patients who have tuberculosis or are living with someone who has tuberculosis). Empiric treatment with pyridoxine should be considered in such cases (see below).

Symptoms

- Anorexia
- Nausea and vomiting
- Dizziness
- Elevated temperature
- Altered mentation
- Slurred speech
- Photophobia and blurred vision
- Symptoms usually occur within 2 hours of ingestion.

Signs

- The classic triad of acute INH neurotoxicity is coma, metabolic acidosis, and refractory seizures.
- Hyperpyrexia, hyperreflexia, tachypnea, tachycardia, hypotension, and altered mental status are common.
- Other manifestations include nystagmus, mydriasis, ataxia, and cyanosis.
- Seizures are usually generalized tonic-clonic seizures.

Workup

- INH toxicity can be difficult to diagnose and commonly is identified after the multidrug-resistant seizures are terminated with pyridoxine.
- Glycosuria, hyperglycemia, and an anion-gap metabolic acidosis (mean pH ~7.05) are typical laboratory findings.
- Electrolytes, glucose, magnesium, and calcium should be

checked to identify other causes of seizure unless it is clear from the history that INH is the etiologic agent.
- An ECG and acetaminophen and aspirin levels should be obtained to screen for co-ingestants if an intentional overdose is suspected.
- Liver enzymes should be measured to screen for INH hepatotoxicity.

Comments and Treatment Considerations

All patients should be admitted to a monitored critical care area. Ingestion of 80 to 150 mg/kg usually results in severe seizures and a high mortality. Pyridoxine is the specific antidote for neurotoxicity after INH ingestion and can be dosed as 1 gram of pyridoxine per gram of INH ingested or a 5 g repeat dosing regimen if the amount ingested is unknown.

Since most patients become symptomatic and rapidly decline within 2 hours of ingestion, treatment must be rapid and aggressive. Rapid administration of activated charcoal with or without initial decontamination (i.e., lavage) is required. Alkalinization has been used to correct profound acidosis. Hemodialysis removes INH but is usually unnecessary because pyridoxine is a safe and effective antidote for INH toxicity.

REFERENCES[www]

Brent J, Vo N, Kulig K, Rumack BH: Reversal of prolonged isoniazid-induced coma by pyridoxine, *Arch Intern Med* 150:1751, 1990.

Olson KR, Kearney TE, Dyer JE, et al: Seizures associated with poisoning and drug overdose, *Am J Emerg Med* 11:565, 1993.

Roberts JR: Drug-induced seizure disorders: isoniazid, *Emerg Med News* 18:6, 1996.

[www]Additional references are available on the following web site: www.signsandsymptoms.com.

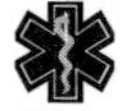

THEOPHYLLINE TOXICITY

Although theophylline use is decreasing as other therapies for asthma and emphysema are increasingly being recognized as more efficacious, it still remains one of the five leading causes of drug-induced seizures. Because of a narrow toxic-therapeutic ratio and multiple drug interactions, theophylline toxicity is common. Of those individuals taking theophylline, the incidence of toxicity has been reported to be as high as 20%. Theophylline toxicity can be acute, acute-on-chronic, or chronic. Seizures are more common with chronic toxicity. Seizures associated with theophylline can be prolonged and fatal. Mortality as high as 60% has been reported.

Symptoms

- GI: anorexia, nausea, vomiting, and abdominal pain
- Tremor
- Anxiety or agitation
- Palpitations
- The symptoms of a serious chronic overdose are frequently subtle and nonspecific and may lead to a missed diagnosis.

Signs

- Agitation, confusion, and tremor are common and frequently precede seizures.
- Seizures may be focal or generalized, are frequently refractory, and portend a very high risk of morbidity and mortality. Seizures can occur without concomitant gastrointestinal or cardiac toxicity.
- Other common signs of toxicity include tachycardia, cardiac arrhythmias, hypotension, and hyperventilation.

Workup

- In acute ingestions, the severity of the toxicity tends to correlate with the peak serum level. Serum levels, however, are less predictive of toxicity in acute-on-chronic or chronic exposures.
- Seizures may occur with therapeutic serum theophylline levels.
- Since theophylline has multiple sustained-released formulas and drug interactions, serum levels are of limited use in guiding the initial treatment and therapy.

- Serial levels measured 2 hours apart will show if a peak level has been reached.
- Electrolytes, glucose, and an ABG should be checked because these patients are usually acidotic, hypokalemic, and hypoglycemic. All these abnormalities must be corrected because they worsen the signs of theophylline toxicity.
- Consider obtaining baseline calcium, PT/PTT, platelets, and a CBC in the event that extracorporeal drug removal is necessary.

Comments and Treatment Considerations

All patients with suspected theophylline toxicity must have intravenous access and critical care monitoring. Theophylline is effectively eliminated with charcoal hemoperfusion (HP). Any seizure or cardiac event associated with theophylline toxicity should prompt the initiation of HP. Theophylline is eliminated somewhat less effectively with hemodialysis (HD), but HD is an acceptable alternative if HP is unavailable.

For less severe toxicity, multidose activated charcoal is the treatment of choice. The predictors of major toxicity vary depending on the type of overdose, with peak serum levels being the best predictor in acute overdose and age over 60 being the main predictor in chronic overmedication. Benzodiazepines and phenobarbital are the drugs of choice for treating theophylline-induced seizures, which may be difficult to control.

REFERENCES[www]

Chu NS: Caffeine- and aminophylline-induced seizures, *Epilepsia* 22:85, 1981.

Olson KR, Kearney TE, Dyer JE, et al: Seizures associated with poisoning and drug overdose, *Am J Emerg Med* 11:565, 1993.

Roberts JR: Drug-induced seizures: theophylline, *Emerg Med News* 19:4, 1997.

[www]Additional references are available on the following web site: www.signsandsymptoms.com.

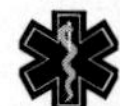

STIMULANT-INDUCED SEIZURES

Stimulants (including cocaine, amphetamines, phencyclidine, and ephedrine) account for approximately 30% of drug-induced seizures. As illicit and prescription stimulants continue to become more widely used, seizures associated with these substances continue to increase in frequency. Stimulants are more likely than other drugs to produce brief, self-limited seizures. Cocaine is the most common stimulant that produces seizures. Other stimulant medications present in a similar manner to cocaine intoxication. Other forms of cocaine-induced neurotoxicity include subarachnoid hemorrhage, cerebral infarction, vasculitis, TIAs, and toxic delirium. Many of these can be complicated by seizures (e.g., subarachnoid hemorrhage), and therefore a complete investigation is required.

See Chapter 32, Toxic Ingestion, Approach to.

REFERENCES[www]

Choy-Kwong M, Lipton RB: Seizures in hospitalized cocaine users, *Neurology* 39:425, 1989.

Ernst AA, Sanders WM: Unexpected cocaine intoxication presenting as seizures in children, *Ann Emerg Med* 18:774, 1989.

Hart JB, Wallace J: The adverse effects of amphetamines, *Clin Toxicol* 8:179, 1975.

Jerrard DA: "Designer drugs" —a current perspective, *J Emerg Med* 8:733, 1990.

Kaye BR, Fainstat M: Cerebral vasculitis associated with cocaine abuse, *JAMA* 258:2104, 1987.

Levine SR, Brust JCM, Futrell N, et al: Cerebrovascular complications of the use of the "crack" form of alkaloidal cocaine, *N Engl J Med* 323:699, 1990.

Mody CK, Miller BL, McIntyre HB, et al: Neurologic complications of cocaine abuse, *Neurology* 38:1189, 1988.

Olson KR, Kearney TE, Dyer JE, et al: Seizures associated with poisoning and drug overdose, *Am J Emerg Med* 11:565, 1993.

Roberts JR: Cocaine-related seizures, *Emerg Med News* 19:8, 1997.

Roberts JR: Drug-induced seizures: round up the usual suspects, *Emerg Med News* 19:9, 1997.

[www]Additional references are available on the following web site: www.signsandsymptoms.com.

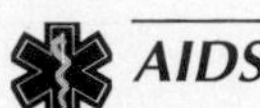

AIDS

HIV must be considered as a diagnostic possibility in any patient with a new-onset seizure. CNS disease is seen in most AIDS patients during the course of their illness. In 10% to 20% of AIDS patients, CNS disease is the initial manifestation of AIDS. Up to 50% of AIDS patients with seizures have no specific CNS lesion identified, and the seizure is presumed to be caused by HIV infection. Secondary causes of seizures include toxoplasmosis, cryptococcal meningitis, herpes encephalitis, syphilis, lymphoma, and tuberculosis. Toxoplasmosis is the most common opportunistic infection that causes seizures in AIDS patients.

Symptoms

- The most common CNS symptoms in HIV-positive patients are seizures, altered mentation, headache, or neuropathy.

Signs

- The examination can range from normal to very abnormal.
- Patients with AIDS-related seizures often have other signs of AIDS (thrush, wasting, Kaposi's lesions, and so forth).
- Most patients with a secondary CNS infection as the cause of seizure have a focal neurologic examination.

Workup

- A CT scan with and without contrast (or MRI if available) is the initial test.
- If the CT scan is normal, a lumbar puncture is required. Fluid should be sent for routine testing, as well as for the following: VDRL, AFB, India ink, cryptococcal antigen, herpes PCR, fungal cultures, and viral cultures. Opening and closing pressures are crucial because these may be the only abnormalities in early cryptococcal meningitis. Coccidioidomycosis titers and toxoplasmosis and cryptococcal antigens should also be obtained.

Comments and Treatment Considerations

Seizures can usually be controlled with intravenous benzodiazepines. Intravenous phenytoin or barbiturates are useful for prolonged, refractory, or repeated seizures.

REFERENCES[www]

Berger JR, Moskowitz L, Fischl M, et al: The neurologic complications of AIDS: frequently the initial manifestation, *Neurology* 34(suppl 1):134, 1984.

Goldschmidt RH, Dong BJ: Current report—HIV treatment of AIDS and HIV-related conditions, *J Am Board Fam Pract* 7:155, 1994.

Hollander H: Cerebrospinal fluid abnormalities and abnormalities in individuals infected with human immunodeficiency virus, *J Infect Dis* 158:855, 1988.

McArthur JW: Neurologic manifestations of AIDS, *Medicine* 66:407, 1987.

Wong MC, Suite NDA, Labar DR: Seizures in HIV infection, *Neurology* 39(suppl):428, 1989.

Wong MC, Suite NDA, Labar DR: Seizures in human immunodeficiency virus infection, *Arch Neurol* 47:640, 1990.

[www]Additional references are available on the following web site: www.signsandsymptoms.com.

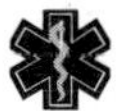

ECLAMPSIA AND PREGNANCY-RELATED SEIZURES

The most common cause of seizures in pregnancy is idiopathic epilepsy. Approximately 0.5% of women of childbearing age have epilepsy. Between 20% to 40% of women have an increase in seizure frequency when they become pregnant. Fewer than 15% of women with their first seizure in pregnancy have gestational seizures; the remaining have idiopathic epilepsy.

Although other conditions must be considered, eclampsia is the likely cause of seizures in pregnant patients with preeclampsia who have a new onset of seizures in their third trimester or in the early postpartum period. Eclampsia is rare (<1% incidence) in the United States, but has a maternal mortality rate above 10%. The hallmark of preeclampsia, which is more common, is (relative) hypertension with proteinuria or edema. Risk factors for eclampsia include chronic hypertension, nulliparity, a family history of eclampsia, multiple gestations, molar pregnancies, diabetes, extremes of age, and fetal hydrops. Seizures before the third trimester or more than 48 hours postpartum are far less likely to be due to eclampsia. Seizures in pregnant women also can be caused by the same conditions found in nonpregnant patients.

Comments and Treatment Considerations

Eclampsia should be considered in any pregnant woman who has seizures and is past 20 weeks' gestation. Obstetric consultation should be obtained immediately, since delivery of the fetus is the definitive therapy.

Aggressive seizure control with magnesium (4 g IV over 10 to 20 minutes followed by 2 g/1 hr) and standard measures such as benzodiazepine administration (if needed) are indicated. Deep tendon reflexes (DTRs) should be monitored, as a loss of reflexes generally precedes ventilatory arrest caused by hypermagnesemia. Antidote for hypermagnesemia is 10 to 20 ml of calcium gluconate 10% solution IV. Hypertension is often initially treated with hydralazine 5 to 10 mg IV (may repeat).

See Preeclampsia and Eclampsia in Chapter 16, Hypertension.

REFERENCES[www]

Aminoff MJ, Simon RP: Status epilepticus: causes, clinical features, and consequences in 98 patients, *Am J Med* 69:657, 1980

Chelsey C: History and epidemiology of preeclampsia-eclampsia, *Clin Obstet Gynecol* 27:801, 1984.

Clifford DB: Seizures in pregnancy, *Am Fam Physician* 29:271, 1984.

Hachinski V: Magnesium sulfate in the treatment of eclampsia, *Arch Neurol* 154:267, 1988.

Kaplan P, Lesser R, Fisher R: No, magnesium sulfate should not be used in treating eclamptic seizures, *Arch Neurol* 45:1361, 1988.

Knight AH, Rhind EJ: Epilepsy and pregnancy: a study of 153 pregnancies in 59 patients, *Epilepsia* 16:99, 1976.

Livingston S: Etiologic factors in adult convulsions: an analysis of 689 patients whose attacks began after 20 years of age, *N Engl J Med* 254:1211, 1956.

Philbert A, Dam M: The epileptic mother and her child, *Epilepsia* 23:85, 1982.

Schmidt D, Canger R, Avanzini G, et al: Changes of seizure frequency in pregnant epileptic women, *J Neurol Neurosurg Psychiatry* 46:751, 1983.

Will A, Lewis K, Hinshaw D, et al: Cerebral constriction in toxemia, *Neurology* 37:1555, 1987.

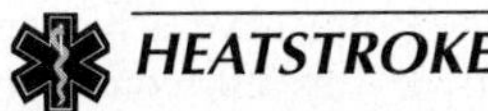

HEATSTROKE

See Chapter 12, Fever (Elevated Temperature).

CHAPTER 28

Seizure, Pediatric

RICHARD SONNER

Seizures in children may be self-limited and have a benign prognosis or may represent a medical or surgical condition associated with significant morbidity and mortality. Care must be taken to distinguish between seizures caused by a serious condition requiring emergent treatment and simple "febrile seizures," commonly seen in young children, for which minimal intervention is indicated. Seizures from trauma or toxic exposure may indicate child abuse or neglect, and a poor prognosis is likely if they are not correctly and promptly identified.

Treatment of seizures is directed by the age of the child and the most likely cause. The general approach to patients who are seizing begins with evaluation and stabilization of the ABCs. Serum glucose should be rapidly assessed or presumptively treated (1 to 4 ml/kg of D25 IV; for neonates: 10 ml/kg of D10 IV). Infants without a history of seizures should receive pyridoxine 100 mg IV. Naloxone (Narcan) (0.1 mg/kg/dose IV up to 2 mg/dose) should be given if narcotic exposure is a possibility, and thiamine (100 mg IV) should be considered for those with a history of alcoholism or malnutrition. The optimal treatment of pediatric seizures is age dependent and controversial. Benzodiazepines (e.g., lorazepam 0.05 to 0.1 mg/kg, maximum 4 mg; diazepam 0.2 to 0.3 mg/kg, maximum 4 mg), phenobarbitol (10 mg/kg IV/IM over 5 to 10 minutes, maximum 120 to 150 mg per dose, may repeat), or phenytoin (18 to 20 mg/kg IV over 10 to 20 minutes) may be used alone or in combination when needed. If intravenous access is not possible, diazepam may be given rectally (0.5 mg/kg, repeat at 0.25 mg/kg if needed). Airway management may be necessary because these agents can cause significant respiratory depression or apnea. Paraldehyde may be considered next, followed by general anesthesia with EEG monitoring for seizures unresponsive to treatment.

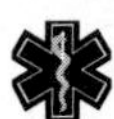 MENINGITIS AND ENCEPHALITIS

Seizures associated with fever may represent a benign event or be symptomatic of central nervous system infection. Simple febrile seizures are generalized seizures associated with fever, occurring in 2% to 5% of children 6 months to 5 years of age, lasting less than 15 minutes and not recurring within 24 hours. Thus a focal or prolonged seizure or a seizure that is complicated by Todd's (postictal) paralysis raises suspicion of underlying cerebral disease. Between 2% and 5% of children with fever and seizures have meningitis, whereas 13% to 16% of children with meningitis have seizures. Information about antibiotic use should be solicited, since antibiotics can mask symptoms and signs of meningitis.

Early administration of antibiotics in the ED after blood and urine cultures are obtained (but often before LP if there will be any delay) is indicated. Symptoms and signs of meningitis may be minimal or absent in children under 12 months and subtle in children between 12 and 18 months. Postictal state is usually very short in simple febrile seizures; a prolonged altered level of consciousness suggests another cause. In addition to bacterial causes of meningitis, viral, mycobacterial, and fungal CNS infections can cause seizure. It is particularly important to consider herpes encephalitis in patients with a CSF pleocytosis with negative gram stain, especially in children with focal neurologic findings or coma, since early antiviral treatment is indicated. Mycobacterial or fungal infection should be suspected in patients with a very low CSF glucose without an identifiable bacterial cause.

See Meningitis and Encephalitis in Chapter 15, Headache, and Chapter 13, Fever in Children Under 2 Years of Age.

Symptoms

- Altered level of consciousness
- Paradoxic irritability

- Vomiting
- Complex seizure features (focal, prolonged, or recurrent)

Signs

- Fever
- Lethargy +++
- Irritability +++
- Vomiting +++
- Nuchal rigidity ++
- Bulging fontanel ++
- Kernig's sign ++
- Brudzinski's sign ++
- Petechiae ++
- "Toxic appearing" ++
- Headache ++
- Apnea +
- Coma +
- Central nervous system infection may also present with focal neurologic signs, cyanosis, hypotension, grunting respirations, or rash.

REFERENCES

Al-Eissa YA: Lumbar puncture in the clinical evaluation of children with seizure associated with fever, *Pediatr Emerg Care* 11:347, 1995.

American Academy of Pediatrics: Practice parameter: the neurodiagnostic evaluation of the child with a first simple febrile seizure, *Pediatrics* 97:769, 1996.

Rosenberg NM, Meert K, Marino D, De Baker K: Seizures associated with meningitis, *Pediatr Emerg Care* 8:67, 1992.

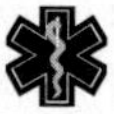

TOXIC INGESTIONS

Toxic causes of seizures in all age groups reported to a poison control center included antidepressants (29%), cocaine and other stimulants (29%), diphenhydramine and other antihistamines (7%), theophylline (5%), and isoniazid (5%). The diagnosis is primarily made based on exposure history, associated symptoms, and physical examination (toxidrome). A patient's current medications could be a potential cause of seizure; exposure to other medicines or toxins at home should be considered, as well as the possibility of intentional overdose.

See Chapter 32, Toxic Ingestion, Approach to, and Chapter 27, Seizure, Adult.

REFERENCES

Kunisaki TA, Augenstein WL: Drug and toxin-induced seizures, *Emerg Med Clin North Am* 12:1027, 1994.

Mott SH, Packer RJ, Soldin SJ: Neurologic manifestations of cocaine exposure in childhood, *Pediatrics* 93:557, 1994.

Olson KR, Kearney TE, Dyer JE, et al: Seizures associated with poisoning and drug overdose, *Am J Emerg Med* 12:392, 1994.

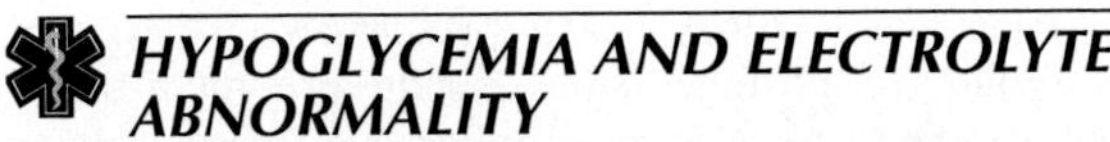

HYPOGLYCEMIA AND ELECTROLYTE ABNORMALITY

Pediatric patients with seizure occasionally have clinically significant abnormalities in glucose, electrolytes, calcium, or magnesium. Hypoglycemia is not uncommon in infants who have systemic stress because of hepatic dysfunction. Neonates and children with status epilepticus are also more likely to have serum chemistry abnormalities. In children under 1 year of age with status epilepticus, the most common disorders are hyponatremia and hypernatremia (23%), hypoglycemia (5%), and hypocalcemia (2%). Water intoxication related to inappropriate dilution of formula may be the cause of electrolyte abnormalities and seizures in infants.

Symptoms

- Vomiting
- Diarrhea
- Poor feeding

Signs

- Prolonged seizures
- Altered mental status
- Clinical evidence of dehydration or shock
- Hypothermia (rectal temperature < 36.5° C) ++++ in infants with hyponatremic seizures

Workup

- Serum chemistry studies are useful in neonates or young infants, children with status epilepticus, and those with a history of metabolic or gastrointestinal disease.

- Serum chemistry studies are very unlikely to be abnormal in patients whose mental status and physical examination are normal.

Comments and Treatment Considerations

Seizures due to metabolic abnormalities often respond better to correction of the metabolic defect than to anticonvulsant drug use. Retrospective studies have shown that when serum chemistry abnormalities are detected in clinically well children who have had seizures, test results rarely change management. Prolonged postictal state should prompt a search for causes of altered mental status other than recent seizure. Infants without previous history of seizure should receive pyridoxine 100 mg IV.

REFERENCES

Lacroix J, Deal C, Gauthier M, et al: Admissions to a pediatric intensive care unit for status epilepticus: a 10-year experience, *Crit Care Med* 22:827, 1994.

Nypaver MM, Reynolds SL, Tanz RR, Davis AT: Emergency department laboratory evaluation of children with seizures: dogma or dilemma? *Pediatr Emerg Care* 8:13, 1992.

Phillips SA, Shanahan RJ: Etiology and mortality of status epilepticus in children, *Arch Neurol* 46:74, 1989.

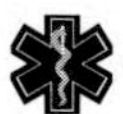

CHILD ABUSE AND HEAD TRAUMA

Homicide is the leading cause of injury-related death in infants (children under 1 year of age), with death most often resulting from head injury. Child abuse accounts for approximately 60% of head injuries and 95% of intracranial injuries in infants. Brain trauma represents up to 40% of injuries in abused children. Posttraumatic seizures are seen in 5% of minor head injuries and 35% of major head injuries in children. A history of trauma can be difficult to obtain from young children and can be misrepresented by caretakers. A complete physical examination includes a search for bony and soft tissue injuries. Suspected child abuse must be reported to the appropriate legal authorities.

See Chapter 18, The Irritable Child and Vomiting.

Signs

- Basilar skull fracture (Battle sign, hemotympanum, otorrhea) or focal neurologic abnormalities (focal motor deficit, pupillary asymmetry) predict +++ chance of abnormal head CT.
- Glasgow coma score <13 correlates with abnormal head CT in +++ of children with head trauma.
- Infants with shaken baby syndrome may not suck or swallow well, may not follow movements, smile, or vocalize, and usually have retinal hemorrhages ++++.
- Respiratory difficulty or bradycardia may occur in children with severe brain injury.
- Cervicoencephalic soft tissue injury confirms trauma; associated injuries may demonstrate abuse.

Workup

- Head CT (bone and soft tissue) is indicated in all children with posttraumatic seizures.
- X-ray of cervical spine should be obtained if cervical spine injury cannot be ruled out clinically.

REFERENCES

American Academy of Pediatrics: Shaken baby syndrome: inflicted cerebral trauma, *Pediatrics* 92:872, 1993.

Hahn YS, Fuchs S, Flannery AM, et al: Factors influencing posttraumatic seizures in children, *Neurosurgery* 22:864, 1988.

Ramundo ML, McKnight T, Kempf J, Satkowiak L: Clinical predictors of computed tomographic abnormalities following pediatric traumatic brain injury, *Pediatr Emerg Care* 11:1, 1995.

CHAPTER 29

Shortness of Breath

VICTOR A. CANDIOTY

The patient with respiratory distress requires immediate and simultaneous diagnosis and management. Rapid clinical assessment localizes the anatomic area involved in most patients able to "move air" and allows the emergency physician to proceed down a logical course of therapy. In patients who are not ventilating, immediate resuscitation following the traditional ABCs supersedes all other actions and is beyond the scope of this chapter.

Stridor is the audible sound of air flowing through a large airway that has been critically narrowed by either an intrinsic or extrinsic cause. Obstruction at or above the larynx typically produces stridor on inspiration. Stridor audible during both inspiration and exhalation indicates obstruction of the trachea. Foreign bodies of the oropharynx or hypopharynx, croup, epiglottitis, acute allergic reactions, and retropharyngeal abscesses or masses can produce stridor. Respiratory sounds confined to exhalation usually localize the obstruction to a point below the carina and represent bronchospasm or airway secretions.

Although dyspnea may be the result of several factors, pulmonary dysfunction leading to a sensation of shortness of breath may be considered in the following categories:

1. Mechanical ("lung pump") dysfunction—airway obstruction, pneumothorax, loss of chest wall integrity, and muscle weakness
2. Primary stimulation of pulmonary receptors—asthma, pneumonia, congestive heart failure (CHF), possibly pulmonary embolism
3. Problems with gas exchange leading to rise of carbon dioxide or fall in oxygen in the blood.

Pulmonary pathology may be primary to the respiratory system, secondary to cardiac disease, or a complication of systemic illness or toxic exposure (e.g., acute respiratory distress syndrome, or ARDS). In addition, metabolic acidosis can cause a compensatory rise in minute ventilation that may lead to dyspnea, particularly in patients with limited pulmonary reserve.

PNEUMOTHORAX, CARDIAC TAMPONADE, MYOCARDIAL INFARCTION, AND PULMONARY EMBOLISM

See Chapter 7, Chest Pain.

PULMONARY EDEMA

Pulmonary edema is characterized by hypoxia, decreased lung compliance, increased work of breathing, and bilateral pulmonary infiltrates on chest x-ray. The most common cause of pulmonary edema encountered in the ED is cardiac dysfunction leading to CHF. Severe disease processes such as sepsis, smoke inhalation, trauma, pulmonary contusion, pneumonia, or salicylate toxicity can cause noncardiogenic pulmonary edema (ARDS).

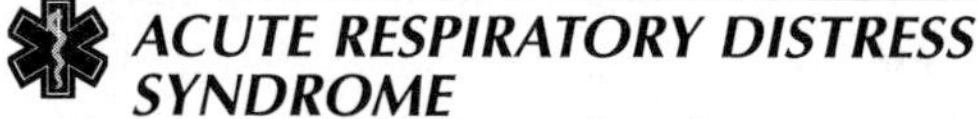

ACUTE RESPIRATORY DISTRESS SYNDROME

The following criteria define the syndrome of ARDS:

1. Clinical evidence of respiratory distress
2. Chest x-ray revealing diffuse air space disease (pulmonary edema)
3. Hypoxia that is difficult to correct with oxygen supplementation (shunt)
4. Pulmonary capillary occlusion (wedge) pressure <18 mm Hg (absence of cardiogenic pulmonary edema [CHF])
5. Total thoracic static compliance <40 ml/cm of water

Symptoms

- Dyspnea
- Dry (nonproductive) cough
- Retrosternal discomfort
- Agitation
- Onset over hours to days

Signs

- Hypoxia (common) progressing to respiratory failure
- Tachypnea
- Coarse crackles with bronchial breath sounds (although chest examination may be relatively unimpressive for the abnormalities seen on chest x-ray)
- Signs of serious underlying disease, often including multisystem organ dysfunction

Workup

- Chest x-ray (abnormal). It may be difficult to differentiate radiographically between cardiogenic and noncardiogenic pulmonary edema. However, generally in ARDS (1) the cardiac silhouette is normal; (2) diffuse, bilateral infiltrates tend to be more peripheral, uneven, and patchy +++ versus the even and perihilar ("batwing") pattern characteristic of cardiogenic pulmonary edema; and (3) pleural effusions are less frequent than in cardiogenic pulmonary edema.
- Arterial blood gases: severe hypoxemia (PaO_2 <50 mm Hg) that is difficult to correct with supplemental O_2 (increased dead space, increased right-to-left shunting, and maldistribution of ventilation)
- Pulmonary artery catheter occlusion (wedge) pressures are normal or near-normal (<18 mm Hg).

Comments and Treatment Considerations

The pathophysiology of ARDS is currently the subject of intense research. It is unclear exactly what triggers the cascade of events that manifests as ARDS.

Treatment, especially in the ED, is predominantly supportive. Assisted mechanical ventilation should be provided early in the course of ARDS to maximize oxygen delivery to all organ systems. Positive end-expiratory pressure (PEEP) is adjusted to the inflection point of the pressure-volume curve of the lung, typically 12.5 to 15 cm H_2O. PEEP works to improve oxygenation, increase functional residual capacity (FRC), decrease physiologic shunt, and improve lung compliance.

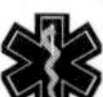 CONGESTIVE HEART FAILURE

Acute exacerbation of CHF is typically caused by cardiac ischemia, although a hypertensive emergency and, less commonly, cardiomyopathy can also cause acute CHF.

Symptoms

- Shortness of breath at rest is the major presenting symptom ++++.
- Paroxysmal nocturnal dyspnea +++
- Orthopnea ++
- Cough
- Fatigue
- Symptoms of myocardial ischemia are common: angina, diaphoresis, and decreased exercise tolerance.

Signs

The presence of physical findings in CHF tends to be more specific than sensitive.

- Vital signs (abnormal): tachycardia, normal or elevated blood pressure, hypotension indicative of cardiac decompensation (shock)
- Wet crackles
- S3 gallop (common in systolic dysfunction), representing rapid ventricular filling associated with impaired ventricular function ++ (>90% specific)
- S4 gallop (common in diastolic dysfunction), representing diminished ventricular compliance
- Peripheral edema ++ (80% specific)
- Jugular venous distention ++ (>90% specific)
- Hepatojugular reflux ++ (>90% specific)

Workup

- Chest x-ray: abnormal
- Enlarged cardiac silhouette
- Symmetric redistribution of pulmonary blood flow ("bat-wing" pattern)
- ECG is neither sensitive nor specific: ischemic changes or arrhythmia may be present.
- Electrolyte and renal function tests: rule out renal failure or significant electrolyte abnormality due to widespread use of diuretics and ACE inhibitors. Total body magnesium depletion is common in patients who are taking diuretics and frequently is not reflected in serum magnesium. Repletion of magnesium facilitates potassium repletion.

Comments and Treatment Considerations

Initial management includes establishing intravenous access, oxygen supplementation, and continuous monitoring of cardiac rhythm and pulse oximetry. Pharmacologic treatment should be directed to treating the underlying cause of CHF, which is often cardiac ischemia (see Chapter 7, Chest Pain). Treatment with nitrates decreases cardiac preload, which improves CHF symptoms directly in addition to improving coronary blood flow. Intravenous loop diuretics (furosemide) are frequently used and are indicated in the setting of fluid overload. ACE inhibitors have become the primary outpatient medical treatment for CHF and may be used for acute exacerbations. In patients with cardiogenic pulmonary edema, administration of a small dose of morphine sulfate may reduce catecholamines and lead to vasodilation and venodilation. Morphine may be particularly effective in patients with a high pulse-pressure product. Bilevel positive airway pressure (BIPAP) may be an effective adjunct to medical therapy in the acute setting because it improves oxygenation and ventilation in cardiogenic pulmonary edema, thus avoiding intubation in a significant percentage of patients.

REFERENCES[www]

Bukata WR: The pharmacologic management of heart failure, 1994, *Emerg Med Acute Care Essays* 19:3, 1995.

[www]Additional references are available on the following web site: www.signsandsymptoms.com.

Desai SR, Hansell OM: Lung imaging in the adults respiratory distress syndrome: current practice and new insights, *Intensive Care Med* 23:7, 1997.

Garber BG, Hebert PC, Yelle JD, et al: Adult respiratory distress syndrome: a systematic overview of incidence and risk factors, *Crit Care Med* 24:687, 1996.

Harlan WR, Oberman A, Grimm R, Rosati RA: Chronic congestive heart failure in coronary artery disease: clinical criteria, *Ann Intern Med* 86:133, 1977.

Peruzzi WT, Franklin ML, Shapiro BA: New concepts and therapies of adult respiratory distress syndrome, *J Cardiothorac Vasc Anesth* 11:771, 1997.

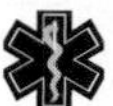

ANAPHYLAXIS, ANAPHYLACTOID REACTIONS, AND ANGIOEDEMA

Anaphylaxis is a life-threatening, rapid, type I hypersensitivity reaction mediated by IgE, causing local and systemic responses to multiple organ systems. Anaphylactoid reactions refer to non-IgE hypersensitivity events that are similar in clinical presentation. Angioedema refers to the deep cutaneous and visceral tissue swelling that accompanies an allergic response.

The following are common causes of anaphylaxis:

- Drugs, especially antibiotics (penicillin is the most common cause of anaphylaxis)
- Insect bites or stings, especially from *Hymenoptera*, snakes, and fire ants
- Foods, especially peanuts, nuts, egg whites, and shellfish; preservatives, especially sulfites
- Plants
- Chemicals
- Latex
- Exercise, especially when coupled with certain foods or drugs
- Immunotherapy

ACE inhibitors can cause a bradykinin-mediated angioedema in 0.2% of patients (70% within the first week, but can occur at any time). Anaphylactoid reactions can be caused by neuromuscular blockers and radiocontrast dyes (iodinated more common than lower-osmolar agents).

The severity of the allergen response depends on the delivery of the allergen; parenteral is most rapid.

Symptoms

Usually peak within 15 to 30 minutes of exposure

- History of known allergen exposure
- Pruritus or tingling, rash or swelling, flushing ++++
- Hoarseness, sensation of throat tightness
- Rhinorrhea, bronchorrhea
- Nausea, vomiting, abdominal cramps
- Dizziness, syncope, near-syncope
- Dyspnea, chest tightness

Signs

May occur in combination or isolation

- Urticaria (pruritic) or angioedema (nonpruritic)++++; preferential edema of lips, tongue, uvula, eyes, and hands
- Distributive shock—hypotension, tachycardia; may occur in the absence of urticaria or angioedema
- Stridor, wheeze, retractions, tachypnea
- Respiratory failure from laryngeal edema

Workup

- None required in the ED; immunodiagnostic skin testing as an outpatient

Comments and Treatment Considerations

Airway maintenance, epinephrine, diphenhydramine, and intravenous fluids are the critical interventions for emergent allergic reactions.

Epinephrine may be given subcutaneously (adults: 0.3 ml of 1:1000 solution; children 0.01 ml/kg), although for severely vasoconstricted patients, absorption may be erratic. IV epinephrine may be used in cases of airway swelling, severe bronchospasm, or cardiovascular collapse. Epinephrine (adults: 0.1 mg; i.e., 100 μg) should be administered using a diluted solution (10 ml of a solution made with 1 ml of 1:10,000 epinephrine solution in 9 ml of NS; or 1 ml of epinephrine 1:10,000 ampule if time does not permit further dilution) given over 1 to 4 minutes.

Diphenhydramine (adults: 50 mg IV or IM; children: 1 mg/kg IV or IM) should be given. Combination H1 and H2 blocker therapy should be considered, since it may be more effective than HI therapy alone.

Intravenous or oral steroids (e.g., methylprednisolone 1 mg/kg) are indicated, although they do not work immediately.

Patients with wheezing may benefit from beta-2 agonist aerosols.

Patients taking beta-blockers can be refractory to standard therapy and may require glucagon 1 mg IV over 5 minutes.

Angioedema not responding to standard therapy and associated with a predominance of gastrointestinal symptoms without urticaria or hypotension may be due to hereditary angioedema, a C1-esterase inhibitor deficiency.

Reassessment is mandatory. Patients with a clinically significant episode, particularly those with respiratory compromise, should be admitted for observation. Those with symptom resolution who successfully complete a period of observation may be safely discharged with antihistamine treatment for a few days and close follow-up. Since recurrence of symptoms without repeat exposure occurs in 5% to 10%, most within 72 hours, a short course of steroids may also be indicated. One should be especially alert to the possibility of recurrent symptoms in patients who have ingested an allergen and in whom absorption of the allergen may be ongoing for several hours. An epinephrine self-injector device (EpiPen) and instructions for its use should be given to patients who are discharged after a serious allergic reaction.

REFERENCES[www]

Atkinson TP, Kaliner MA: Anaphylaxis, *Med Clin North Am* 76:841, 1992.

Fisher M: Fortnightly review: treatment of acute anaphylaxis, *BMJ* 311:731, 1995.

Yunginger JW: Anaphylaxis, *Ann Allergy* 69:87, 1992.

[www]Additional references are available on the following web site: www.signsandsymptoms.com.

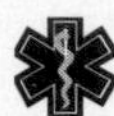

ASTHMA

Factors to consider in the evaluation of asthma patients include the patient's appearance and ability to speak, increased recent inhaler use, recent use of steroids, and a history of previous asthma attacks requiring intubation or hospital admission. Very acutely ill asthmatics may not move enough air to wheeze and may have relatively normal PCO_2 as they tire. Hypoxia generally precedes the development of hypercapnia.

The diagnosis of asthma must be made cautiously in older patients, since their wheezing may be caused by cardiac disease.

See Chapter 7, Chest Pain.

Symptoms

- Dyspnea
- Wheezing
- Cough
- Chest tightness
- Inability to sleep

Signs

- Expiratory wheezing
- Hyperinflation
- Rhonchi
- Prolonged expiration
- Pulsus paradoxus 10 to 25 mm Hg

Reliable markers of severe illness include the following:

- Abnormal vital signs (RR >25, pulse >110, bradycardia, hypotension)
- Diaphoresis
- Accessory muscle use
- "Silent" chest
- Feeble respiratory effort, broken sentences, or exhaustion
- Cyanosis, confusion, coma (life-threatening signs)

Workup

Pulmonary function: serial measurement of pulmonary function during treatment is strongly encouraged, because clinical markers in all but very severe cases may not reliably indicate severity of disease. Patients with severe asthma frequently have peak expiratory flow rate (PEFR) values of 20% to 30% of predicted, improving only to 50% to 60%, at which point they may become asymptomatic.

ABG: routine ABG is unnecessary because patients are treated on the basis of the clinical presentation. Hyperventilation associated with an asthma attack should lead to a decreased PCO_2 (respiratory alkalosis). Hypercapnia (or normal PCO_2) occurs when patients are no longer able to ventilate adequately, thus confirming a clinical diagnosis of respiratory failure. Hypoxia is common in even mild to moderate asthma as a result of ventilation-perfusion mismatch.

Chest x-ray: indications include clinical suspicion of pneumonia, pneumothorax, pneumomediastinum, clinical deterioration despite aggressive treatment, or suspicion of cardiac asthma.

Spirometry or peak flow (PEFR) provides objective data regarding severity and response to treatment. In adults, PEFR <40% of known baseline, <100 L/min before treatment or <300 L/min after treatment are markers of severe disease.

CBC and electrolytes are of little value in patient management.

ECG: indicated if underlying cardiac disease and in those suspected of being theophylline toxic. Sinus tachycardia is common, and RV strain (rightward axis and RVH) or P pulmonale may be seen.

Comments and Treatment Considerations

Oxygen should be provided for all patients. Beta-agonists such as albuterol (2.5 to 5.0 mg in 3 ml normal saline) by inhalation are the mainstay of treatment of acute asthma. Repeated dosing by inhalers with a spacer or through nebulization should be given and titrated to a clinical response. Continuous nebulization has been shown to be more effective in relieving obstruction, decreasing admission rates, and shortening respiratory therapy time in children and adults with severe obstruction.

Systemic corticosteroids should be used early in patients with severe disease, those with minimal or no improvement after initial beta-adrenergic therapy, and those with peak flows

<50% of predicted after 1 hour of therapy. Intravenous administration provides no advantage over oral routes. Although inhaled corticosteroids have become the first-line agents in the treatment of chronic asthma, their role in acute treatment is less clear.

Anticholinergics by inhalation (e.g., ipratropium bromide) act to inhibit parasympathetically mediated bronchoconstriction. Inhaled anticholinergics, however, have been shown to be inferior to beta-adrenergics in asthmatics. These agents may have a role in conjunction with beta-adrenergics, where the combination produces greater improvement than that achieved by either class of medication alone.

Volume and free water deficits should be addressed with either oral or intravenous fluid since the extra work of breathing and increased minute ventilation increase insensible losses.

Helium-oxygen mixtures (Heliox), which have lower density than the nitrogen-oxygen mixture in ambient air, decrease turbulent air flow and may improve the delivery of oxygen to alveoli for gas exchange. Diffusion of CO_2 is more rapid, theoretically improving the respiratory acidosis associated with respiratory muscle fatigue and air trapping. Heliox mixtures are given in 70:30 or 80:20 ratios by a tight-fitting mask or through mechanical ventilators. Their greatest theoretical benefit is in patients with upper airway obstruction (e.g., laryngospasm).

Administration of intravenous nonselective adrenergic agents such as epinephrine is currently reserved for patients with impending respiratory failure who deteriorate despite treatment with continuous nebulization, as complications may occur.

Because severe asthma is characterized by significant increases in airway resistance and air trapping, the initiation of mechanical ventilation is associated with potential complications, especially barotrauma (pneumothorax and pneumomediastinum). The ability to achieve adequate alveolar ventilation (and a normal $Paco_2$) for patients in respiratory failure is often limited in status asthmaticus. Consequently, new ventilator strategies are being used that call for "permissive hypercapnia," that is, the deliberate underventilation of the patient. Thus the $Paco_2$ is allowed to rise while adequate Pao_2 is maintained. Permissive hypercapnia requires deep sedation and paralysis.

REFERENCES

Abou-Shala N, MacIntyre N: Emergent management of acute asthma, *Med Clin North Am* 80:677, 1996.

Beasley R, Miles J, Fishwick D, Leslie H: Management of asthma in the hospital emergency department, *Br J Hosp Med* 55:253, 1996.

Bukata WR: Asthma guidelines, 1997, *Emerg Med Acute Care Essays* 21:5, 1997.

Kardon EM: Acute asthma, *Emerg Med Clin North Am* 14:93, 1996.

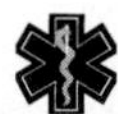

CHRONIC OBSTRUCTIVE PULMONARY DISEASE

Chronic obstructive pulmonary disease (COPD) is a general term that encompasses three distinct diseases: emphysema, chronic bronchitis, and asthma. These diseases frequently coexist, especially in the elderly, with the individual components of airway destruction and collapse (emphysema), airway inflammation (chronic bronchitis), and airway reactivity (asthma) combining in varying degrees to create obstructive pulmonary symptoms and respiratory distress. Emphysema and chronic bronchitis are discussed in detail here.

Symptoms and Signs (Table 29-1)

Workup

- Cardiac monitor and continuous pulse oximeter
- Chest x-rays, if CHF or pneumonia is suspected
- ABG to assess acid-base status, if deteriorating clinically or in extremis
- ECG, if concern for acute cardiac disease

Comments and Treatment Considerations

The minimum FiO_2 required to maintain mentation or O_2 saturation >85% to 90% should be used. Occasionally, intubation may be required, since supplemental oxygen, although required in cases of very low oxygen saturations, may lead to hypoventilation.

Inhaled beta-agonists (albuterol) are used in conjunction with anticholinergics (ipratropium bromide) to treat any component of reversible bronchospasm that exists.

Table 29-1 Symptoms and Signs of Emphysema and Chronic Bronchitis

Emphysema	Chronic Bronchitis
Symptoms	
"Pink puffer"	"Blue bloater"
Dyspnea (marked) with minimal exertion progressing to shortness of breath at rest	Dyspnea absent
Anorexia, insomnia, weight loss suggest decompensation.	Vigorous cough, productive
Signs	
Thin, alert, anxious	Wheezes
"Tripod" position	Rhonchi
Tachypneic	Basilar rales
	Progression to acute ventilatory failure: CO_2 narcosis, altered mental status, coma
	Right heart failure: peripheral edema, jugular venous distention, hepatojugular reflux, hepatomegaly, RV heave, S_3, S_4, holosystolic murmur of tricuspid insufficiency, $P_2 > A_2$
	Cor pulmonale and chronic ventilatory failure (late findings)

Corticosteroids, although not effective during the brief period the patient is in the ED, provide antiinflammatory activity, enhance the effect of beta-agonists, and should be initiated promptly. Prednisone 60 mg orally or methylprednisolone 125 mg intravenously, if the patient is unable to take oral medications, are equally efficacious and are given for a 5-day "pulse," or longer course with a gradual taper as indicated.

Antibiotic therapy is indicated in patients who demonstrate evidence of bacterial infection and in those with chronic bronchitis whose sputum changes in quality or quantity. Sputum culture has proven not to be cost effective. First-line agents covering *Streptococcus pneumoniae*, *Haemophilus influenzae,* and *Moraxella (Branhamella) catarrhalis* include trimethoprim-sulfamethoxazole, amoxicillin, tetracycline, and doxycycline. The more costly agents, such as the macrolides, cephalosporins, amoxicillin-clavulanate, or expanded-spectrum quinolones, can be used in patients considered to be more severely ill or requiring hospitalization.

REFERENCES

Celli B: Current thoughts regarding treatment of chronic obstructive pulmonary disease, *Med Clin North Am* 80:589, 1996.

Chapman K: Therapeutic approaches to chronic obstructive pulmonary disease: an emerging consensus, *Am J Med* 10(suppl 1A):55, 1996.

Mandavia DP, Dailey RH: Chronic obstructive pulmonary disease. In Rosen P, Barkin RM, Hockberger RS, et al, editors: *Emergency medicine: concepts and clinical practice*, ed 4, St Louis, 1997, Mosby.

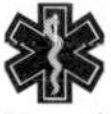

ASPIRATED FOREIGN BODIES

Foreign body (FB) aspiration is the most common cause of in-home accidental death in children under 6 years old. FBs of both the upper esophagus and tracheobronchial tree can present with airway symptoms, with FBs of the latter accounting for 10% to 15% of all cases. However, symptoms may subside or be absent with passage of an FB into the airways. Delayed wheezing or stridor may be seen with FBs of the mainstem bronchus. A coin is the most common esophageal FB, whereas peanuts and sunflower seeds are the most commonly aspirated FBs of the respiratory tree. Rubber balloons are common causes of asphyxiation.

Symptoms

- Choking ++++
- Coughing ++++
- Gagging

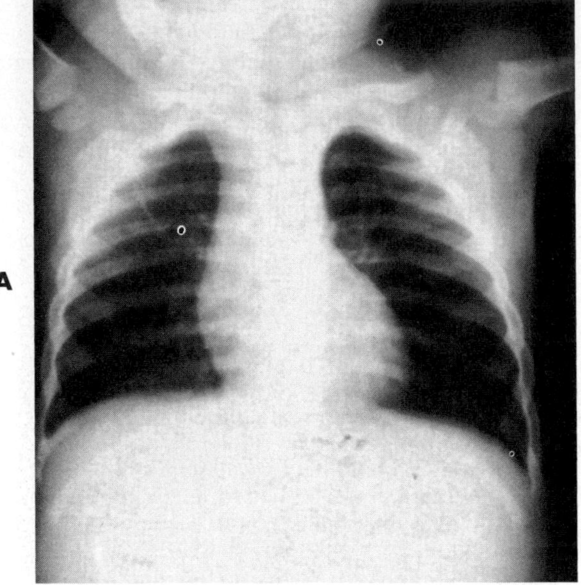

Fig. 29-1 **A,** "Normal inspiratory" chest film in a child with a left mainstem bronchus foreign body. (From Rosen P, Barkin RM, Hockberger RS, et al, editors: *Emergency medicine: concepts and clinical practice,* ed 4, St Louis, 1997, Mosby.)

Signs

- Auscultation (abnormal) ++++
- Inspiratory stridor implies FB location at or above the larynx.
- Inspiratory and expiratory stridor suggests obstruction in the trachea. Expiratory stridor implies obstruction below the carina.
- Inability to vocalize

Workup

- Soft tissue lateral x-ray of the neck is positive for an FB +++
- Chest x-rays (abnormal) ++++
- Air in the esophagus

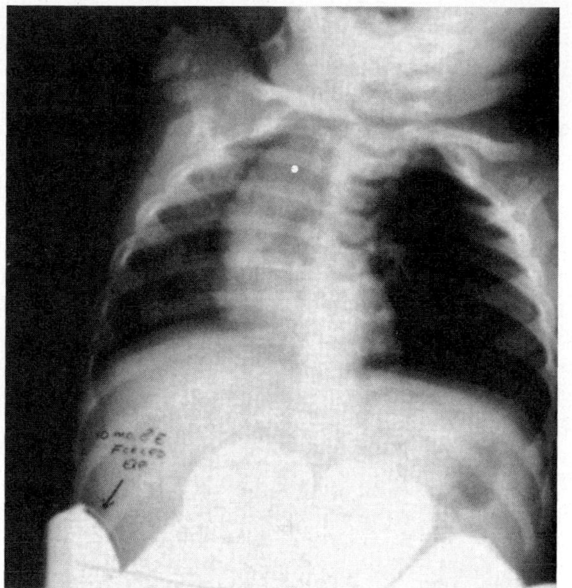

Fig. 29-1, cont'd B, Forced expiratory view showing expanded lung on left with shift of mediastinum to uninvolved right side.

- Visible FB shadow
- Hyperinflation of affected side on exhalation (Fig. 29-1)
- Mediastinal shift away from FB side
- Persistent hyperinflation on decubitus chest x-ray, with affected side "down" owing to air trapping
- Bronchoscopy or endoscopy or CT scan may be helpful if plain films are nondiagnostic.

Comments and Treatment Considerations

A common location for airway FBs is in a mainstem bronchus, usually the right, producing cough, unilateral wheezing, and stridor. Recurrent stridor or wheezing may indicate an FB that is changing position in the airway (stridor when moving proximally and wheezing when moving distally).

FB aspiration in children is often misdiagnosed as pneumonia (27%). Overall, the mean interval from aspiration to removal is 19 days. Removal of tracheal FBs requires laryngoscopy or bronchoscopy under general anesthesia because of edema of the airway from the FB itself or chemical pneumonitis in cases of food aspiration. Respiratory care (antibiotics, steroids, O_2, cool mist or chest physiotherapy) is often necessary for 24 to 72 hours after FB removal, as indicated.

For esophageal FBs endoscopic removal under general anesthesia has been the traditional method of choice, although retrograde retrieval with a Foley catheter under fluoroscopy or antegrade passage into the stomach (bougienage) are alternative removal methods. Button batteries retained in the esophagus must be immediately removed because of the risk of severe esophageal damage or perforation.

REFERENCES[www]

Conners G: A literature-based comparison of three methods of pediatric esophageal coin removal, *Pediatr Emerg Care* 13:154, 1997.

Hoeve LJ, Rombout J, Pot DJ: Foreign body aspiration in children: the diagnostic value of signs, symptoms, and preoperative examination, *Clin Otolaryngol* 18:55, 1993.

Marais J, Mitchell R, Wightman AJ: The value of radiographic assessment for oropharyngeal foreign bodies, *J Laryngol Otol* 109:452, 1995.

[www]Additional references are available on the following web site: www.signsandsymptoms.com.

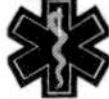

EPIGLOTTITIS

See Chapter 30, Sore Throat.

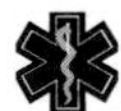

CROUP

Croup, or laryngotracheobronchitis, is a common respiratory infection affecting children from 6 months to 3 years of age (peak incidence, 2 years). The most important concern of the emergency physician is to distinguish between croup, which is typically viral in origin and self-limited, and epiglottitis, which is generally bacterial in origin, requires antibiotic treatment, and more often leads to airway compromise. Croup results from glottic and subglottic mucosal edema and is associated with a characteristic "barking seal" cough. Bacterial tracheitis is a rare, very serious infection that may produce a cough similar to that produced by croup. Patients are acutely ill and require intravenous antibiotic therapy with close airway monitoring in an ICU setting.

Symptoms

- Gradually increasing URI symptoms, mild fever, and nonproductive cough over 2 to 3 days
- Symptoms worse at night
- Paroxysmal, "barking" cough often accompanied by inspiratory stridor and dyspnea (predominant symptom)
- Symptomatic improvement with exposure to cool, damp air

"Spasmodic" croup variant

- Abrupt onset without antecedent URI symptoms
- Year-round incidence
- Possibly a result of airway hyperreactivity caused by viruses, allergens, or possible genetic predispositions

Signs

- Barking cough
- Inspiratory stridor
- Hoarseness
- Signs of respiratory distress vary depending on degree of obstruction and include tachypnea, intercostal and suprasternal retractions, tachycardia, nasal flaring, and cyanosis.

Workup

- Clinical presentation is usually sufficient to make the diagnosis.
- X-rays: Anteroposterior view of neck may show a marked narrowing of the subglottic trachea ("steeple sign"). Direct laryngoscopy may be necessary to rule out epiglottitis, although the patient should be moved to the operating room before manipulation if epiglottitis is a serious consideration.

Comments and Treatment Considerations

Treatment should begin with a cool mist vapor by mask or blow-by as tolerated. Most children show improvement. Any increase in agitation may result in worsening symptoms.

Steroids have been shown to be beneficial for croup, with positive responses noted as early as 1 hour after administration. Dexamethasone (0.6 mg/kg IM) has been shown to be superior to inhaled budesonide. A single dose usually is sufficient, although a short course of outpatient steroids may be considered. In patients with severe symptoms, nebulized, racemic epinephrine (<20 kg: 0.25 ml; 20 to 40 kg: 0.5 ml; >40 kg: 0.75 ml of a 2.25% solution diluted to 4 ml total volume) has been proven to be effective in decreasing subglottic edema and obstruction, although standard L-epinephrine (5 ml of 1:1000 solution) delivered by nebulizer is also effective. Observation for 2 hours after administration of epinephrine is generally sufficient to reveal which children are at risk for deterioration and which can be safely discharged home.

REFERENCES

Bukata WR: Croup, bacterial tracheitis, and epiglottitis, *Emerg Med Acute Care Essays* 17:4, 1993.

Croup. In Harwood-Nuss AL, Linden CH, Luten RC, et al, editors: *The clinical practice of emergency medicine,* Philadelphia, 1991, JB Lippincott.

Geelhoed GC: Croup, *Pediatr Pulmonol* 23:370, 1997.

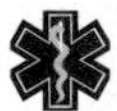

HYPOXIA

Decreased Pa_{O_2} (partial pressure of oxygen in the plasma) can be caused by the following pathologic processes:

- Hypoventilation from any cause
- V/Q mismatch (e.g., PE, pneumonia, asthma, COPD, interstitial lung disease, CHF)
- Shunt (e.g., congenital heart disease)
- Diffusion abnormalities (e.g., interstitial inflammation or edema)
- Reduced Fi_{O_2} (fraction of O_2 in inspired gas; e.g., altitude, fire in an enclosed space)

Immediate management of hypoxia entails administration of supplemental oxygen sufficient to achieve an oxygen saturation of approximately 90%. In patients with COPD and chronic hypercapnia, supplemental oxygen may result in a rise in $PaCO_2$ and lead to ventilatory arrest. Therefore the least amount of oxygen needed to achieve adequate oxygenation should be provided. In critically ill patients with chest pain or altered mental status and hypoxia, administration of 100% oxygen by non-rebreather mask is suggested. If severe acidosis results, endotracheal intubation and mechanical ventilation are necessary.

See Chapter 7, Chest Pain.

DECREASED OXYGEN DELIVERY AND IMPAIRED OXYGEN UTILIZATION

Most oxygen delivered to tissues is carried by hemoglobin. Therefore decreased blood flow (due to hypotension or embolism), anemia, or pathologic conditions that affect oxygen-hemoglobin binding properties (e.g., carbon monoxide, methemoglobin, abnormal hemoglobin) can dramatically reduce oxygen available to tissues even in the presence of a normal PaO_2. Other conditions directly disrupt the ability of cells to use delivered oxygen (e.g., cyanide poisoning).

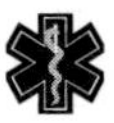

CONGENITAL HEART DISEASE

The most common form of congenital heart disease (CHD) is a ventricular septal defect, which occurs in 30% to 40% of all children with CHD. Half of patients with CHD are diagnosed in the first week of life, and the vast majority by 1 year of age. The exact abnormalities are numerous, but are divided into two basic categories—cyanotic and acyanotic—depending on whether an extrapulmonary right-to-left shunt is present.

The treatment of respiratory distress resulting from congenital heart anomalies in the ED setting is extremely limited and often consists only of maximizing oxygen delivery and, in cases of first presentation of disease, obtaining emergent echocardiography to define the abnormality. All patients should be placed on a cardiac monitor with continuous pulse oximetry monitoring, and 100% FiO_2 should be delivered to maximize oxygenation.

Patients with CHD surviving into adulthood who have cardiopulmonary decompensation are becoming more common. Evaluation and management must be tailored to the individual case, given the variability in the original defects and the nature of the corrective procedures. In general, however, initial management of adult survivors of CHD with heart failure is similar to that for adults with acquired cardiac disease and similar symptoms. Prompt cardiac consultation is recommended.

See Cardiac Disease: Structural Defects and Arrhythmias in Chapter 18, The Irritable Child and Vomiting.

REFERENCES

Harris MA, Valmorida JN: Neonates with congenital heart disease. I. Overview, *Neonatal Netw* 15:81, 1996.

Hoffman J: Congenital heart disease: incidence and inheritance, *Pediatr Clin North Am* 37:25, 1990.

McNamara D: Value and limitations of auscultation in the management of congenital heart disease, *Pediatr Clin North Am* 37:93, 1990.

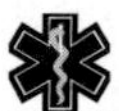

AIR EMBOLISM

Undissolved intravascular air can occur as an arterial gas embolus (AGE) or venous gas embolus (VGE). Volumes of 100 to 300 ml are considered fatal; in canine models, 0.5 to 1.0 ml/kg causes 40% mortality.

AGE can occur from rapid ascent during dives (a form of "the bends"), intrathoracic trauma, hydrogen peroxide ingestion, other pressurized gas inhalation, or a VGE that crosses from right to left through a foramen ovale or ventricular septal defect. AGEs travel to cerebral arteries (most common), coronary arteries, or spinal arteries, causing strokes, ischemia, infarction, dysrhythmias, or paralysis.

VGE can occur as a complication of central venous catheterization, penetrating and blunt chest trauma, high-pressure mechanical ventilation after chest trauma, thoracocentesis, hemodialysis, and a variety of surgical procedures. It can cause immediate hypoxia, hemodynamic collapse (thought to be from obstruction of the right pulmonary outflow tract), and death. Venous gas bubbles are commonly observed after diving and are most often asymptomatic. (Divers are also at risk for pneumothorax if ascent is made without exhalation of expanding lung gases.) Lethality of air emboli depends on rate and volume of embolized air and position of the patient at the time. Higher rates and volumes and sitting position increase mortality.

Symptoms

AGE

Neurologic symptoms often overshadow cardiopulmonary symptoms; in sport divers, symptoms most frequently occur within 10 minutes of surfacing ++++, but may be delayed.

- Loss of consciousness +++
- Dyspnea +++
- Limb paralysis or numbness +++
- Severe headache ++
- Aphasia or dysarthria ++
- Hemoptysis ++
- Seizures

VGE

- Breathlessness, dyspnea
- Chest pain
- Sense of impending death

Signs

AGE

Cerebral embolism:

- Neurologic signs: altered mental status, focal deficits, seizure
- Pulmonary signs: crepitus, unequal breath sounds (pneumothorax)

Coronary embolism:

- Dysrhythmias

VGE

Depends on the rate of embolus formation. All signs are nonspecific, especially in multiple trauma scenarios, which makes diagnosis difficult.

- Sudden gasp, wheeze
- Rapid, shallow respirations followed by apneic period
- Tachycardia
- Hypotension, cardiovascular collapse if severe
- Loss of consciousness; altered mental status
- Unexplained decrease in P_{ETCO2} and O_2 saturation
- The only specific sign, a "mill-wheel" murmur, is an uncommon and late sign, present only after cardiovascular deterioration has begun ++++

Workup

AGE

- MRI is very sensitive for cerebral lesions ++++; CT is almost as sensitive
- Transesophageal echocardiography (TEE) and Doppler ultrasound are the most sensitive in detecting air emboli as they occur (as little as 0.02 ml/kg and 0.25 ml, respectively) +++++ ; these are very sensitive and record bubbles that have no clinical significance.
- TEE is best for detecting air in the left ventricle.
- Initial chest x-rays are often normal ++
- ALT, AST, and LDH are significantly higher in AGE than routine decompression sickness.
- Elevated CPK ++++

Comments and Treatment Considerations

AGE

Consider the possibility of an cerebral air embolism in anyone with altered mental status or neurologic symptoms following a compressed air dive. One third of divers who suffer loss of consciousness have a fatal outcome. Those who have spontaneous recovery can relapse ++. In addition to ACLS care, 100% O_2 by NRB should be given while arranging for recompression and hyperbaric therapy. Lidocaine 5 mg/kg may protect against high intracranial pressure in cerebral air emboli. Naloxone 2 mg/kg bolus followed by a 2 mg/kg/hr infusion, and doxycycline, through leukocyte inhibition, have each shown evidence of protection against cortical ischemic effects.

VGE

Provide patients with oxygen and place them in the left lateral decubitus position (to prevent air from entering the right ventricular outflow track) while arranging for emergent hyperbaric therapy. Aspiration of intracardiac air may be considered in emergent circumstances. Thoracotomy is both diagnostic and therapeutic for suspected air embolism in penetrating thoracic injury.

REFERENCES[www]

Glenski JA, Cucchiara RF, Michenfelder JD: Transesophageal echocardiography and transcutaneous O_2 and CO_2 monitoring for detection of venous air embolism, *Anesthesiology* 64:541, 1986.

Hardy KR: Diving-related emergencies, *Emerg Med Clin North Am* 15:223, 1997.

Palmon SC, Moore LE, Lundberg J, et al: Venous air embolism: a review, *J Clin Anesth* 9:251, 1997.

[www]Additional references are available on the following web site: www.signsandsymptoms.com.

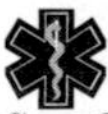

CARBON MONOXIDE

See Chapter 15, Headache.

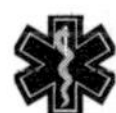

METHEMOGLOBIN

See Chapter 22, Mental Status Change and Coma.

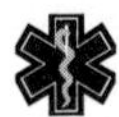

CYANIDE

See Chapter 22, Mental Status Change and Coma.

CHAPTER 30

Sore Throat

GREGG GREENOUGH

The history and physical examination are key to diagnosing the specific entities that are manifested by sore throat. Rarely do laboratory tests (e.g., electrolytes, blood counts, or throat cultures) assist in management decisions. The most worrisome conditions to consider are epiglottitis, retropharyngeal, parapharyngeal, or peritonsillar abscesses, and Ludwig's angina. All can cause sudden airway obstruction and asphyxia or lead to sepsis. Deep space infections can rapidly spread down fascial planes and into contiguous spaces, causing carotid invasion and hemorrhage, jugular vein thrombosis, mediastinitis, pericarditis, and empyema. Retropharyngeal abscesses can cause vertebral osteomyelitis, transverse myelitis, and atlantoaxial subluxation. Treatment focuses on administration of appropriate antibiotics and surgical drainage of abscesses after confirming that the airway is secure (beware of acute airway obstruction, particularly in children with epiglottis).

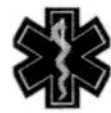

EPIGLOTTITIS

Epiglottitis should be suspected in patients who have a severe sore throat and odynophagia but a normal oropharyngeal examination. Stridor, a change in voice, and tenderness over the thyroid cartilage also are of concern. Dyspnea, when present, is a serious symptom because of the potential for airway compromise. As the number of children receiving *Haemophilus influenzae* type B immunization rises, the percentage of cases occurring in adults will continue to grow. Antecedent cough or symptoms of an upper respiratory infection (URI) usually are not present in most cases. Also consider the possibility of bacterial tracheitis, a dangerous condition that may be confused with croup. (See Croup, in Chapter 29, Shortness of Breath).

Symptoms
Children

- Fever ++++
- Dysphagia +++
- Worsening sore throat +++
- Dyspnea ++++

Adults and older children

- Sore throat ++++
- Dysphagia ++++
- Anterior neck tenderness ++++
- Fever ++

Most children but few adults need an artificial airway established. Predictors of airway intervention include sitting erect, stridor, and shorter time to symptom onset (<8 hours).

Signs
Children

- Fever ++++
- Stridor ++++
- Drooling +++
- Muffled voice ++++
- Tripod position with neck extended
- Children less than 2 years old may look less toxic and be less symptomatic. Half may have a barking cough resembling croup.

Adults

- Neck tenderness ++++
- Dyspnea +++
- Posterior pharyngitis ++
- Fever ++
- Dysphonia ++
- Stridor ++
- Sitting erect ++
- Drooling ++

Workup

- Children with a high likelihood of having epiglottitis and who are not at risk of immediate airway compromise should be taken to the operating room for evaluation and treatment. X-rays or other measures that cause agitation should generally not be performed in the ED, since patients with epiglottitis are at risk for acute airway obstruction. Although one study of children found that use of a tongue depressor for visualization was safe, younger children should proceed directly to the operating room for any diagnostic or therapeutic procedure.

- Lateral x-rays of soft tissue of neck: ++++ in adults, +++ in children (Fig. 30-1). They are not adequately sensitive to rule out epiglottitis.
- Indirect laryngoscopy in adults and older children ++++
- Direct laryngoscopy +++++
- Blood and throat cultures have low yield.

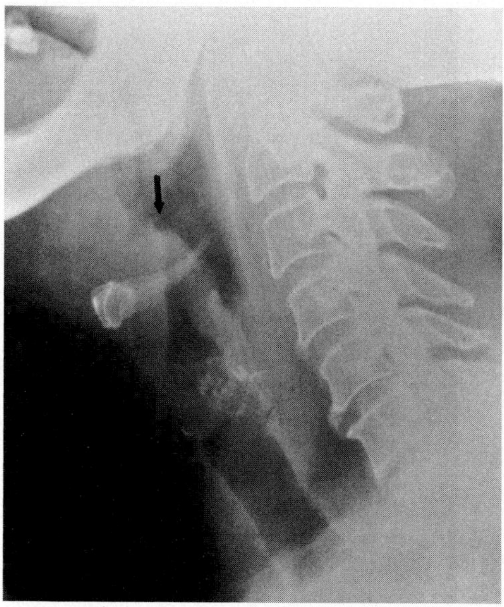

Fig. 30-1 Epiglottitis. Upright lateral view of neck. Enlarged abnormal epiglottis *(arrow)*. (Courtesy Michael Zucker, MD, Los Angeles.)

- Leukocytosis is common but nonspecific and does not change management.

Comments and Treatment Considerations

Third-generation cephalosporins should be given early. Most adults do not need airway intervention and generally only require observation in an ICU setting. Children with epiglottitis generally require emergent intubation to protect the airway.

REFERENCES

Frantz TD, Rasgon BM, Quesenberry CP: Acute epiglottitis in adults: analysis of 129 cases, *JAMA* 272:1358, 1994.

Gorelick MH, Baker MD: Epiglottitis in children, 1979 through 1992: effects of *Haemophilus influenzae* type b immunization, *Arch Pediatr Adolesc Med* 148:47, 1994.

Mayo-Smith MF, Spinale JW, Donskey CJ, et al: Acute epiglottitis: an 18-year experience in Rhode Island, *Chest* 108:1640, 1995.

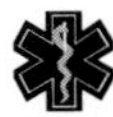

RETROPHARYNGEAL ABSCESS

Retropharyngeal abscess (RPA) is a disease seen primarily in children less than 6 years of age. This diagnosis (as well as the others discussed in this chapter) is suspected in a patient with sore throat and dysphagia that are subjectively more severe than the objective findings noted on examination. RPA is especially of concern in a child who appears ill and has limited neck mobility. Among patients with RPA, 60% had an antecedent HEENT infection (URI, pharyngitis, and otitis or mastoiditis); 40% had a history of foreign body or trauma. Adults more often have a history of intraoral procedure, foreign body or trauma, or poor dentition.

Symptoms

- Fever ++++
- Neck swelling +++
- Poor oral intake +++
- Sore throat +++
- Drooling
- Dysphagia
- Odynophagia

Signs

- Cervical adenopathy +++
- Posterior pharyngeal "bulge" or swelling +++
- Stridor ++
- Neck stiffness ++
- Atraumatic torticollis may occur and confers an increased risk of atlantoaxial subluxation.

Workup

- X-rays of soft tissue of neck ++++ : using prevertebral width criteria (>7 mm at C2 in all patients, >14 mm in children, and >22 mm in adults at C6 as abnormal) (Fig. 30-2)

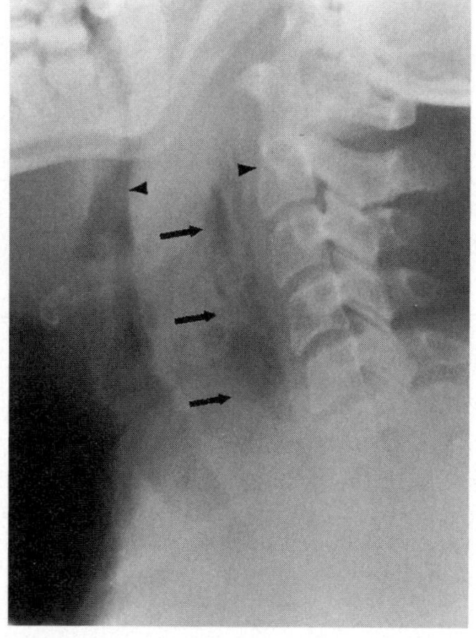

Fig. 30-2 Prevertebral/retropharyngeal abscess. Upright lateral view of neck. Prevertebral soft tissue swelling *(arrowheads)* and gas *(arrows)*. (Courtesy Michael Zucker, MD, Los Angeles.)

- CT with contrast ++++ can localize the abscess, help differentiate between abscess and cellulitis, and demonstrate atlantoaxial subluxation.
- Ultrasound has been shown in small studies to find abscesses as well as CT and may better differentiate abscess from cellulitis than CT.
- MRI may be used.

Comments and Treatment Considerations

ENT consultation is required. Antibiotic treatment should include coverage of mixed aerobic-anaerobic infection (e.g., penicillin 24 million units daily divided q4-6h and metronidazole 1 g load then 0.5 g q6h). Abscesses need to be incised and drained.

REFERENCES

Bank DE, Krug SE: New approaches to upper airway disease, *Emerg Med Clin* 13:473, 1995.

Tannebaum RD: Adult retropharyngeal abscess: a case report and review of the literature, *J Emerg Med* 14:147, 1996.

Thompson JW, Cohen SR, Reddix P: Retropharyngeal abscess in children: a retrospective and historical analysis, *Laryngoscope* 98:589, 1988.

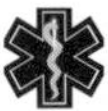

LUDWIG'S ANGINA

Ludwig's angina is a progressive cellulitis of the floor of the mouth that may lead to tongue displacement and airway obstruction. The infection begins in the submandibular space and may extend to the soft tissues of the mouth and neck. Ludwig's angina commonly originates from a dental infection after a recent dental procedure. Other causes include penetrating injury of the mouth floor, mandibular fracture, sialadenitis, and recent intravenous drug injection into neck veins. Diagnosis is primarily clinically based, and early recognition is important because the infection can rapidly lead to airway compromise.

Symptoms

- Dental pain ++++ (especially mandibular second or third molar)
- Neck swelling +++
- Dysphagia +++
- Neck pain +++
- Dyspnea and stridor ++
- Dysphonia ++
- Tongue swelling ++
- Sore throat ++

Signs

- Submandibular swelling with brawny induration +++++ (Fig. 30-3)
- Elevated, protruding tongue +++++
- Fever ++++
- Trismus +++
- Generally no fluctuance or lymphadenopathy

Workup

- The diagnosis should be apparent during clinical examination.
- Lateral x-ray of soft tissue of neck ++++ : submandibular soft tissue swelling
- CT with contrast: for stable patients; helps differentiate cellulitis (the majority of cases) from abscess, the latter requiring surgical drainage
- X-ray panoramic view may identify a dental focus of infection.
- Blood cultures are generally not helpful.

Comments and Treatment Considerations

Typical causative organisms are *Streptococcus viridans, Staphylococcus aureus, S. epidermidis,* and anaerobes. Greater than 50% of infections are polymicrobial, and aggressive treatment with intravenous antibiotics (e.g., penicillin 24 million units daily divided q4-6h and metronidazole 1 g load then 0.5 g q6h) is usually effective. Surgical intervention and early antibiotic therapy have obviated the need for tracheostomy in most patients.

REFERENCES

Har-El G, Aroesty JH, Shaha A, et al: Changing trends in deep neck abscess, *Oral Surg Oral Med Oral Pathol* 77:446, 1994.

Juang YC, Cheng DL, Wang LS, et al: Ludwig's angina: an analysis of 14 cases, *Scand J Infect Dis* 21:121, 1989.

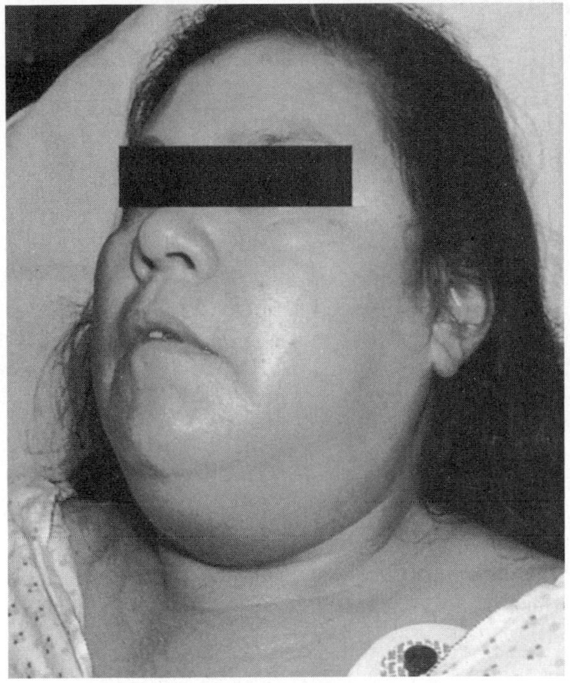

Fig. 30-3 Submandibular swelling with brawny induration. (Courtesy Jeffrey Finkelstein, MD.)

Moreland LW, Corey J, McKenzie R: Ludwig's angina: report of a case and review of the literature, *Arch Intern Med* 148:461, 1988.

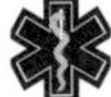 *PARAPHARYNGEAL ABSCESS*

Parapharyngeal abscess (PPA) is a rare cause of deep space infection. It is caused by dental infection (30%), peritonsillar abscess (PTA), pharyngeal infections, mastoiditis, or parotitis and may spread rapidly and extend into the mediastinum and soft tissues of the neck, leading to airway obstruction, erosion into the carotid artery, suppurative mediastinitis, and sepsis.

Symptoms

- Pain and swelling of the upper neck +++++
- Fever ++++
- Odynophagia ++++
- Trismus +++
- Sore throat
- Torticollis (rare)
- History of recent dental problem

Signs

- Displacement of lateral pharyngeal wall toward the midline
- Brawny or erythematous lateral neck swelling
- Palpable, usually nonfluctuant tender mass below the angle of the mandible ++++
- Stridor +++
- Respiratory distress (rare)

Workup

- CT of neck and cervical spine in patients with stable airways; if evidence of mediastinitis, include entire thorax
- Posteroanterior and lateral neck x-rays show nonspecific soft tissue swelling.
- WBC and blood cultures do not influence management.

Comments and Treatment Considerations

Attention is given to airway management first. Patients with PPA need to be admitted to the hospital for surgical drainage or CT-guided aspiration and intravenous antibiotics. The first dose of antibiotics (e.g., high-dose penicillin 24 million units daily divided q4-6h and metronidazole 1 g load then 0.5 g q6h) should be initiated in the ED.

REFERENCES

DeMarie S, Tham R, van der Mey AGL, et al: Clinical infections and non-surgical treatment of parapharyngeal space infections complicating throat infection, *Rev Infect Dis* 2:975, 1989.

Ortiz JA, Hudkins C, Kornblut A: Adenitis, adenopathy, and abscesses of the head and neck, *Emerg Med Clin North Am* 5:359, 1987.

Sethi DS, Stanley RE: Parapharyngeal abscesses, *J Laryngol Otol* 105:1025, 1991.

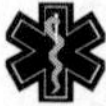 *PERITONSILLAR ABSCESS*

Peritonsillar abscess (PTA) is diagnosed through clinical examination and most commonly results from tonsillitis. Large abscesses may displace the uvula laterally and lead to respiratory compromise if not treated. PTA is rare in individuals under 6 years and over 40 years. Peritonsillar cellulitis (PTC) has a similar presentation, but no fluctuance is noted on physical examination.

Symptoms

- Odynophagia +++++
- Sore throat +++++
- Dysphagia ++++
- Drooling ++++
- Otalgia ++++
- Voice change ++++
- Fever +++
- History of recent tonsillitis +++ or prior PTA ++
- Length of symptoms, age, and degree of fever do not help differentiate PTA from PTC.

Signs

- Unilateral peritonsillar edema and fluctuance +++++
- Trismus ++++
- Uvular deviation to the opposite side of the abscess with inferior or medial displacement of the tonsil
- Exudative tonsillitis ++

Workup

- Diagnosis is generally established by clinical examination.
- Needle aspiration of abscess can confirm diagnosis and also be therapeutic.
- Contrast CT +++++ may be used if other nonlocalized infections are a diagnostic consideration.
- Intraoral ultrasound can distinguish between PTA and PTC +++++ but is rarely needed.
- WBC, blood, and abscess cultures do not influence management.

Comments and Treatment Considerations

PTA should be suspected in patients with symptoms more

severe than would be expected with usual tonsillitis or with a sore throat that worsens despite treatment.

Success rates of needle aspiration followed by oral antibiotics are similar to those for incision and drainage (80% to 90%). Possible complications include carotid artery laceration and pulmonary aspiration of pus.

Despite high rates of beta-lactamase-producing anaerobes in PTA (up to 50% in two studies), penicillin is effective in the majority after a drainage procedure. Clindamycin or metronidazole may be added for treatment failures (10%).

REFERENCES

Ophir D, Bawnik J, Poria Y: Peritonsillar abscess: a prospective evaluation of outpatient management by needle aspiration, *Arch Otolaryngol Head Neck Surg* 114:661, 1988.

Patel KS, Delis V, Oyarzabal M: Clinical differentiation of peritonsillar cellulitis from abscess, *Adv Otorhinolaryngol* 47:172, 1992.

Snow DG, Campbell JB, Morgan DW: The management of peritonsillar sepsis by needle aspiration, *Clin Otolaryngol* 16:245, 1991.

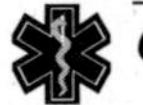

CROUP

See Chapter 29, Shortness of Breath.

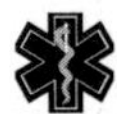

DIPHTHERIA

Diphtheria is a rare disease in the United States due to immunization. Although diphtheria can infect the skin or respiratory tract, pharyngeal disease leading to airway compromise is the most immediately life-threatening complication. Diphtheria produces an exotoxin that can cause cardiovascular, neurologic, and renal dysfunction.

Symptoms

- Sore throat
- Low-grade fever
- Dysphagia
- Croupy cough (in children with laryngeal involvement)

Signs

- Exudative membrane: a thin, leathery, exudative tonsillar, uvular, palatal, pharyngeal, or nasal membrane, varying in color from light gray to black, that may bleed profusely if removed, is the *sine qua non* of respiratory disease +++.
- Intrinsic and extrinsic eye muscle dysfunction, dysphonia, or other signs of neurologic deficit may be present.

Workup

- Throat culture (request culture for diphtheria) +++++
- Plasma clearance rate helps differentiate toxic from nontoxic strains.

Comments and Treatment Considerations

Treatment consists of antitoxin therapy and erythromycin, although some resistance to erythromycin has been noted. Airway management is the highest priority when compromised. Neurologic dysfunction is generally self-limited.

REFERENCES[www]

Harnisch JP, Tronca E, Nolan CM, et al: Diphtheria among alcoholic urban adults: a decade of experience in Seattle, *Ann Intern Med* 111:71, 1989.

Karzon DT, Edwards KM: Diphtheria outbreaks in immunized populations, *N Engl J Med* 318:41, 1988.

Rakhmanova AG, Lumio J, Groundstroem K, et al: Diphtheria outbreak in St Petersburg: clinical characteristics of 1860 adult patients, *Scand J Infect Dis* 28:37, 1996.

[www]Additional references are available on the following web site: www.signsandsymptoms.com.

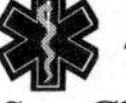 MYOCARDIAL INFARCTION

See Chapter 7, Chest Pain.

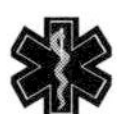 THYROIDITIS

Thyroiditis can cause anterior neck pain; see Chapter 24, Palpitations and Tachycardia.

CHAPTER 31

Syncope and Near-Syncope

ERIC SAVITSKY and RICHELLE COOPER

Syncope is defined as an acute, transient loss of consciousness with loss of postural tone and accounts for approximately 3% of all ED visits. Near-syncope should be approached in a similar fashion to syncope, as both entities share similar etiologies. The differential diagnosis is broad, ranging from benign to life-threatening conditions. History and physical examination obtained in the ED are the most useful diagnostic tools. The cause is determined in only a small minority of patients in whom the ED workup is nondiagnostic. However, even benign causes for syncope can lead to falls and significant injury, particularly in the elderly.

Approximately 50% to 60% of cases of syncope have an identifiable cause. Causes of syncope can be divided into two etiologic categories: cardiogenic and noncardiogenic. One-year mortality for cardiogenic syncope is 18% to 35% if untreated, as opposed to 6% for noncardiogenic syncope. Seizures also are characterized by transient loss of consciousness. In practice, distinguishing between an unwitnessed seizure and a syncopal event may be difficult. Certain features of the history and physical examination, such as a preceding aura, postictal period, or neurologic abnormality, make a diagnosis of seizure more likely. When a clear differentiation between a syncopal event and a seizure is not possible, patients are often hospitalized and evaluated for both conditions.

See Chapter 27, Seizure, Adult, Chapter 28, Seizure, Pediatric, and Chapter 36, Weakness and Fatigue.

CARDIOGENIC SYNCOPE

Important categories of cardiogenic syncope include arrhythmias, left ventricular outflow obstruction, right ventricular compromise, and pump failure. (Fig. 31-1).

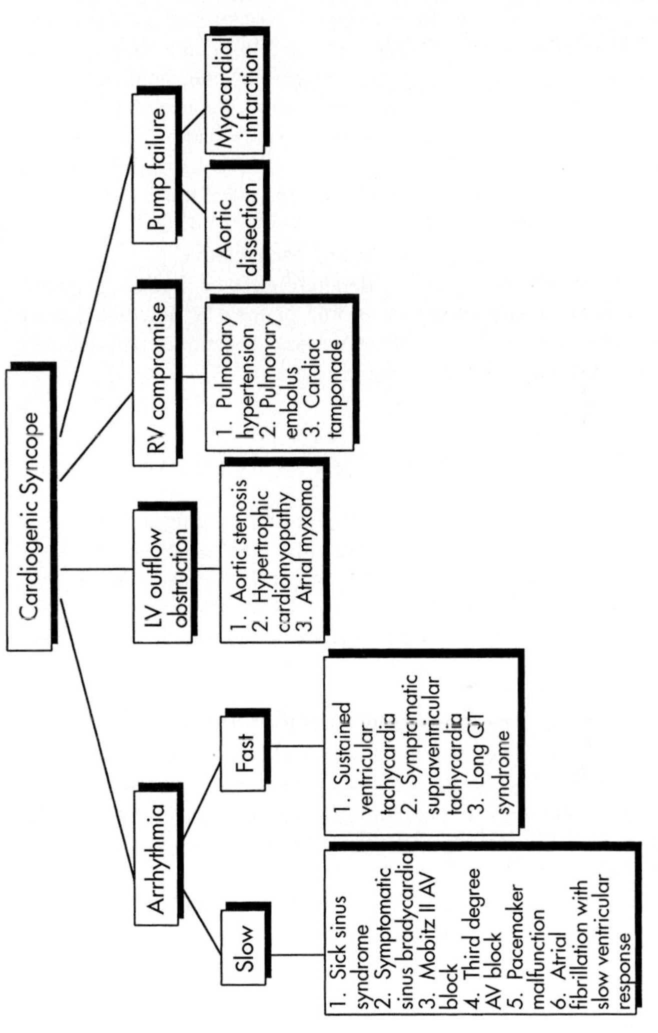

Fig. 31-1 Categories of cardiogenic syncope.

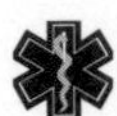

ARRHYTHMIAS

Arrhythmias are the most dangerous cause of syncope and near-syncope. Tachyarrhythmias capable of inducing syncope include sustained ventricular tachycardias and rapid supraventricular tachycardias. Bradyarrhythmias associated with syncope include sick sinus syndrome, sinus pause >3 seconds, sinus bradycardia <40 bpm, Mobitz II AV block, third-degree AV block, pacemaker malfunction, and atrial fibrillation with a slow ventricular response.

See Chapter 24, Palpitation and Tachycardia.

Symptoms and signs vary depending on the rhythm. Syncope may occur while sitting or supine or may be associated with exertion. Patients may report weakness, fatigue, palpitations, chest discomfort, or dyspnea.

Workup

- Initial monitoring yields a diagnosis in 2% to 11% of syncope patients.
- In preselected populations, 24-hour monitoring will diagnose an arrhythmia in 14% of patients. Cardiac event and loop recorders are twice as likely to produce diagnostic rhythm strips as compared to continuous 48-hour monitoring.
- Electrophysiologic studies are warranted in only a small percentage of patients.

Comments and Treatment Considerations

In a study of patients with syncope and a history of pacemaker use, only 6.5% of the time was pacemaker malfunction the cause of syncope. These patients often have underlying cardiac disease and should be admitted for evaluation of cardiogenic syncope.

Patients with a prolonged QT interval should be considered at high risk for cardiogenic syncope and evaluated accordingly.

Patients at risk for coronary artery disease who have unexplained syncope should be evaluated for cardiogenic syncope. If no cause is found after initial evaluation, they should be admitted to a telemetry unit for further evaluation.

REFERENCES[www]

Clark PI, Glasser SP, Spoto E: Arrhythmias detected by ambulatory monitoring: lack of correlation with symptoms of dizziness and syncope, *Chest* 77:722, 1980.

Gibson TC, Heitzman MR: Diagnostic efficacy of 24-hour electrocardiographic monitoring for syncope, *Am J Cardiol* 53:1013, 1984.

Kinlay S, Leitch JW, Neil A, et al: Cardiac event recorders yield more diagnoses and are more cost-effective than 48-hour Holter monitoring in patients with palpitations: a controlled clinical trial, *Ann Intern Med* 124:16, 1996.

[www]Additional references are available on the following web site: www.signsandsymptoms.com.

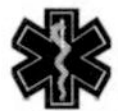

MYOCARDIAL INFARCTION

Comments and Treatment Considerations

Syncope is a presenting complaint in a small minority of all myocardial infarctions. Many patients over the age of 70 do not report chest pain during MI. In patients over the age of 85, dyspnea is the most common complaint during myocardial infarction, followed by chest pain, syncope, stroke, or altered mental status.

See Chapter 7, Chest Pain.

REFERENCES[www]

Bayer AJ, Chadha JS, Farag RR, et al: Changing presentation of myocardial infarction with increasing old age, *J Am Geriatr Soc* 34:263, 1986.

Bosker G: Assessment and triage of elderly patients with acute coronary ischemia, *Emerg Med Reports* 9:25, 1988.

Brady WJ: Missing the diagnosis of acute MI: challenging presentations, electrocardiographic pearls, and outcome—effective management strategies, *Emerg Med Reports* 18:91, 1997.

[www]Additional references are available on the following web site: www.signsandsymptoms.com.

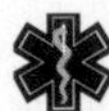

AORTIC DISSECTION

Syncope occurs in about 5% to 10% of cases of aortic dissection and may indicate aortic rupture or cardiac tamponade. Isolated syncope without other symptoms and signs is uncommon.

See Chapter 7, Chest Pain.

REFERENCES[www]

Rigolin VH, Harrison JK, Wilson JS, et al: Update on aortic dissection, *Emerg Med Reports* 17:35, 1993.

Slater EE, DeSanctis RW: The clinical recognition of dissecting aortic aneurysm, *Am J Med* 60:625, 1976.

Spittell PC, Spittell JA, Joyce JW, et al: Clinical features and differential diagnosis of aortic dissection: experience with 236 cases (1980 through 1990), *Mayo Clin Proc* 68:642, 1993.

[www]Additional references are available on the following web site: www.signsandsymptoms.com.

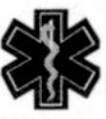

TRANSIENT ISCHEMIC ATTACKS

Transient ischemic attacks (TIAs) refer to cerebrovascular insufficiency leading to transient neurologic dysfunction. Typically, symptoms associated with vertebrobasilar artery insufficiency accompany the syncopal event. Basilar artery insufficiency may produce "drop attacks." TIAs are characterized by sudden, brief periods of paresis that cause the patient to fall down. Drop attacks are not true syncopal events because consciousness is not lost.

See Chapter 8, Dizziness (Vertigo), and Chapter 36, Weakness and Fatigue.

REFERENCES

Baloh R: Vertebrobasilar insufficiency and stroke, *Otolaryngol Head Neck Surg* 112:114, 1995.

Fields WS, Lemak NA: Joint study of extracranial arterial occlusion, VII subclavian steal—a review of 168 cases, *JAMA* 222:1139, 1972.

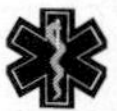

PULMONARY EMBOLUS

Syncope occurs in up to 10% of patients with pulmonary embolus. In these patients syncope is a sign of massive pulmonary embolus, with commonly more than 50% of the pulmonary circulation obstructed. Patients typically have marked acute right ventricular overload. Two-dimensional echocardiography may be helpful in these patients.

See Chapter 7, Chest Pain.

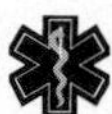

CARDIAC TAMPONADE

See Chapter 7, Chest Pain.

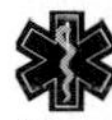

SUBARACHNOID HEMORRHAGE

Up to 50% of patients have a transient loss of consciousness after rupture of an intracranial aneurysm. These patients commonly exhibit other signs and symptoms of subarachnoid hemorrhage, which can be elicited during a careful history and physical examination.

See Chapter 15, Headache.

REFERENCES[www]

Fontanarosa PB: Recognition of subarachnoid hemorrhage, *Ann Emerg Med* 18:1199, 1989.

Sawin PD, Loftus CM: Diagnosis of spontaneous subarachnoid hemorrhage, *Am Fam Physician* 55:145, 1997.

Vermeulen M: Subarachnoid haemorrhage: diagnosis and treatment, *J Neurol* 243:496, 1996.

[www]Additional references are available on the following web site: www.signsandsymptoms.com.

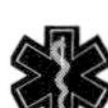

ECTOPIC PREGNANCY

See Chapter 34, Vaginal Bleeding.

AORTIC STENOSIS

Symptoms

- Angina
- Dyspnea
- Orthopnea
- Peripheral edema
- Syncope
- Symptoms are often exertional.

Signs

- Cardiac auscultation: normal S1, soft A2 or single S2, loud S4, and a harsh crescendo-decrescendo systolic murmur at the right upper sternal border radiating to the carotids. Loudness of the murmur may diminish and length may increase as the stenosis becomes more severe.
- Classic delayed and diminished carotid upstrokes are often not present in the elderly because of the inelasticity of the vascular system in this population.
- Narrow pulse pressure may be noted.

Workup

- ECG commonly shows evidence of left ventricular hypertrophy and possibly left atrial enlargement.
- Echocardiography is a rapid diagnostic test that can demonstrate abnormal valve function and estimate gradients across the valve.
- Chest x-rays are nondiagnostic. A calcified aortic valve is often seen in the elderly but often indicates benign aortic sclerosis.
- Cardiac catheterization is the gold standard for determining the degree of stenosis and valve area.

Comments and Treatment Considerations

Mean survival after the onset of angina is 5 years, after the onset of syncope, 3 years, and after congestive heart failure (CHF) symptoms, 2 years.

Symptoms typically develop when the valve area is less than 1 to 1.5 cm^2 and valve gradients exceed 50 mm Hg.

The incidence of sudden death is high once symptoms develop. Any patient with a suspected aortic stenosis related syncope should be hospitalized pending a cardiologist's evaluation.

Caution should be taken when treating angina or symptoms of congestive heart failure (CHF), because overdiuresis or nitrate-induced preload reduction may lead to dramatic and potentially irreversible hypotension.

REFERENCES[www]

Ross J Jr, Braunwald E: Aortic stenosis, *Circulation* 38(suppl):61, 1968.

Wilson JS, Hearne SE, Harrison JK, et al: How to recognize—and manage—aortic stenosis in the elderly, *J Crit Illness* 9:42, 1994.

[www]Additional references are available on the following web site: www.signsandsymptoms.com.

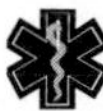

HYPERTROPHIC CARDIOMYOPATHY

Hypertrophic cardiomyopathy is a condition characterized by an hypertrophied, nondilated left ventricle. It is the most common cause of sudden death in young athletes.

Symptoms

- Dyspnea +++
- Angina +++
- Syncope ++
- Symptoms typically are exertional.

Signs

- Cardiac auscultation: mimics aortic stenosis with normal S1, normal S2, and dynamic crescendo-decrescendo, harsh systolic murmur that is heard best between the apex and left sternal border. The murmur is classically accentuated with decreased preload (standing or Valsalva) and is softer with increased preload (squatting).
- Carotid upstrokes are brisk, unlike aortic stenosis.

Workup

- ECG may show evidence of left ventricular hypertrophy. Q waves in the precordial leads +++ represent depolarization of the hypertrophied myocardial septum.
- Chest x-rays demonstrate cardiomegaly +++
- Two-dimensional echocardiography: definitive, demonstrating a thickened ventricular wall with hyperdynamic ejection and abnormal relaxation phase
- Holter monitoring frequently detects arrhythmias, often ventricular +++.
- Stress testing may also be valuable because of the exertional nature of symptoms.

Comments and Treatment Considerations

The etiology of hypertrophic cardiomyopathy–related syncope is multifactorial and may be associated with outflow obstruction, arrhythmia, or ischemia.

Inherited and sporadic forms of this disease exist. This diagnosis is often not considered in the elderly; however, one third of cases occur in patients over 60 years of age.

REFERENCES[www]

Baughman KL: Hypertrophic cardiomyopathy, *JAMA* 267:846, 1992.

Lipsitz LA: Syncope in the elderly, *Ann Intern Med* 99:92, 1983.

Spirito P, Seidman CE, McKenna WJ, et al: The management of hypertrophic cardiomyopathy, *N Engl J Med* 336:775, 1997.

[www]Additional references are available on the following web site: www.signsandsymptoms.com.

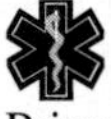

PULMONARY HYPERTENSION

Primary pulmonary hypertension occurs in familial and sporadic forms and has been linked to the use of certain diet pills. Secondary pulmonary hypertension occurs as a result of many disorders including COPD, chronic hypoventilation, sleep apnea, left ventricle dysfunction, mitral stenosis, small multiple pulmonary emboli, and congenital cardiac shunts. Women represent the majority of cases of primary pulmonary hypertension. Symptoms tend to be present for some time, up to 1 to 3 years before diagnosis.

Symptoms

- Dyspnea +++ is the most common presenting symptom and occurs in all patients as the disease progresses.
- Syncope or near-syncope +++ , particularly with exertion
- Fatigue ++
- Chest pain ++
- Raynaud's phenomenon +

Signs

- Cardiac auscultation: loud P2; may have a systolic ejection murmur, S3 or S4
- Signs of right ventricular failure (late)

Workup

- Electrocardiography often shows evidence of right ventricular hypertrophy.
- Chest x-rays may demonstrate right ventricular hypertrophy and often reveal enlarged central pulmonary arteries.
- Echocardiography will rule out valvular and congenital cardiac lesions, as well as provide an estimate of pulmonary artery systolic pressure.
- Right heart catheterization is diagnostic for pulmonary hypertension.

Comments and Treatment Considerations

Patients with pulmonary hypertension and right ventricular dysfunction are at increased risk for pulmonary thromboembolic events, which may also cause syncope.

REFERENCES[www]

Hughes JD, Rubin JL: Primary pulmonary hypertension: an analysis of 28 cases and a review of the literature, *Medicine* 65:56, 1986.

Rubin JL: Primary pulmonary hypertension, *N Engl J Med* 336:111, 1997.

[www]Additional references are available on the following web site: www.signsandsymptoms.com.

NONCARDIOGENIC SYNCOPE

Noncardiogenic syncope can be subdivided into several categories (Fig. 31-2).

NEUROCARDIOGENIC (VASOVAGAL) SYNCOPE

Symptoms

- A history of identifiable triggering events, including pain, emotional stress, or anxiety related to "fight-or-flight" situations. Previous history of similar episodes.
- Presyncopal or prodromal phase lasting a few seconds to a few minutes is often reported.
- Symptoms during the prodrome include a sense of lightheadedness +++, diaphoresis ++, headache or visual changes ++, epigastric discomfort, nausea, and vomiting ++.

Signs

- Normal physical examination is most often noted.
- Decreased heart rate and low blood pressure are noted if the patient is still symptomatic.

Workup

- Complete history and physical examination to rule out life-threatening causes of syncope
- Head-upright, tilt-table testing is advocated by some to confirm diagnosis; however, the accuracy of these tests is controversial.

Comments and Treatment Considerations

The diagnosis of vasovagal disorder in new-onset syncope should be made with hesitation in patients at risk for cardiac disease.

Episodes typically occur while the patient is standing and are uncommon in the supine or seated position.

Patients should be warned that syncope might recur when they are exposed to similar inciting triggers. The syncopal event can be aborted if the patient lies down during the prodromal phase.

All patients undergoing ED procedures should be placed in a protective position because vasovagal syncope may occur.

REFERENCES[www]

Grubb BP, Kosinski D: Current trends in etiology, diagnosis, and management of neurocardiogenic syncope, *Curr Opin Cardiol* 11:32, 1996.

Kapoor W: Evaluation and management of the patient with syncope, *JAMA* 268:2553, 1992.

[www]Additional references are available on the following web site: www.signsandsymptoms.com.

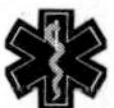

CAROTID SINUS SYNCOPE

Carotid sinus syncope is carotid sinus hypersensitivity leading to episodes of acute decrease in blood pressure. Attacks of syncope are precipitated by shaving, sudden turning of the head, or a tight collar and typically occur in elderly patients.

Workup

- Carotid massage: The patient is placed in the supine position, with ECG and blood pressure monitoring, and the carotid artery is massaged for 5 to 40 seconds. A decline in systolic blood pressure of >50 mm Hg or asystole >3 seconds is considered diagnostic. This test is infrequently done in the ED setting. Both carotids should not be massaged simultaneously.

Comments and Treatment Considerations

Carotid sinus hypersensitivity is found in 5% to 25% of patients without symptoms, and only 5% to 33% of these individuals have spontaneous symptoms.

These patients often have a history of either a tissue scar or a neck tumor arising from the carotid body, parotid gland, thyroid gland, or lymph node.

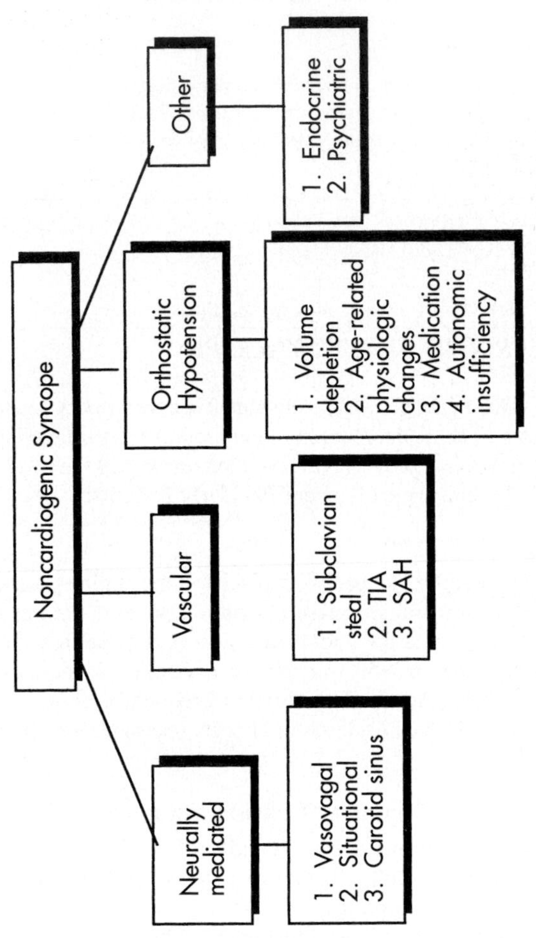

Fig. 31-2 Categories of noncardiogenic syncope.

REFERENCES[www]

Kapoor WN: Syncope in older persons, *J Am Geriatr Soc* 42:426, 1994.
Lipsitz LA: Syncope in the elderly, *Ann Intern Med* 99:92, 1983.

[www]Additional references are available on the following web site: www.signsandsymptoms.com.

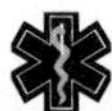

ORTHOSTATIC HYPOTENSION

In orthostatic hypotension, syncope occurs immediately after rising from a sitting or supine position and often is associated with weakness, diaphoresis, headache, visual changes, and epigastric discomfort.

See Hypovolemia in Chapter 36, Weakness and Fatigue.

REFERENCES[www]

Atkins D, Hanusa B, Sefcik T, et al: Syncope and orthostatic hypotension, *Am J Med* 91:179, 1991.
Hanlon JT, Linzer M, Macmillan NJP, et al: Syncope and presyncope associated with probable adverse drug reactions, *Arch Intern Med* 150:2309, 1990.
Kapoor W: Syncope in older persons, *J Am Geriatr Soc* 42:426, 1994.

[www]Additional references are available on the following web site: www.signsandsymptoms.com.

CHAPTER 32

Toxic Ingestion, Approach to

MICHAEL J. BURNS and RICHARD OH

An estimated 5 million poison exposures occur annually in the United States. Not infrequently, the ED physician is faced with an uncooperative, unreliable, or unresponsive poisoned patient and is required to rapidly assess the severity of illness, make a diagnosis, and provide sound initial treatment, often without the results of complete history or extensive laboratory tests. A systematic and consistent approach to the evaluation and treatment of poisoning is therefore necessary. Evaluation involves poisoning recognition, identification of agents involved, assessment of severity, and prediction of toxicity. Treatment involves the provision of supportive care, prevention of poison absorption, and, when necessary, the administration of antidotes and enhancement of poison elimination. The tempo, sequence, methods, and priorities of treatment are determined by the agent(s) involved and the presenting and predicted severity of poisoning.

STEPWISE APPROACH TO ALL POISONED PATIENTS

1. ABCs with ACLS measures as necessary
2. Maintain in-line cervical immobilization in those with suspected co-existing trauma
3. IV, O_2, cardiac monitoring, ECG
4. Rapid initial screening physical examination: vital signs (including pulse oximetry and rectal temperature), mental status, and pupillary assessment
5. For those with altered mental status:
   a. Thiamine 100 mg IV (alcoholic or at risk for vitamin deficiency)
   b. Dextrostick or empiric glucose administration. Dose: adult 50 ml of D50 IV; child 2 to 4 ml/kg D25 IV

   c. Consider naloxone (0.1 to 2.0 mg IV). Doses up to 10 mg necessary for certain synthetic opioids (e.g., propoxyphene).
6. Consider flumazenil (0.1 to 1.0 mg) only in those with known isolated benzodiazepine ingestion who have CNS or respiratory depression and ECG reveals QRS <100 msec (i.e., severe CA unlikely). May precipitate seizures in those with mixed ingestion (e.g., TCA), underlying seizure disorder, or those treated with a complete coma-reversing dose (e.g., acute benzodiazepine withdrawal). Flumazenil is *not* recommended for routine use.
7. Endotracheal intubation for those who remain in severe respiratory distress or are unable to protect their airway
8. Detailed history and physical examination (see Symptoms and Signs)
9. Directed toxicologic laboratory evaluations (see Workup)
10. Initiate patient decontamination (e.g., removal of contaminated clothing, topical irrigation, activated charcoal [AC], gastric lavage, whole bowel irrigation [WBI], and endoscopic or surgical removal). Gastric lavage may be considered but is rarely indicated for most toxic ingestions (see Comments and Treatment Considerations).
11. Antidote administration as indicated (see Table 32-3)
12. Enhanced elimination techniques (e.g., forced diuresis, urinary pH manipulation, multidose AC, hemodialysis, hemoperfusion, hemofiltration, exchange transfusion, hyperbaric oxygen [HBO]) (see Table 32-4)
13. Supportive care

SYMPTOMS AND SIGNS

Symptoms obtained by history and signs by physical examination may be used to establish and confirm a diagnosis of poisoning. A group of signs and symptoms that are often associated with a particular poison or type of poison is referred to as a *toxidrome*. Familiarity with common toxidromes is important to the practicing ED physician and allows for clinical recognition of toxin patterns (Table 32-1).

Text continued on p. 434

Table 32-1 Toxidromes

Toxidrome	Symptoms	Signs	Examples of Toxic Agents
Sympathomimetic	Agitation Hallucinations Headache Nausea, vomiting Palpitations Paranoia Tremors	CNS: **Agitation**, hyperalert, delirium, seizures, **coma** VS: **Hypertension**, widened pulse pressure, **tachycardia,** widened pulse pressure, tachypnea, hyperpnea, hyperthermia Pupils: **Mydriasis** Other: **Diaphoresis**, tremors, hyperreflexia, flushed or pale skin	Cocaine Amphetamines Ephedrine Pseudoephedrine Phenylpropanolamine Theophylline Caffeine Albuterol Methylphenidate
Anticholinergic	Agitation Hallucinations Mumbling speech Unresponsive	CNS: **Agitation**, **delirium**, hypervigilance, mumbling speech, hallucinations, coma VS: Hyperthermia, **tachycardia**, hypertension, tachypnea Pupils: **Mydriasis** Other: **Dry flushed skin**, **dry mucous membranes**, decreased bowel sounds, urinary retention, myoclonus, choreoathetosis, picking behavior, seizures (rare)	Antihistamines Tricyclic antidepressants Cyclobenzaprine Orphenadrine Antiparkinson agents Antispasmodics Phenothiazines Atropine Scopolamine

		Mnemonic: "**Hot as a hare, blind as a bat, dry as a bone, red as a beet, mad as a hatter**"	Belladonna alkaloids (e.g., Jimson weed)
Hallucinogenic	Hallucinations Perceptual distortions Depersonalization Synesthesia Agitation	CNS: **Hallucinations**, depersonalization, agitation VS: Hyperthermia, tachycardia, hypertension, tachypnea Pupils: Mydriasis (usually) Other: Nystagmus	Phencyclidine LSD Mescaline Psilocybin Designer amphetamines (e.g., MDMA, MDEA, STP, DOM)
Opioid	Lethargy Confusion Unresponsive	CNS: **Lethargy**, coma, confusion VS: Hypothermia, bradycardia, hypotension, hypopnea, **bradypnea** Pupils: **Miosis** (usually) Other: Hyporeflexia, pulmonary edema, **needle marks**	Heroin Morphine Meperidine Methadone Oxycodone Hydrocodone Fentanyl Hydromorphone Diphenoxylate Loperamide Propoxyphene Pentazocine

Terms in **bold** are common findings.

Continued.

Table 32-1 Toxidromes—cont'd

Toxidrome	Symptoms	Signs	Examples of Toxic Agents
Sedative-hypnotic	Confusion Stupor Unresponsive Slurred speech	CNS: **Lethargy**, coma, confusion, dysarthria, ataxia VS: Hypothermia, bradycardia, hypotension, hypopnea, **bradypnea** Pupils: Miosis (usually) Other: Hyporeflexia, nystagmus	Benzodiazepines Barbiturates Carisoprodol Meprobamate Glutethimide Alcohols Zolpidem
Cholinergic	Confusion Unresponsive SOB Cramps Nausea, vomiting Diarrhea Weakness Seizures Drooling	CNS: **Agitation**, coma, confusion, seizures VS: **Bradycardia**, hypertension or hypotension, tachypnea or bradypnea Pupils: **Miosis** (not universal) Other: **Salivation, urinary and fecal incontinence**, diarrhea, **emesis**, **diaphoresis**, **lacrimation**, GI cramps, bronchoconstriction, muscle fasciculations, weakness	Organophosphate and carbamate insecticides Nerve agents Nicotine Pilocarpine Physostigmine Edrophonium Bethanechol Urecholine Neostigmine Pyridostigmine

Serotonin syndrome	Lethargy Confusion Agitation Tremulous	CNS: Agitation, lethargy, coma, **confusion**, delirium VS: **Hyperthermia**, tachycardia, hypertension, tachypnea Pupils: Mydriasis Other: Tremor, myoclonus, hyperreflexia, clonus, diaphoresis, flushing, trismus, rigidity, diarrhea	MAOIs alone or with: SSRIs, meperidine, dextromethorphan, TCAs, L-tryptophan, trazodone, nefazodone
Cyclic antidepressant	Confusion Agitation Unresponsive Slurred speech	CNS: Lethargy, coma, confusion, seizures VS: Hyperthermia, **tachycardia**, hypertension then hypotension, hypopnea Pupils: **Mydriasis** Other: **Dry skin**, **myoclonus**, choreoathetosis, cardiac arrhythmias and conduction disturbances	Amitriptyline Nortriptyline Imipramine Clomipramine Desipramine Doxepin Trimipramine
Sympatholytic	Lethargy Confusion Unresponsive	CNS: Lethargy, confusion, coma, seizures (uncommonly) VS: **Bradycardia**, hypotension, bradypnea, hypopnea Pupils: **Miosis** (often)	Alpha-adrenergic antagonists (e.g., prazosin) Beta-blockers (e.g., propranolol) Calcium channel blockers (e.g., verapamil, diltiazem) $Alpha_2$-adrenergic agonists (e.g., clonidine)

Terms in **bold** are common findings.

Continued.

Table 32-1 Toxidromes—cont'd

Toxidrome	Symptoms	Signs	Examples of Toxic Agents
Digitalis and other cardiac glycosides	Anorexia Nausea Vomiting Diarrhea Lethargy Weakness Dizziness Vertigo Visual disturbances (xanthopsia, chromatopsia) Syncope	CNS: Normal or lethargy and confusion VS: Bradycardia, hypotension Pupils: Normal Other: **Cardiac arrhythmias** and **conduction disturbances**	Digoxin Digitoxin *Digitalis purpurea* (foxglove) *Digitalis lantana* *Nerium oleander* (oleander) *Thevetia peruviana* (yellow oleander) *Convallaria majalis* (lily of the valley) *Urginea maritima* (red squill)

Extrapyramidal Dystonia Akathisia Parkinsonism	Anxious Inability to talk	CNS: Alert and oriented, anxious, dysarthria, mutism VS: Normal Pupils: Normal Other: **Oculogyric crisis**, **facial grimacing, torticollis,** buccolingual spasm, tremor, rigidity, involuntary movements, opisthotonus, bradykinesia, masked facies, akathisia	Antipsychotics (e.g., haloperidol, phenothiazines, molindone) Antiemetics (e.g., droperidol, prochlorperazine, metoclopramide)

Terms in **bold** are common findings.

HISTORY

- May be unreliable when obtained from patient; corroborate with family, friends, police, prehospital personnel, patient's physician, and pharmacist
- Thoroughly search exposure environment for pill bottles, suicide note, drug paraphernalia
- Obtain time, route, and location of exposure, reason for exposure
- Inquire specifically about OTC drugs
- Correlate history with physical examination and ancillary test results

PHYSICAL EXAMINATION

1. Vital signs, mental status, skin findings, and pupillary signs are most useful and allow for patient classification into a state of physiologic stimulation or depression.
2. Physiologic stimulation (increased P, BP, RR, T, agitation, seizures, and mydriasis) commonly occurs from:
   a. Sympathomimetics
   b. Anticholinergics
   c. Central hallucinogens
   d. Drug withdrawal states
3. Physiologic depression (decreased P, BP, RR, T, lethargy, coma, and miosis) commonly occurs from:
   a. Sympatholytics
   b. Cholinergics
   c. Opiates
   d. Sedative-hypnotics and alcohols
4. Mixed physiologic effects from:
   a. Polydrug overdoses
   b. Metabolic poisons (e.g., hypoglycemic agents, salicylates, cyanide)
   c. Heavy metals (e.g., arsenic, iron, lead, lithium, mercury)
   d. Membrane-active agents (e.g., volatile inhalants, antiarrhythmics, local anesthetic agents)
   e. Agents with multiple mechanisms of action (e.g., cyclic antidepressants)

WORKUP

- Ancillary studies may be useful to confirm, establish, or refute poisoning diagnosis. Tests ordered should be guided by history and physical examination.
- ECG is recommended for all intentional poisonings or those involving cardiotoxic agents. ECG provides clues for diagnosis (e.g., sinus tachycardia and QRS prolongation for CA poisoning).
- Symptomatic patients or those with unreliable or unknown history should minimally have measurements of serum electrolytes (calculate anion gap), BUN, creatinine, glucose, urinalysis.
- Routine urine pregnancy testing is recommended in women of childbearing age.
- ABG, co-oximetry, serum osmolality, and lactate measurements are recommended in patients with acid-base, cardiovascular, neurologic, or respiratory disturbances.
- An anion gap metabolic acidosis should prompt measurement of serum Ca^{2+}, creatinine, glucose, ketones, lactate, osmolality, salicylates, toxic alcohols, and examination of the urine for crystals.
- Liver function tests and PT (INR) should be performed for acetaminophen or other hepatotoxic agent ingestions.
- Toxic screening should minimally include serum measurements of acetaminophen and salicylate in those with intentional poisoning or uncertain history.
- Comprehensive toxic screening is rarely necessary or indicated, particularly when patients are asymptomatic or have clinical findings consistent with history. A toxicologic screen for drugs of abuse is also generally unnecessary.
- At times, obtaining quantitative levels of toxins is necessary to determine or predict the severity of poisoning and guide treatment (see the box on p. 436).

COMMENTS AND TREATMENT CONSIDERATIONS

Management strategies are dictated by the poison involved, presenting and predicted severity of illness, and time of presenta-

DRUGS FOR WHICH QUANTIFICATION OF LEVEL MAY BE USEFUL	
Acetaminophen	Methanol
Carboxyhemoglobin	Ethylene glycol
Methemoglobin	Antiepileptic agents
Digoxin	Carbamazepine
Lithium	Phenytoin
Theophylline	Valproic acid
Salicylate	Heavy metals
Paraquat	Lead
Iron	Mercury

tion in relation to time of exposure. Supportive care in conjunction with decontamination procedures is sufficient for the majority of patients.

POISON DECONTAMINATION (Table 32-2)

- The sooner decontamination is performed, the more effective it is in preventing poison absorption.
- For dermal and ocular exposures, contaminated clothing and particulate matter should be immediately removed, and exposed areas should be irrigated copiously with normal saline or tap water.
- For inhalation exposures, the patient should be immediately removed from the contaminated area and given supplemental oxygen.
- GI decontamination is recommended for all poison ingestions unless the exposure was clearly nontoxic. AC administration alone is the preferred means of GI decontamination for the majority of poison ingestions.
- AC does not effectively adsorb heavy metals, inorganic ions, corrosives, boric acid, hydrocarbons, alcohols, and essential oils.
- Gastric lavage (in addition to AC) may be useful for life-threatening ingestions (e.g., obtunded patients, lethal toxin not bound by AC) if it can be performed within 60 minutes of ingestion.

Table 32-2 Gastrointestinal Decontamination Methods

Method	Indications	Contraindications	Dosing/Technique	Complications
Activated charcoal	Consider for all poison ingestions unless clearly nontoxic	Bowel obstruction or perforation Depressed mental status and unprotected airway (intubate first) Relative: corrosive and low-viscosity hydrocarbon ingestions	1 g/kg AC or 10:1 (g:g) AC to toxicant	Nausea and vomiting Abdominal cramps Diarrhea (with sorbitol) Constipation (aqueous suspensions) Aspiration
Gastric lavage	Consider for obtunded patient or patient with life-threatening ingestion; can be performed within 60 min of ingestion Consider for life-threatening ingestion of agent not bound by AC	Corrosive ingestion Low-viscosity hydrocarbon ingestion Depressed mental status and unprotected airway (intubate first) Patient noncompliance Significant esophageal or gastric pathology	Left lateral decubitus or supine 24-28 Fr tube (pediatric); 36-40 Fr tube (adults) Gravity instillation and drainage of up to 5 L of tap water or NS	Aspiration Esophageal perforation Tracheal lavage GI bleeding Hypoxia and hypercapnia Laryngospasm Fluid and electrolyte disturbance

Continued

Table 32-2 Gastrointestinal Decontamination Methods—cont'd

Method	Indications	Contraindications	Dosing/Technique	Complications
Syrup of ipecac	Home or prehospital setting Alert patient within 15-60 min of ingestion	CNS depression Corrosive ingestion Low-viscosity hydrocarbons Agent that may rapidly compromise airway Debilitated patients Third-trimester pregnancy	0-6 mo: No SOI 6-12 mo: 10 ml 12 mo – 12 yr: 15 ml (may repeat) >12 yr: 30 ml (may repeat)	Protracted vomiting (delays administration of AC or antidotes) Lethargy Aspiration
Whole bowel irrigation	Consider for toxic foreign bodies (e.g., cocaine and heroin drug packets), SR or EC drug preparations, heavy metals (e.g., As, Fe, Li, Hg, Zn), and suspected drug concretion	Bowel obstruction, perforation, bleeding, or ileus Depressed mental status Unprotected airway (intubate first)	Polyethylene glycol EG-3350 (e.g., CoLyte) NGT administration recommended 1-6 yr: 500 ml/hr 6-12 yr: 1 L/hr >12 yr: 1-2 L/hr	Nausea and vomiting Abdominal cramps and bloating Aspiration

Cathartics	Adjunct to AC (first and only dose)	Bowel obstruction, perforation, ileus Electrolyte imbalance Hypotension Mg cathartics to those with renal failure	Sorbitol (70%): 1 g/kg or 1-2 ml/kg for all >2 yr Magnesium citrate: 4 ml/kg $MgSO_4$: 250 mg/kg	Nausea, vomiting, diarrhea Abdominal cramps and bloating Dehydration Hypotension Hypernatremia Hypermagnesemia Viscus perforation Aspiration
Endoscopic surgery	Pharmacobezoars Heavy metals in stomach Surgery for those with suspected ruptured cocaine packets	Endoscopy should *not* be used to remove drug packets (high risk for iatrogenic rupture)		
Dilution	Corrosive ingestion	Vomiting patient	5 ml/kg milk or water (up to 250 ml)	Vomiting and increased toxic exposure

- Many believe whole bowel irrigation (WBI) is useful for patients who have ingested heavy metals (e.g., arsenic, iron, and lithium), drug packets ("body stuffer" or "body packer"), sustained-release or enteric-coated preparations, or those who are suspected to have drug concretions (pharmacobezoars).
- Syrup of ipecac is *not* recommended for hospital use.

ANTIDOTES

Antidotes are not commonly available for most toxic agents and are used in only about 1% of poison exposures. Common antidotes and their doses are listed in Table 32-3. It is appropriate to administer an antidote when the expected benefits of therapy outweigh its associated risk.

ENHANCED ELIMINATION TECHNIQUES (Table 32-4)

In approximately 1% of poison exposures it becomes necessary to accelerate the removal of absorbed toxins using enhanced elimination techniques. In a few selected cases, an aggressive approach to elimination can be lifesaving. Enhanced elimination techniques should be considered when a patient fails to or is unlikely to respond to maximal supportive care and the predicted benefit of the intervention outweighs its risks of complications. Consultation with a toxicologist is recommended.

SUPPORTIVE CARE

Supportive care is frequently all that is necessary to effect good patient outcome.

Hypertension

If treatment is needed, hypertension is best treated initially with nonspecific sedation (e.g., benzodiazepines). When it is associated with end-organ dysfunction, hypertension is best treated with calcium channel blockers (e.g., verapamil), phentolamine, or a combination of nitroprusside with a beta-blocker. Beta-blockers should not be used alone in sympathomimetic states (e.g., cocaine), since they may precipitate unopposed alpha-adrenergic vasoconstriction.

Text continued on p. 448

Table 32-3 Common Antidotes

Poison	Antidote(s)	Dose
Acetaminophen	*N*-Acetylcysteine (Mucomyst 20%)	Initial oral dose: 140 mg/kg, then 70 mg/kg q4h × 17 doses
Anticholinergic agents*	Physostigmine (Antilirium)	Initial dose: 0.5-2.0 mg slow IV over 3-5 min; children: 0.02 mg/kg
Benzodiazepines*	Flumazenil (Romazicon)	Initial dose: 0.1-0.2 mg IV over 30-60 sec, repeat 0.1-0.2 mg IV every minute prn up to 1.0 mg
β-Blockers	Glucagon	Initial dose: 5-10 mg IV bolus, then 2-10 mg/hr IV infusion; children: 50-150 μg/kg IV bolus initially, then 0.07 mg/kg/hr IV
	Calcium	Calcium chloride 10%: 1 gm (10 ml) IV; repeat as necessary
	Insulin + dextrose	Insulin load: 0.5 U/kg IV bolus, then 0.5-1.0 U/kg/hr IV; dextrose 10% IV infusion (with KCL), titrate to euglycemia
Calcium channel blockers	Calcium	Calcium chloride 10%: 1-4 g (10-40 ml) IV; repeat as necessary; children: 20 mg/kg initially

*Risks may outweigh benefits; consultation with a toxicologist before therapy is strongly recommended.

Continued.

Table 32-3 Common Antidotes—cont'd

Poison	Antidote(s)	Dose
	Glucagon	Initial dose: 5-10 mg IV bolus, then 2-10 mg/hr IV infusion
	Insulin + dextrose	Insulin load: 0.5 U/kg IV bolus, then 0.5-1.0 U/kg/hr IV
Carbon monoxide	Oxygen ± hyperbaric chamber	100% oxygen by ventilator or NRB high-flow oxygen by tight-fitting facemask
Crotalid Snakebite[†]	Wyeth Polyvalent *Crotalidae* antivenin (equine)	Mild: 3-5 vials; moderate: 6-10 vials; severe: 10-20 vials
		Mix reconstituted antivenin in 1000 ml NS over 4-6 hr
Cyanide	Amyl nitrate pearls	One ampule by inhalation for 15 sec every 3 min until IV access
	Sodium nitrite (3% solution)	10 ml (300 mg) IV over 3 min; children: 0.33 ml/kg IV
	Sodium thiosulfate (25%)	50 ml (12.5 g) IV over 10 min; children: 1.65 ml/kg IV
Digoxin (cardiac glycosides)	Digoxin Immune Fab (Digibind)	Number of mg ingested × 0.8 ÷ 0.6 = number of vials needed
		Digoxin concentration (in ng/ml) × 5.6 × kg (weight) ÷ 600 = number of vials
		Empiric dose: 10 vials (acute poisoning); 1-3 vials (chronic)
		Reconstitute Digibind in NS and administer IV over 5-30 min

Ethylene glycol methanol	Ethanol 10% in D5W[†] hemodialysis	Initial load: 10 ml/kg IV of 10% ethanol over 30 min, then 1.5 ml/kg IV infusion (titrate drip to serum ethanol 100 mg/dl); double to triple infusion during hemodialysis
	Fomepizole (4-methylpyrazole) (Antizol)[†] hemodialysis	Initial load: 15 mg/kg IV over 30 min, then 10 mg/kg every q12h IV over 30 min (re-bolus during HD)
Heparin	Protamine sulfate	1 mg neutralizes 90-115 mg heparin; initial dose: 1 mg/min to total dose 200 mg in 2 hr
Hydrofluoric acid	Calcium gluconate	Topical Ca gluconate gel 3% applied for 1-2 days *or* intradermal or SQ Ca gluconate injection 5% at burn site (0.5 ml per cm^2 burn area
		Regional intravenous (Bier block): 10 ml 10% in 40 ml NS injected locally in venous system × 20-30 min
		Intraarterial Ca gluconate 10%: 10-20 ml in 40 ml NS over 4 hr; repeat as necessary until pain relief
Iron	Deferoxamine (Desferal)	15 mg/kg/hr IV infusion until urine color clears or patient clinically well (not to exceed 6 g/24 hr)

[†] Consultation with a toxicologist is recommended.

Consultation with a toxicologist should be sought if the practitioner is unfamiliar with the therapy for any specific ingestion.

Continued.

Table 32-3 Common Antidotes—cont'd

Poison	Antidote(s)	Dose
Isoniazid	Pyridoxine (vitamin B6)	Initial dose: 1 g pyridoxine for every g INH ingested or empiric 5 g IV over 10 min if amount ingested unknown
Lead†	2,3-dimercaptosuccinic acid [DMSA] (Succimer); 100 mg capsules	30 mg/kg po in three divided doses × 5 days, then 20 mg/kg in twice daily doses × 14 days; repeat therapy prn after 2 week rebound
Mercury† Arsenic† Lead† Gold†	British antilewisite, dimercaprol (BAL); in peanut oil	Initial dose: 4-6 mg/kg IM q4-6h × 2 days
Methemoglobinemia	Methylene blue (1% solution)	Initial dose: 1-2 mg/kg (0.1-0.2 ml/kg) IV over 5 min; repeat prn
Opiates	Naloxone (Narcan) Others: nalmefene, naltrexone	Initial dose: 0.1-2.0 mg IV push (opioid-dependent patients should receive 0.1 mg IV every 30-60 sec until clinical response); synthetic opiates may need up to 10 mg for initial reversal dose; children 0.1 mg/kg IV initially

Organophosphates Carbamates Nerve agents	Atropine	Initial dose: 0.5-2.0 mg IV; repeat every 3-5 min until sweat and secretions clear; children: 0.05 mg/kg IV
	Pralidoxime [2-PAM] (Protopam)	Initial dose: 1 g IV over 15 min, then IV infusion of 3-4 mg/kg/hr for 24-72 hr or until clinical toxicity resolves; children: 25-50 mg/kg IV initially
Sulfonylurea	Octreotide (Sandostatin) + dextrose	Initial dose: 50-100 μg SQ or IV, then 50g q12h until euglycemia maintained without supplemental dextrose; children: 1-2 μg/kg SQ initially
Tricyclic antidepressants	Sodium bicarbonate ($NaHCO_3$)	Initial dose: 1-2 ampules (50-100 mEq) IV push, then IV infusion to maintain blood pH 7.45-7.55 and $Pco_2 \cong 30$ mm Hg (usual drip: 3 amps $NaHCO_3$ in 1 L D5W infused at 200-250 ml/hr); children: 1 mEq/kg IV bolus initially

*Risks may outweigh benefits; consultation with a toxicologist before therapy is recommended.

† Consultation with a toxicologist is recommended.

Consultation with a toxicologist should be sought if the practitioner is unfamiliar with the therapy for any specific ingestion.

Table 32-4 Enhanced Elimination Techniques

Technique	Dosing Technique Requirements	Complications	Agents for which Effective
Multiple-dose AC	0.5-1.0 g/kg AC q2-4h Requires bowel sounds	Nausea, vomiting, diarrhea, constipation, bowel obstruction and infarction, aspiration	Carbamazepine, **phenobarbital**, **theophylline**, quinine, nadolol, dapsone, meprobamate, salicylates, valproate, SR and EC preparations
Forced diuresis	Isotonic fluid (e.g., NS) at 500 ml/hr Requires normal kidney and cardiac functioning Requires urinary catheterization	Fluid overload, pulmonary edema	Barium, bromides, chromium, cisplatin, iodide, fluoride, calcium, lithium, potassium
Urinary alkalinization	D5W or 1/2 NS + 50-150 mEq $NaHCO_3$/L at 500 ml/hr initially Goal: urine flow 3 ml/kg/hr and urinary pH $\geq$ 7.5	Fluid overload, pulmonary edema, cerebral edema, hypernatremia, hypokalemia, alkalemia, ionized hypocalcemia	Chlorpropamide, **salicylates**, barbiturates, methotrexate, fluoride, sulfonamides

Hemodialysis	Requires poison with molecular weight <500 d, low protein binding, high water solubility, low endogenous clearance, small volume of distribution	Hypotension, bleeding, hypothermia, air embolus, central venous access complications	Barbiturates, bromides, chloral hydrate, **alcohols**, **lithium**, procainamide, theophylline (hemoperfusion better), **salicylates**, atenolol, sotalol
Hemoperfusion	Requires drug to be bound by AC	Charcoal embolization, hypocalcemia, hypoglycemia, thrombocytopenia, leukopenia, hypotension, bleeding, hypothermia	Barbiturates, meprobamate, glutethimide, phenytoin, carbamazepine, valproate, **theophylline**, disopyramide, paraquat, procainamide, *Amanita* mushrooms, methotrexate
Hemofiltration	Can be run continuously	Clotting of filter, bleeding	Aminoglycosides, vancomycin, metal chelate complexes, procainamide
Exchange transfusion	Double or triple volume exchanges usually performed	Transfusion reactions, ionized hypocalcemia, hypothermia	Arsine, sodium chlorate, methemoglobinemia, sulfhemoglobinemia, neonatal drug toxicity

Hypotension

Hypotension may occur as many poisons deplete endogenous catecholamine stores. Intravenous fluids are the first-line treatment, and pressors (e.g., norepinephrine) rarely may be needed. Antidotes and other specific treatments should be used as indicated.

Agitation

Agitation is generally best treated with benzodiazepines, supplemented as needed with neuroleptics. Physostigmine may be appropriate for some patients with agitated delirium secondary to the anticholinergic syndrome.

Ventricular Arrhythmias

Standard doses of antiarrhthymics are recommended for treatment of ventricular arrhythmias. Sodium bicarbonate (1 to 2 mEq/kg IV bolus) is indicated for wide complex tachycardias from tricyclic antidepressant overdose and other membrane-active agents; antidotal treatment should be followed as indicated.

Bradyarrhythmias with Hypotension

Treatment of bradyarrhythmias with hypotension is drug specific. Standard doses of atropine are recommended. Calcium and glucagon are given to those with calcium channel blockers and beta-blocker poisoning; digoxin Fab fragments should be given to those with digoxin poisoning (see Table 32-3 for dosing).

Seizures

Generally, seizures are best treated with benzodiazepines followed by phenobarbital. Pyridoxine is indicated for INH-induced seizures (see Table 32-3 for dosing).

SPECIAL CASES

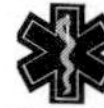

CYCLIC ANTIDEPRESSANTS

The clinical presentation of poisoning from cyclic antidepressants varies widely because of complex pharmacologic factors.

Symptoms

- Lethargy to coma, seizures

Signs

- Mydriasis (anticholinergic) or miosis (alpha-adrenergic blockade)
- Dry skin
- Tachycardias
- Lethargy to coma
- Seizures
- Agitated delirium (occasionally)
- Hypotension
- Hypertension (mild, early)

Workup

- ECG may show cardiac conduction disturbances (e.g., prolonged QRS, R in aVR [rightward axis of terminal 40 ms of limb lead QRS]). Wide complex tachycardias (both SVT with aberrant conduction and VT) and VF can occur.

Comments and Treatment Considerations

All but the most trivial poisonings require close cardiac monitoring, since patients can rapidly deteriorate in the first few hours after ingestion. If patients remain or become asymptomatic after 4 to 6 hours of observation, they are unlikely to have a complication related to CA ingestion.

Death most commonly is caused by refractory hypotension or ventricular arrhythmia. A QRS >100 ms or R in aVR >3 mm predicts serious toxicity and warrants close monitoring and sodium bicarbonate administration. Sodium bicarbonate (overcomes fast sodium channel blockade) in 1 to 2 mEq/kg boluses is recommended until arterial pH is 7.50 to 7.55 to decrease the toxic cardiac effects (attenuates conduction disturbance and provides positive inotropic effects). Hyperventilation is recommended in those requiring intubation as adjunctive therapy to sodium bicarbonate.

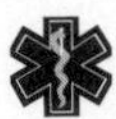

ACETAMINOPHEN

Acetaminophen (APAP) is one of the most common causes of pharmaceutically associated poisoning and death in the United States annually. Shortly following acetaminophen overdose, patients are often asymptomatic; therefore an APAP level should be obtained with all suspected ingestions. Administer empiric *N*-acetylcysteine (NAC) to patients (1) who may have ingested a toxic amount of APAP *and* (2) for whom the estimated time of ingestion is close to or greater than 8 hours and delay while waiting for a level may or will result in treatment beginning greater than 8 hours after ingestion.

Symptoms

- Early (first 24 hours): initial toxicity is often mild or overlooked, consisting of anorexia, nausea, vomiting, and malaise.
- Late (24 to 72 hours after ingestion): symptoms of liver failure (e.g., recurrent nausea, vomiting, and malaise, abdominal pain, lethargy, confusion)

Signs

- Early: none
- Late (24 hours): right upper quadrant tenderness
- Signs of fulminant hepatic and multiorgan system failure (e.g., confusion, coma, tachypnea, jaundice, asterixis) may ensue from 24 to 96 hours in those not treated or treated too late.

Workup

- Plasma APAP concentrations measured from 4 to 24 hours after acute single overdose can be plotted on the modified Rumack-Matthew nomogram to predict the risk of subsequent hepatotoxicity and need for NAC antidotal treatment (Fig. 32-1). Perform baseline and daily BUN/creatinine, LFTs, PT/INR.

Comments and Treatment Considerations

Those with a level greater than the line connecting 150 μg/ml at 4 hours and 5 mg/L at 24 hours ("possible hepatic toxic-

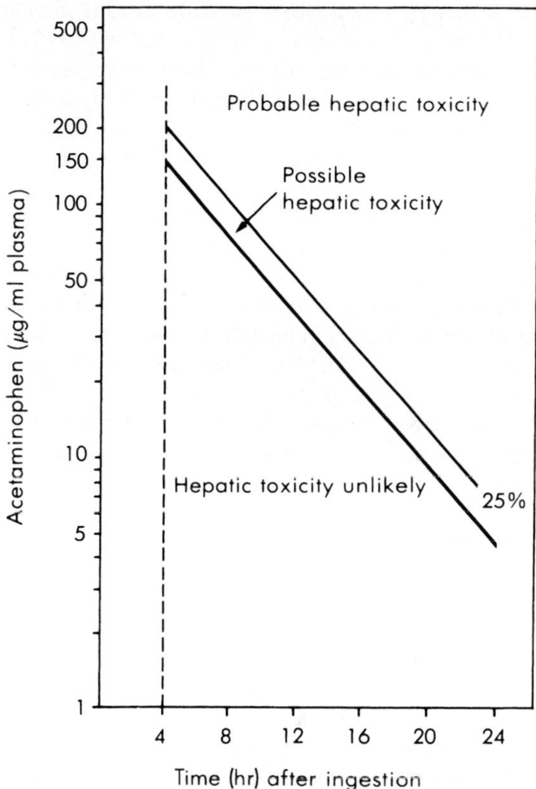

Fig. 32-1 Rumack-Matthew nomogram for acetaminophen poisoning. (From Rumack BH, Matthew H: Pediatrics 55:871, 1975.)

ity" line) currently receive antidotal therapy with NAC in the United States (see Table 32-3 for dosing). Treatment is almost 100% effective at preventing APAP toxicity if is initiated within 8 hours of ingestion. Effectiveness progressively diminishes with the further delay of treatment. A decision to initiate or forgo antidotal treatment in (1) those with multiple subtoxic ingestions, (2) those who have ingested sustained-release preparations (e.g., Tylenol ER), or (3) those more susceptible to hepatotoxicity (e.g., hepatic disease, alcoholics) should be made in conjunction with a medical toxicologist. In addition, consider toxicologic consultation in admitted patients when abbreviated treatment is being considered (<72-hour treatment)

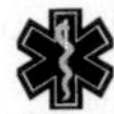

SALICYLATES

Salicylates are a common cause of poisonings in the United States. Salicylates are readily available in OTC products such as aspirin, Pepto-Bismol (bismuth subsalicylate), and oil of wintergreen (methyl salicylate). Salicylate poisoning is frequently misdiagnosed, particularly when chronic poisoning exists. Symptoms and signs are often nonspecific, and erroneous diagnoses such as "sepsis," "altered mental status," "gastroenteritis," or "CHF" are not infrequently made.

Symptoms

- Mild or early poisoning (1 to 12 hours after acute ingestion): nausea, vomiting, abdominal pain, headache, tinnitus, dizziness, fatigue
- Moderate or intermediate poisoning (12 to 24 hours after ingestion): fever, sweating, deafness, lethargy, confusion, hallucinations, breathlessness
- Severe or late poisoning (greater than 24 hours after acute ingestion or unrecognized, untreated chronic ingestion): coma, seizures, fever

Signs

- Mild or early: lethargy, ataxia, mild agitation, hyperpnea, mild abdominal tenderness
- Moderate or intermediate: fever, asterixis, diaphoresis, deafness, pallor, confusion, slurred speech, disorientation, agitation, hallucinations, tachycardia, tachypnea, orthostatic hypotension
- Severe or late: dehydration, coma, seizures, hypothermia or hyperthermia, tachycardia, hypotension, respiratory depression, pulmonary edema, arrhythmias, papilledema

Workup

- Obtain electrolytes, glucose, BUN/creatinine, urinalysis (particularly urine pH), ABG, salicylate level; LFTs, CBC, PT/INR, and calcium, for severe poisoning
- Acid-base disturbances: respiratory alkalosis (mild or early poisoning), respiratory alkalosis with metabolic acidosis (moderate or intermediate poisoning), and metabolic acidosis with or without respiratory acidosis (severe or late poisoning).
- Serum salicylate concentration, in conjunction with history (acute or chronic ingestion) and severity and phase of poisoning, determines appropriate treatment strategy.

Comments and Treatment Considerations

History of salicylate ingestion can be difficult to elicit, especially in cases of chronic ingestion, when the combination of confusion, hyperthermia, tachypnea, and dehydration may easily be confused with sepsis. Treatment requires GI decontamination (multidose AC), correction of acid-base, fluid, and electrolyte disturbances, and enhanced elimination with serum alkalinization (see Table 32-4). Hemodialysis is indicated for those with severe toxicity (e.g., [SA] >100 mg/dl in acute and >60 mg/dl in chronic poisoning, altered mental status, refractory acid-base disturbances, and deterioration despite maximal supportive care).

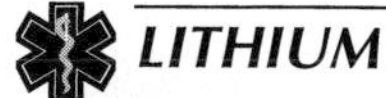

LITHIUM

Symptoms

- Mild or early: nausea and vomiting
- Moderate or intermediate: agitation, confusion, lethargy, slurred speech
- Severe or late: marked confusion, coma, seizures

Signs

- Mild or early: dysarthria, ataxia, tremor, muscle weakness, hyperreflexia
- Moderate or intermediate: confusion, agitation, hypertonia, myoclonus
- Severe or late: coma, seizures, muscle rigidity, cardiovascular collapse

Workup

- Lithium level, electrolytes, BUN/creatinine, and ECG. Lithium level, in conjunction with history (acute or chronic ingestion) and neurologic exam (e.g., mental status) is used to determine severity of poisoning and appropriate treatment strategy.

Comments and Treatment Considerations

Treatment involves restoration of sodium and water balance (rehydration with intravenous normal saline in dehydrated patients) and hemodialysis for those with severe poisoning.

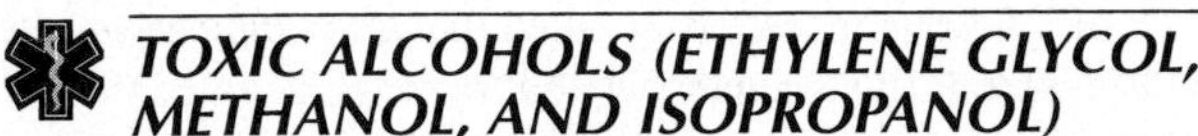

TOXIC ALCOHOLS (ETHYLENE GLYCOL, METHANOL, AND ISOPROPANOL)

Poisoning by ethylene glycol and methanol requires early diagnosis and treatment to prevent accumulation of their toxic acid metabolites and subsequent development of profound metabolic acidosis and end-organ complications.

Symptoms

- Early (1 to 12 hours): anorexia, nausea, vomiting, abdominal pain, headache, vertigo, weakness, lethargy, coma
- Late (6 to 36 hours): progressive visual disturbances (e.g., blurred vision, diplopia, scotomata, "snowfields," tunnel vision, blindness), shortness of breath, confusion, lethargy, seizures, coma, hematemesis, flank pain

Signs

- Early: CNS inebriation (e.g., slurred speech, nystagmus, lethargy, coma, ataxia)
- Late: progressive visual field and acuity deficits, optic disc hyperemia, papilledema, mydriasis nonreactive to light, confusion, agitation, delirium, coma, myoclonus, tetany, seizures, tachypnea, hyperpnea, ketotic breath, sinus tachycardia, hypertension or hypotension.

Workup

- Serum electrolytes, BUN/creatinine, glucose, amylase, calcium, ketones, osmolality, lactate, ABG, urinalysis, and solvents (e.g., ethanol, ethylene glycol, isopropanol, and methanol)
- Early: Elevated osmolal gap without anion gap (common); possibly urine fluorescence with Wood's lamp in ethylene glycol poisoning (fluorescein in some commercial antifreezes)
- Late: Elevated anion gap with or without elevated osmolal gap (common)
- Normal osmolal gap (early or late) does not exclude toxic alcohol poisoning.
- Ketosis (serum and urinary acetone) without acidosis is commonly seen in isopropanol poisoning.
- Serum hypocalcemia, urinary calcium oxalate crystals, ATN (microscopic hematuria, proteinuria, oliguria), elevated BUN/creatinine, bronchopneumonia on chest x-ray, and cerebral edema demonstrated by head CT may be seen in ethylene glycol poisoning.

Comments and Treatment Considerations

Conventional treatment of ethylene glycol and methanol poisoning includes sodium bicarbonate administration for metabolic acidosis, ethanol or fomepizole (4-MP) infusion to inhibit metabolism to toxic acid metabolites (see Table 32-3 for dosing), vitamin administration (e.g., folinic acid, folate, thiamine, pyridoxine) to enhance toxic metabolite elimination, and hemodialysis to rapidly remove toxic alcohol and its metabolites. Fomepizole or ethanol therapy is indicated for those with suspected ingestion by history or laboratory data (e.g., ethylene glycol or methanol levels >20 mg/dl or osmolal gap >10 mOsm/L). Hemodialysis is indicated for those with (1) ethylene glycol or methanol levels >50 mg/dl, (2) pH ≤ 7.20, and (3) significant end-organ toxicity (e.g., renal insufficiency, visual impairment, or seizures).

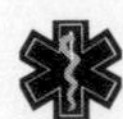

TOXIC TIME BOMBS

Both actual and predicted toxic effects determine patient disposition. Certain poisons produce delayed toxic manifestations, usually secondary to toxic metabolites, and few, if any, early signs may be present following lethal doses of these agents. If history, physical examination, or initial laboratory testing is suggestive of delayed toxicity, a prolonged period of observation or treatment is required, even if the patient is initially well appearing (see the box below).

POISONS WITH DELAYED CLINICAL TOXICITY

Acetaminophen
Pennyroyal oil
Carbon tetrachloride
Mushrooms
- *Amanita* (amatoxin)
- *Lepiota* (amatoxin)
- *Gyromitra* (gyromitrin)
- *Cortinarius* (orellanine/orelline)

Toxic alcohols
- Ethylene glycol
- Methanol

Sustained-release preparations
- Calcium-channel blockers
- Beta-blockers
- Lithium
- Theophylline

Enteric-coated preparations
- Aspirin

MAOIs
Drug packet ingestion (heroin, cocaine)
Oral hypoglycemic agents
Lomotil
Methylene chloride (metabolized to CO)
Paraquat /diquat
Cyanogenic glycosides
Warfarin /superwarfarin
- Brodifacoum

Elapid snake envenomation
Antimetabolites
- Colchicine
- Methotrexate
- Alkylating agents

Fat-soluble organophosphate insecticides
Ergotamines
Heavy metals
- Lead
- Thallium
- Mercury

REFERENCES

American Academy of Clinical Toxicology, European Association of Poisons Centres and Clinical Toxicologists: Position statements, *J Toxicol Clin Toxicol* 35:695, 1997.

Hoffman RS, Goldfrank LR: The poisoned patient with altered consciousness: controversies in the use of a "coma cocktail," *JAMA* 274:562, 1995.

Kulig K, Bar-Or D, Cantrill SV, et al: Management of acutely poisoned patients without gastric emptying, *Ann Emerg Med* 14:562, 1985.

Litovitz TL, Smilkstein M, Felberg L, et al: 1996 Annual report of the American Association of Poison Control Centers Toxic Exposure Surveillance System, *Am J Emerg Med* 15:447, 1997.

Pond SM, Lewis-Driver DJ, Williams GM, et al: Gastric emptying in acute overdose: a prospective randomised controlled trial, *Med J Aust* 163:345, 1995.

Proudfoot A: Acute poisoning: principles of management, *Med Int* 61:2499, 1989.

CHAPTER 33

Trauma and Burns, Approach to

CHARLES POZNER, HILARIE CRANMER, and RESA LEWISS

TRAUMA

Accidental injuries are the leading cause of death for ages 1 to 44 and the fourth leading cause overall in United States. If suicide and homicide are included, trauma and unintentional injury are together the third leading cause of death for all U.S. residents. Of all accidental deaths, 50% die at the scene of major vessel or neurologic injury, 30% die within the first few hours of irreversible shock or intracranial hematomas, and 20% die days or weeks later of sepsis or multiorgan failure. Therefore the initial management of trauma is one of the most important and basic functions for which the emergency physician (EP) must become proficient and efficient. One of the EP's most important responsibilities is to recognize when the patient requires another venue, be it the operating room, the interventional radiology suite, or transfer to another facility, for the most appropriate management.

PREHOSPITAL CARE

The initial phase of management of trauma patients begins at the scene of the accident.

- Stabilization and prevention of additional injury: airway and ventilation, spine immobilization, hemorrhage control
- Data collection: mechanism, estimated blood loss
- Expeditious transport: ideal duration of treatment at trauma scene is 10 minutes or less.
- Advanced notification allows for assembly of trauma team, anticipation of patients' needs, preparation for procedures, timely consultations, operating room preparedness, blood bank and critical care units readiness

- Initiation of treatment: timely placement of IV line, needle thoracostomy for tension pneumothorax, MAST trousers (use generally limited to unstable patients with pelvic fractures)
- Triage: determination of appropriate hospital destination based on initial patient assessment

OVERVIEW OF EVALUATION OF MULTIPLY INJURED PATIENTS

Although described sequentially, many of the following steps are performed simultaneously. Once detected, immediately life-threatening processes must be attended before progressing with a detailed evaluation. On arrival at the resuscitation suite, the following items must be ensured:

1. Team in place, leader identified, responsibilities assigned
2. EMS report: mechanism, age, injuries, prehospital therapy, status changes
3. Airway, IV (two large-bore/proximal), 100% O_2 mask, cardiac and O_2 saturation monitors
   - Airway management. *Assumptions:* cervical injury (if altered mental status, head injury, or clinical suspicion), full stomach. *Definitive airway management* for airway protection or obstruction, respiratory failure, closed head injury (hyperventilation), persistent hypotension, refractory agitation (to facilitate evaluation)
   - Breathing: adequacy of ventilation with bilateral breath sounds
   - Circulation: check pulses, consider immediate interventions
   - Hemorrhage: pressure, elevation, pressure points, MAST (pelvic fractures)
   - Disability: Glasgow coma score, pupils, movement of all extremities, posturing
   - Exposure: undress, front and back, protect against hypothermia

RESUSCITATION

Surgical intervention plays the primary role in the management of exsanguinating hemorrhage. Volume resuscitation is only a bridge to this definitive therapy.

- Crystalloid: NS/LR, wide open unless stable; initial 2 L bolus in unstable patients (rapid infuser)
- Blood (O− [or O+ in male or postmenopausal female]): immediate if severe blood loss or unstable after 2 L crystalloid

SCREENING RADIOGRAPHS

Radiographs are obtained concurrently with the head-to-toe examination; team members may wear lead protection to facilitate the process. Chest and pelvic x-rays are usually taken first. Cervical spine x-rays help to diagnose cervical spine fracture, but management may proceed (including intubation with in-line immobilization) if patient instability does not permit immediate x-ray evaluation of the neck. Cervical spine precautions must be followed until the cervical spine is evaluated radiographically (at least three views) and clinically cleared.

- Supine anteroposterior chest x-ray: evaluate for subcutaneous pleural air, deep sulcus (Fig. 7-2) (pneumothorax) plus mediastinal shift (tension pneumothorax); effusion (hemothorax), nasogastric tube, or hollow viscous above hemidiaphragm or abnormal hemidiaphragm (diaphragmatic rupture); wide or abnormal mediastinum (possible aortic injury); air-space consolidation (possible pulmonary contusion)
- Pelvic x-ray: pelvic fractures may be occult sites of major blood loss (unnecessary to obtain in asymptomatic and alert, oriented patients who can be easily examined)
- Lateral cervical spine x-ray: demonstrates many (approximately 85%), but not all, cervical spine fractures. (At least three views are needed.)

  See Chapter 23, Neck Pain and Stiffness.

HEAD-TO-TOE EXAMINATION (SECONDARY SURVEY)

A more thorough and detailed examination is performed after initial stabilization. Initial priorities are placed on identifying life threats. Some injuries may be missed, especially in unconscious patients with head injury or blunt abdominal trauma and in those with dramatic injuries that distract attention from other, potentially more significant injuries.

- HEENT: scalp and cranium, pupils and eyes, orbits, facial integrity, nose (blood/CSF, septal hematoma), oropharynx (teeth, bleeding), ears (otorrhea, hemotympanum, Battle's sign)
- Neck: airway injuries, subcutaneous emphysema, penetration, vascular injuries, stepoffs, jugular venous distention
- Chest: penetration (possible cardiac injury if between right midclavicular line and left anterior axillary line and upper abdomen), abrasions and bruises, open wounds, flail chest, subcutaneous emphysema
- Abdomen: abrasions and bruises (possible underlying injury), abdominal breathing, distention, bruits (possible vascular injury), tenderness, guarding, (normal examination does not rule out abdominal injury)
- Pelvis: instability and fracture (may indicate source of occult bleeding), genitourinary bleeding
- Rectal and urethral examination: tone, prostate, blood, (retrograde urethrogram if meatal blood, "high-riding" prostate, scrotal hematoma)
- Back: stepoffs, penetration, abrasions and bruises (possible retroperitoneal injury)
- Extremities: hemorrhage, deformity, pulses, capillary refill
- Neurologic: LOC, agitation, tone, gross motor or sensory focality, priapism

LABORATORY STUDIES AND TREATMENTS

- Hematocrit (may be normal even with exsanguination; recheck after IV fluid resuscitation)
- Type and crossmatch blood, electrolytes, urinalysis, PT/PTT
- Pregnancy test (women of childbearing age)
- Other "trauma labs": toxicology screen, amylase, liver function tests, ABG, lactate and base deficit; use of these tests is controversial.
- Tetanus prophylaxis
- Prophylactic antibiotics if indicated (e.g., open fractures)
- Foley catheter and nasogastric or orogastric tube: evaluate for genitourinary and gastrointestinal hemorrhage; evacuate bladder and stomach (aspiration risk if spine immobilized)

MANAGEMENT OF THE TRAUMA AIRWAY

Securing the airway and maintaining ventilation are the first priorities for patient survival. Rapid sequence intubation for airway control is the safest for the patient, and care is taken to provide in-line immobilization in patients with potential cervical spine injuries.

Preparation (SOAP)

- **S**uction: on and at bedside
- Pre-**O**xygenation: 100% NRB mask
- **A**irway equipment (tested): BVM, ETT (two sizes), stylet, syringe, laryngoscope, endotracheal CO_2 detector, EDD
- **P**harmaceuticals: sedatives, paralytics, induction agents, intracranial pressure protectors
- Cricothyrotomy equipment immediately available

Advanced Airway Techniques

1. Difficult airway: neck or lower face injury, obese habitus (consider awake intubation with airway anesthesia and sedation)
2. Orotracheal intubation: method of choice
   a. Suspected cervical spine injuries: in-line immobilization
   b. Contraindications: not feasible due to patient anatomy, tracheal disruption
3. Rapid sequence intubation
   a. Consider alternatives to paralysis if anticipate difficulty with bag-valve-mask ventilation and intubation (e.g., large open face or neck wounds, difficult anatomy)
   b. Pretreatment: consider lidocaine (1.5 mg/kg) in head-injured patients
   c. Consider defasciculating dose of nondepolarizing agent (e.g., vecuronium 0.01 mg/kg)
   d. Induction: fentanyl (3 μg/kg) or midazolam (0.1 to 0.3 mg/kg) or etomidate (0.3 mg/kg); etomidate may be drug of choice for head trauma.
   e. Paralysis: succinylcholine (1 to 2 mg/kg): fast onset and offset; contraindications: crush or burn >24 hours, hyperkalemia, chronic neuromuscular disease
   f. If succinylcholine is contraindicated: newer nondepolarizing agent (rocuronium 0.6 mg/kg) or higher dose of

standard nondepolarizing agent (e.g., vecuronium 0.15 mg/kg)
   g. Confirm placement: ETT seen between cords, auscultation, O_2 saturation, ET CO_2 detection, chest x-ray. May also use esophageal detector device. Fogging of tube is unreliable.
4. Nasotracheal intubation
   a. Higher complication and failure rate
   b. Contraindications: respiratory arrest, intracranial hypertension (relative), cribriform plate injury (relative)
5. Surgical airway
   a. Indications: unfeasible or failed intubation
6. Other options: fiberoptic intubation, retrograde intubation, light-wand-guided intubation, Bullard laryngoscope, laryngeal mask airway, Combitube.

HEAD AND NECK INJURIES

Head and neck injuries may be isolated or be associated with multisystem trauma. Aggressive management of shock is essential for patients with multiple injuries. Efforts should be made to rapidly obtain a head CT in all but the most critically unstable patients who require emergent operative management of other injuries. Neurosurgeons may consider a ventriculostomy with intracranial pressure monitoring in the operating room if CT is not possible. Identification of spinal cord injuries is also a priority in patents with multiple injuries; the physical examination may be the only means to detect injury.

Head Trauma

Significant intracranial injuries may show no external signs. The EP must determine if an intracranial injury is present, the extent of that injury, and minimize the progression of secondary injury.

Signs

- Abnormal Glasgow coma score
- Asymmetric or abnormal pupils
- Otorrhea and rhinorrhea
- Loss of skull integrity
- Battle's signs
- Periorbital ecchymoses ("raccoon eyes")
- Posturing

Management

- Head of bed at 30 degrees (if possible)
- Increased intracranial pressure: ventilate (P_{CO_2} 30 to 35 mm Hg); consider mannitol (1.0 g/kg)
- Anticipate coagulopathy
- Seizure prophylaxis: phenytoin 18 mg/kg over 20 minutes
- Open fracture: antibiotic prophylaxis (e.g., cefazolin 1 g)
- Neurosurgical consultation
- Head CT to diagnose intracranial hemorrhage, mass effect, depressed or basilar skull fracture

Facial Trauma

Although airway patency must always be considered in patients with facial trauma, deforming injuries to the face should never distract the EP from attending to other, more serious life-threatening conditions.

Signs

- Hemorrhage
- Enophthalmos, exophthalmos
- Ecchymoses
- Dysconjugate gaze
- Deformity
- Asymmetry
- Instability
- Malocclusion
- Stepoffs
- Crepitus
- Septal hematoma

Management

- CT scan, panoramic view of mandible
- May delay repair (antibiotics)

Special considerations

LeFort fractures

I: Maxilla at nasal fossa

II: Maxilla, nasal bones, medial aspects of orbits

III: Maxilla, zygoma, nasal bones, ethmoids, vomer, lesser bones of the cranial base

Neck Injuries

Life-threatening injuries to the neck may be subtle, leading to dangerous delays in diagnosis. The most immediate risks to life are airway compromise, hemorrhage, and cervical spine injury. Vascular and airway injuries may initially be occult, particularly with blunt trauma.

Blunt Neck Injury

Signs

- Hematoma
- Ecchymosis
- Dyspnea
- Stridor
- Bruit
- Dysphagia
- Focal neurologic deficits
- Subcutaneous emphysema
- Horner's syndrome (miosis, ptosis, anhydrosis)

Management

- Airway: early intubation if risk of airway compromise
- Timely ENT consultation
- Cervical spine and chest x-rays, fiberoptic bronchoscopy, angiography or Doppler of major neck vessels, esophagram, endoscopy
- Hospital admission for observation

Special considerations

Vascular injury (intimal tear, thrombosis, pseudoaneurysm) may present as hemiparesis or be initially asymptomatic

Penetrating Neck Injury

Potential injuries

- Posterior: cord, vertebral artery
- Anterior: vessels, trachea, esophagus

Signs

- Hematoma
- Ecchymosis
- Dyspnea
- Stridor
- Bruit
- Dysphagia
- Focal neurologic deficits
- Subcutaneous emphysema
- Horner's syndrome
- Hemoptysis
- Absent pulse

Management

1. Airway: early intubation if indicated
2. Hemorrhage: pressure, oropharyngeal packing

3. Timely ENT consultation
4. Unstable: operating room
5. Special considerations
   a. Workup if platysma violated (never probe the wound)
   b. Zone I: below cricoid (see Full Workup, below)
   c. Zone II: cricoid to angle of mandible (mandatory surgical exploration is controversial)
   d. Zone III: above angle of mandible (see Full Workup, below)
6. "Full workup" (nonsurgical approach, institution specific)
   a. Lateral neck film (preintubation), chest x-ray
   b. Bronchoscopy, esophagoscopy, esophagography, angiography
   c. Intravenous antibiotics
   d. Hospital admission for observation

THORACIC TRAUMA

The EP must quickly identify and treat all life-threatening conditions and constantly monitor the patient for deterioration during subsequent examination and management. Both blunt and penetrating injuries can cause significant morbidity and mortality. Rapid deceleration may also bring about subtle, although potentially life-threatening, processes (see Tension Pneumothorax, Cardiac Tamponade, and Traumatic Aortic Rupture, in Chapter 7, Chest Pain).

Potential injuries

- Flail chest
- Open chest wound
- Pneumothorax
- Tension pneumothorax
- Hemothorax
- Tracheobronchial tree disruption
- Esophageal injury
- Pulmonary contusion
- Myopericardial (tamponade, myocardial contusion)
- Great vessel injury
- Diaphragmatic injury

Signs

- Dyspnea
- Hypoxemia
- Shock
- Hemoptysis
- Decreased breath sounds
- Tracheal deviation
- Distended neck veins
- Asymmetric chest excursion
- Abrasions
- Contusions
- Dullness, hyperresonance
- Subcutaneous emphysema
- Irregular pulse
- Bowel sounds in chest

Management

1. Assess thoracic integrity, breath sounds, trachea, jugular venous distention
2. Tension pneumothorax
   a. Needle: 14 g 2″, second intercostal space, midclavicular line
   b. Tube: 28 to 36 Fr, fifth intercostal space, anterior-midaxillary line
3. Open pneumothorax: loose dressing (taped on only three sides to prevent tension pneumothorax) as bridge to thoracostomy
4. Hemothorax: decreased breath sounds, hypoxemia
   a. Chest tube: 32 to 38 Fr, fifth intercostal space anterior-midaxillary line, directed posteriorly (may use autotransfuser)
   b. To OR if >1500 ml blood initially, >200 ml/hr bleeding, unresponsive to volume resuscitation, expanding effusion
5. Cardiac tamponade (jugular venous distention, hypotension, tachycardia): pericardiocentesis, OR
6. Pulseless
   a. Rapid IV fluid bolus
   b. Consider needle thoracostomies
   c. *Blunt injury:* thoracotomy rarely indicated
   d. *Penetrating injury:* thoracotomy indicated (if limited time in arrest)
      (1) Incise pericardium, deliver heart, control hemorrhage, cross-clamp aorta, open heart massage
7. Supine anteroposterior chest x-ray
   a. Normal: consider tamponade and other source of shock outside of chest

b. Tension pneumothorax, pneumothorax, hemothorax: thoracostomy
c. Mediastinal abnormality: possible aortic injury
d. Infiltrate: possible pulmonary contusion
e. Pneumomediastinum: possible tracheobronchial injury
f. Abnormal hemidiaphragm (most often left): surgery to repair diaphragm
g. Lower rib fractures: consider abdominal injury

8. ECG
   a. Myocardial contusion: ischemia, arrhythmia

ABDOMINAL AND PELVIC TRAUMA

Mechanism of injury is vitally important in the assessment of abdominal trauma. Blunt trauma can present without any external physical signs, and life-threatening intraabdominal injuries may be overlooked during initial assessment and treatment. In penetrating trauma, it is important to determine whether the peritoneum was violated, as well as the likely path of the penetrating object.

The EP must consider anatomic site, number of wounds, type and size of weapon, and the angle of approach of the weapon. Projectiles often have unpredictable paths and therefore surgical exploration is frequently necessary for assessment of the extent of injury. Because of the characteristics of the diaphragm and its changing position with respiration, penetrating injuries occurring below the nipple line anteriorly and the tip of the scapula posteriorly may directly involve the abdominal cavity. Knife or gunshot wounds may enter the abdomen, traverse the diaphragm, and enter the thorax, or vice versa. Blunt trauma may cause fracture of the pelvis, which may lead to significant hemorrhage. Bladder or urethral injuries may occur in both blunt and penetrating trauma.

Potential injuries

- Solid organ
- Hollow viscous
- Vascular (including mesentery)
- Fracture (pelvis)

Upper: diaphragm, stomach, liver, spleen, gallbladder, bowel

Lower: bowel, colon
Retroperitoneum: pancreas, kidneys, ureters, aorta, IVC, spinal cord, duodenum
Pelvis: fracture, rectum, bladder, blood vessels, genitalia

Signs

- Hemodynamic instability (up to 20% with benign examination)
- Abrasions, contusions
- Penetrating wounds (must log roll)
- Guarding
- Distention
- Hematemesis
- Hematochezia
- Hematuria

Management

I. *Further workup*
   A. Pulseless
      1. *Penetrating wound:* thoracotomy, cross-clamp aorta, OR
      2. *Blunt trauma:* thoracotomy rarely indicated
   B. Hemodynamically unstable, persistent shock: bedside ultrasound or Doppler to confirm abdominal source, if needed, or if penetrating trauma or positive ultrasound
   C. Stable; proposed algorithms
      1. Emergency laparotomy: impaled object, evisceration, peritoneal signs, diaphragm injury, pneumoperitoneum, rectal/NGT blood
      2. Selective treatment
         a. Local exploration: if intact peritoneum, observe; if peritoneum violated, must workup
         b. PL: to OR if gross blood, >100,000 RBCs in blunt trauma (5000 if lower chest wound with possible diaphragm injury), stool/urine, amylase/alkaline phosphatase; observe if negative
         c. CT: positive, to OR if indicated; if negative, observe (add rectal contrast if concern for colon injury)
         d. Laparoscopy
   3. Gunshot wound
      a. Emergency laparotomy: generally performed if peritoneum violated (through-and-through wound, missile on plain film), flank injury

b. Selective management: studied by some who use varying algorithms, including local exploration, DPL (OR if >5000 RBC), CT to identify injury, laparoscopy; observation if negative workup

D. Stable, blunt injury
1. CT: intraperitoneal and retroperitoneal injury; less reliable for hollow viscous injury; may also evaluate head, neck, chest
2. Ultrasound is used as an alternative at some institutions. DPL has been supplanted by CT or ultrasound for stable patients at most institutions.
3. Selective management: stable spleen or liver injuries observed

II. *Special considerations*
A. External pelvic fixation for pelvic fractures leading to hemodynamic instability
B. If unable to control bleeding from pelvic fracture, consider radiographic embolization

EXTREMITY TRAUMA

Vessel, nerve, and orthopedic injury may occur as a result of both penetrating and blunt mechanisms. Open fractures require prompt orthopedic consultation and operative irrigation and fixation. Diminished pulses require emergent relocation and splinting and possible angiography to document integrity of the vasculature. Compartment syndromes must be considered in the setting of extremity trauma.

Potential injuries

- Fracture
- Dislocation
- Laceration
- Puncture
- Crush
- Compartment syndrome
- Neurovascular injury
- Soft injury tissue

Signs

- Deformity
- Hematoma
- Lacerations
- Abrasions
- Pulselessness
- Pain
- Paralysis, paresthesia
- Bruit
- Thrill

Management

1. Reduce and splint major deformities in anatomic position
2. Vascular injury
   a. Risk stratification (proximity not important):
      (1) High risk: pulsatile bleed, absent pulse, shotgun wound, nerve deficit, hematoma, bruit, major tissue defect, delayed capillary refill, ABI <1.00 (see Chapter 10, Extremity Pain and Numbness)
      (2) Low risk: normal examination, ABI >1.00
   b. Workup
      (1) High risk: arteriography; operating room if gross arterial bleeding
      (2) Low risk: observation

Special considerations

- Serial arteriography/duplex scan of minor vessel injury; may be alternative to surgical repair in some cases
- Antibiotics (e.g., cefazolin, gentamicin) for open fractures
- Low threshold for compartment pressure measurement and emergent fasciotomy if indicated

SPINAL CORD INJURY

Sequelae of spinal cord injuries can be devastating. Observe initial cervical spine precautions and document full neurologic examination.

- Spinal immobilization
- Orthopedic and neurosurgical consultation
- Methylprednisolone (Solu-Medrol): 30 mg/kg IV bolus followed by 5.4 mg/kg/hr infusion for patients with spinal cord injury and neurologic deficits

REFERENCES[www]

American College of Surgeons: *Advance trauma life support instructors manual,* Chicago, 1997, American College of Surgeons.

Civil ID, Ross SE, Botehlo G, Schwab CW: Routine pelvic radiography in severe blunt trauma: is it necessary? *Ann Emerg Med* 17:488, 1988.

[www]Additional references are available on the following web site: www.signsandsymptoms.com.

Croce MA, Fabian TC, Menke PG, et al: Nonoperative management of blunt hepatic trauma is the treatment of choice for hemodynamically stable patients: results of a prospective trial, *Ann Surg* 221:744, 1995.

Lorenz HP, Steinmetz B, Lieberman J, et al: Emergency thoracotomy: survival correlates with physiologic status, *J Trauma* 32:780, 1992.

Moore FA, Moore EE: Trauma resuscitation, *Sci Am* 1:3, 1989.

Perry NM, Lewars MD: ABC of major trauma. Radiological assessment—I, *BMJ* 301:805, 1990.

Shaffer MA, Doris PE: Limitation of the cross table lateral view in detecting cervical spine injuries: a retrospective analysis, *Ann Emerg Med* 10:508, 1981.

Shatney CH: Initial resuscitation and assessment of patients with multisystem blunt trauma, *South Med* J 81:501, 1988.

Talucci RC, Shaikh KA, Schwab CW: Rapid sequence intubation with oral intubation in the multiply injured patient, *Am Surg* 54:185, 1988.

BURNS

Burn patients have the same acute care needs as any trauma patient, with attention primarily focused on the ABCs and immediate threats to life or limb. Burn patients require an additional assessment of burn severity based on depth of burn, percentage of body surface area (BSA) affected, location of the burn. Attention to the etiologic agent, presence of inhalational injury, or coexisting illness also must be considered in treatment. Serious burns require specialized burn center management after initial stabilization.

INHALATIONAL INJURY

Inhalational injury may be the most immediately life-threatening manifestation of thermal burns, and initially can be occult. If significant injury to the airway is suspected, the patient should be given humidified 100% O_2 until the airway can be directly visualized or secured by early intubation. Carbon monoxide and cyanide exposure should be investigated. (See Chapter 15, Headache, for carbon monoxide poisoning; for cyanide poisoning, see Chapter 22, Mental Status Change and Coma.)

Symptoms

- Brassy cough
- Hoarse voice

Signs

- Stridor
- Mouth, nose burn
- Airway edema, erythema
- Singed facial, nasal hairs
- Sooty sputum

Workup

- Laryngoscopy or fiberoptic bronchoscopy to look for carbonaceous deposits or other injury associated with significant airway injury requiring intubation
- CO level

Comments and Treatment Considerations

Early intubation is required for patients with symptoms and signs of possible significant airway burn, since edema may make later airway management difficult.

THERMAL SKIN INJURY

Significant burns pose complex problems of fluid balance, thermoregulation, and secondary infection. Initial therapy in the ED beyond the ABCs involves intravenous fluid resuscitation, pain control, wound management, and tetanus immunoprophylaxis. Patients with "major" burns (see below) should receive subsequent treatment at a burn center.

Burn Depth

First degree

- Redness
- Tenderness
- Pain
- No blisters
- Intact two-point discrimination

Second degree

1. Superficial partial thickness
   a. Thin-walled fluid-filled blisters
   b. Pink and moist
   c. Soft
   d. Tender to touch
2. Deep partial thickness
   a. Red and blanched white skin
   b. Thick-walled blisters, often ruptured
   c. Decreased two-point discrimination
   d. Pressure sensation intact
   e. Poor capillary refill and sometimes anesthetic

Third degree (full thickness)

- White, leathery appearance with underlying clotted vessels
- Anesthetic

Fourth degree

- Destruction of skin, subcutaneous tissue, and possibly fascia, muscle, and bone

Body Surface Area Determination

- "Rule of nines" is generally used (Fig. 33-1). The area of the patient's palm represents approximately 1% of BSA.

Severity Categorization

Major burns

Partial-thickness burn >25% BSA in adults or >20% in children under 10 years and adults over 50 years; full-thickness burns >10% BSA; burn of face, eyes, ears, hands, feet, perineum; chemical burns; high-voltage electrical burns; those associated with inhalational injury or major trauma; those sustained by high-risk, co-morbid patients. These patients need admission to a burn unit or transfer to a burn facility after initial stabilization. Admission to a burn unit is also advised for those patients who may have less severe burns but who have special psychosocial or rehabilitative care needs.

Moderate burns

Partial-thickness burn 15% to 25% BSA in adults or 10% to

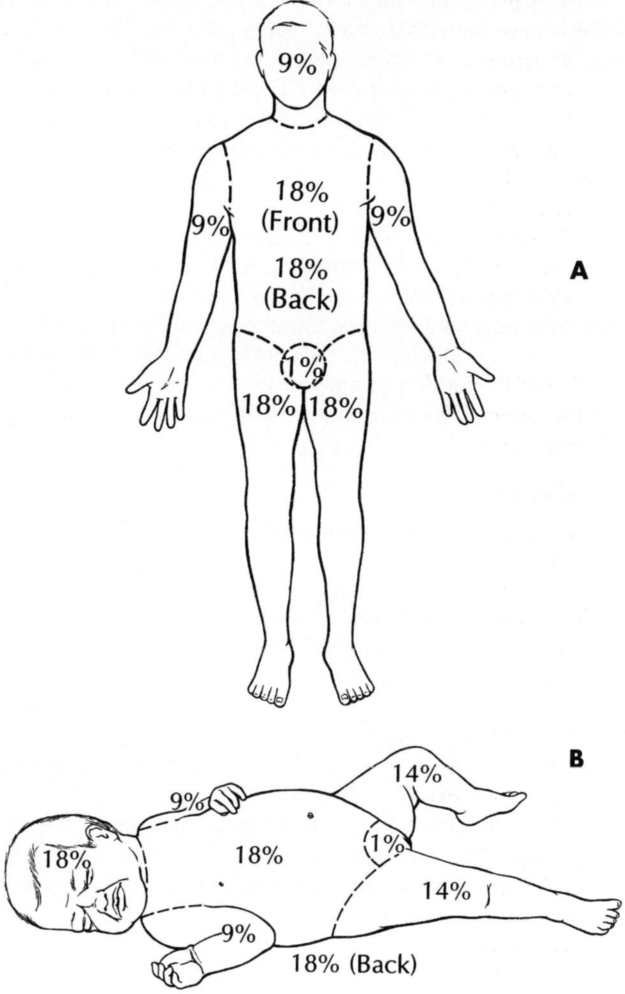

Fig. 33-1 Rule of nines. **A,** Adult. **B,** Infant. (From Rosen P, Barkin RM, Hockberger RS, et al, editors: *Emergency medicine: concepts and clinical practice,* vol 2, ed 4, St Louis, 1998, Mosby.)

20% BSA in children under 10 years and adults over 50 years; full-thickness burn 2% to 10% BSA that does not threaten function or cosmesis of eyes, ears, face, hands, feet, perineum; minor burn in high-risk patient. These patients require admission to the hospital but not necessarily to a burn unit. Specialized surgical consultation is appropriate.

Minor burns

Partial-thickness burn <15% BSA in adults or <10% in children under 10 years and adults over 50 years; full-thickness burn <2% BSA without threat to function or cosmesis. These patients require oral analgesia, mild soap and water cleansing, consideration of blister debridement (except palms and soles), tetanus toxoid immunization, topical antibiotic sterile dressing, and discharge. They need explicit burn care instructions and a wound check in 24 to 48 hours.

Management

1. Patients with major burns should be transfered to a burn center after stabilization and ED treatment.
2. Fluid resuscitation guidelines
   a. Parkland formula: 4 ml/kg/%BSA burned
   b. Lactated Ringer solution: first half over 8 hours and second half over 16 hours
   c. Goal urine output: >0.5 ml/kg/hr (adults); and 1 ml/kg/hr (children)
   d. Foley catheter, nasogastric tube, and central venous line (if indicated)
3. Pain control on basis of burn depth, patient profile, and anticipated interventions
   a. Opiates—pharmacologically advantageous; easy reversal
   b. NSAIDs, acetaminophen
4. Wound management
   a. Tetanus: toxoid booster to all; tetanus immune globulin if status unknown
   b. Escharotomy: for circumferential chest burn that compromises ventilation; vascular compromise of extremity
   c. Cleansing: sterile saline, mild soap
   d. Blisters: consider fluid evacuation except on palms and soles

e. Topical antibacterials: consider silver sulfadiazine, bacitracin
f. Coverage with sterile dry dressing or sterile dry sheets for major burns

ELECTRICAL INJURY

Electrical injuries may cause little external thermal injury and still lead to significant deep conductive burns internally. The extent of injury depends on the duration of contact with the current, the voltage (high, >1000 V; or low, <1000 V), and the type of current (alternating current [AC], more serious because of risk of continuous muscle contraction; versus direct current [DC], less serious because of single muscle spasm). Electrical exposure can cause immediate cardiopulmonary arrest, other cardiac dysrhythmias, a change in mental status, and thermal skin burns. Other injuries include rhabdomyolysis, compartment syndrome, neurologic including intracranial injury, or isolated hand or mouth injury. A high index of suspicion for significant internal injury is required.

CHEMICAL INJURY

Chemical agents continue to burn until the etiologic agent is removed. Therefore immediate removal of the caustic agent (first wipe off a solid chemical) and extensive decontamination (copious irrigation with water, unless contraindicated by nature of chemical) of affected areas is required. The physician should wear appropriate protective attire. The patient's clothes should be removed and placed into a plastic bag. Copious eye irrigation (i.e., liters of normal saline) and thorough ophthalmologic evaluation is required for chemical contact to the eye and should proceed until the corneal pH normalizes and all substances are removed.

REFERENCES[www]

American Burn Association: Hospital and prehospital resources for optimal care of patients with burn injury: guidelines for development and oper-

---

[www]Additional references are available on the following web site: www.signsandsymptoms.com.

ation of burn centers, *J Burn Care Rehabil* 11:97, 1990.

Flint L: What's new in trauma and burns, *J Am Coll Surg* 182:177, 1996.

Hammond JS, Ward CG: High-voltage electrical injuries: management and outcome of 60 cases, *South Med* J 81:1351, 1988.

Mann R, Heimbach D: Prognosis and treatment of burns, *West J Med* 165:215, 1996.

Monafo WW: Initial management of burns, *N Engl J Med* 335:1581, 1996.

Nguyen TT, Gilpin DA, Meyer NA, Herndon DN: Current treatment of severely burned patients, *Ann Surg* 223:14, 1996.

Rockwell WB, Ehrlich HP: Should burn blister fluid be evacuated? *J Burn Care Rehabil* 11:93, 1990.

Rose JK, Herndon DN: Advances in the treatment of burn patients, *Burns* 23(suppl 1):19, 1997.

Schwartz LR: Thermal burns. In Tintinalli JE, Ruiz E, Krome RL, editors: *Emergency medicine: a comprehensive study guide,* New York, 1996, McGraw-Hill.

Staley M, Richard R: Management of the acute burn wound: an overview, *Adv Wound Care* 10:39, 1997.

CHAPTER 34

Vaginal Bleeding

VENA RICKETTS

The most important factor in assessing patients with vaginal bleeding is pregnancy status. History alone is not sufficient; a urine or blood test is mandatory in all cases. Evaluation for ectopic pregnancy is required for female patients with pelvic pain, vaginal bleeding, or syncope and a positive pregnancy test.

Bleeding in nonpregnant women can occasionally be severe and cause hemodynamic compromise. Stable patients who are at risk for chronic pathologic conditions of the pelvis (e.g., cancer) should be referred for outpatient gynecologic follow-up after ED evaluation and treatment.

COMPLICATIONS OF EARLY PREGNANCY

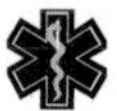

ECTOPIC PREGNANCY

Vaginal bleeding, pelvic pain, or syncope in early pregnancy should be considered indicative of ectopic pregnancy until proven otherwise, since it is the leading cause of maternal death in the first trimester of pregnancy. Patients may be unaware, or not admit, that they are pregnant. Vaginal bleeding is minimal in most ectopic pregnancies. A minority of patients have no vaginal bleeding.

Symptoms

- Pelvic or abdominal pain ++++
- Vaginal spotting ++++
- Amenorrhea +++
- Nausea and vomiting ++
- Dizziness +++

- Asymptomatic ++
- For complaints of shoulder pain, ruptured ectopic pregnancy with blood in the peritoneal cavity should be investigated.

Signs

- Abdominal or pelvic tenderness ++++
- Adnexal tenderness ++++
- Adnexal mass +++. Occasionally an ectopic pregnancy can be found on the opposite side of a palpable adnexal mass (20%). This finding is due to a corpus luteum cyst, which can be misinterpreted as an ectopic pregnancy.
- Hemodynamic compromise if rupture

Workup

- Urine pregnancy test +++++ (most assays)
- Vaginal ultrasound provides better visualization of pelvic structures than abdominal ultrasound.
- Quantitative serum βHCG is a radioimmune assay that becomes positive 8 days after fertilization.
- Serum progesterone level adds no additional information of clinical benefit.
- Rh assay
- Hematocrit with type and crossmatch if clinically indicated

Comments and Treatment Considerations

Since 1970 the incidence of ectopic pregnancy has increased nearly threefold. The incidence of heterotopic pregnancy (intrauterine and coexisting ectopic pregnancy) is now approximately 1:4000.

Unstable patients with ectopic pregnancy require emergent operative management. ED evaluation should be brief and concentrate on patient stabilization (ABCs, two large-bore intravenous lines, and volume resuscitation as needed).

For stable patients, the results of transvaginal ultrasound and serum βHCG are considered. Definitive ultrasonographic identification of intrauterine pregnancy (IUP) can be made at most institutions at a βHCG level of approximately 1500 mIU/ml. For stable patients with a βHCG level below this and without evidence of an IUP or ectopic pregnancy by ultrasound, close obstetric outpatient follow-up with a recheck of βHCG level in 2 days should be considered. The diagnosis of ectopic pregnancy is generally made in patients with a βHCG level below the discriminatory zone with ultrasound evidence of ectopic pregnancy or in those with a βHCG level above the discriminatory zone and without signs of IUP on ultrasound. Treatment of ectopic pregnancy may be medical (methotrexate) or surgical. Obstetric consultation is required.

Mothers who are Rh negative should receive MICRhoGAM 50 μg when <13 weeks into their pregnancy and RhoGAM if >13 weeks.

REFERENCES[www]

Abbott J, Emmans LS, Lowenstein SR: Ectopic pregnancy: ten common pitfalls in diagnosis, *Am J Emerg Med* 8:515, 1990.

Cacciatore B, Stenman UH, Ylostalo P: Diagnosis of ectopic pregnancy: vaginal ultrasonography in combination with a discriminatory serum βHCG levels and vaginal sonography findings, *Br J Obstet Gynaecol* 97:904,1990.

Stovall TG, Ling FW, Andersen RN, Buster JE: Improved sensitivity and specificity of a single measurement of serum progesterone over serial quantitative beta-human chorionic gonadotropin in screening for ectopic pregnancy, *Hum Reprod* 7:723, 1992.

[www]Additional references are available on the following web site: www.signsandsymptoms.com.

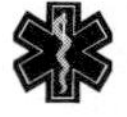

ABORTIONS: THREATENED, COMPLETE, INCOMPLETE, MISSED, AND SEPTIC

Vaginal bleeding is common during early pregnancy, with most pregnancies proceeding to term despite early bleeding (threatened abortion). Spontaneous abortions frequently occur, however. In general, fetal tissue passes without active medical intervention (completed abortion). Completed abortions require follow-up to ensure that the βHCG level returns to 0 (i.e., no ectopic pregnancy or molar pregnancy). Incomplete (open cervical os or ultrasound evidence of retained products) and septic abortions require ED obstetric consultation, whereas some cases of missed abortion can be managed expectantly with close obstetric follow-up. What appears on gross visual examination to be products of conception can actually be a molar pregnancy or a decidual cast associated with an ectopic pregnancy. All presumed products of conception should be sent for pathologic examination (consent is required in some states).

All patients who are Rh negative and have vaginal bleeding in early pregnancy should receive MICRhoGAM.

REFERENCES

Batzofin JH, Fielding WL, Friedman EA: Effect of vaginal bleeding in early pregnancy on outcome, *Obstet Gynecol* 63:515, 1984.

Wilson RD, Kendrick V, Wittmann BK, McGillivary B: Spontaneous abortion and pregnancy outcome after normal first-trimester ultrasound examination, *Obstet Gynecol* 67:352, 1986.

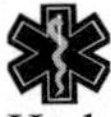

MOLAR PREGNANCY

Hydatidiform mole occurs in 1:200 to 1:2000 pregnancies in the United States. Invasive mole (chorioadenoma destruens) occurs in 1:12,000 pregnancies. This is a progressive form of hydatidiform mole that has invaded the myometrium or other structures. Choriocarcinoma is an epithelial tumor that occurs in 1:40,000 pregnancies. Timely diagnosis of molar pregnancy is important because early treatment is highly effective.

Symptoms

- Molar pregnancy often has no specific clinical characteristics to distinguish it from a normal pregnancy in the early stages of gestation.
- Vaginal bleeding +++++
- Abdominal pain ++

Signs

- Absent fetal heart tone +++++
- Uterine enlargement may be disproportionate to the expected gestational age +++.

- Preeclampsia in pregnancy less than 24 weeks' gestation ++
- Enlarged ovaries due to theca lutein cysts ++
- Hyperemesis gravidarum, which is frequently severe and protracted compared to normal pregnancy ++
- Anemia secondary to vaginal bleeding +++, with occasional manifestation of what appears to be hydatid vesicles from the vagina
- Signs of hyperthyroidism + and pulmonary trophoblastic emboli +

Workup

- Continuous disproportionate rise in serum βHCG levels
- Ultrasonography is the technique of choice to confirm the diagnosis of a mole.
- Rule out metastases (chest x-ray; consider head CT scanning)

Comments and Treatment Considerations

Treatment of hydatidiform mole consists of dilation and curettage. Patients who have vigorous bleeding and a uterine size greater than 20 weeks should be treated in an area where abdominal hysterectomy can be performed in an emergency. Chemotherapy is used for metastatic disease.

REFERENCES

Berkowitz RS, Goldstein DP, DuBeshter B, Bernstein MR: Management of completed molar pregnancy, *J Reprod Med* 32:634, 1987

Szulman AE, Surti U: The syndromes of hydatidiform mole. I. Morphologic evolution of the complete and partial mole, *Am J Obstet Gynecol* 32:20, 1978.

Watson EJ, Hernandez E, Miyazawa K: Partial hydatidiform moles: a review, *Obstet Gynecol* 42:540, 1987.

THIRD TRIMESTER BLEEDING

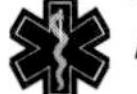

PLACENTAL ABRUPTION

Placental abruption is disruption of the uteroplacental bond that can cause fetal and maternal death. Severe pain, particularly in the setting of cocaine use, should suggest the diagnosis.

Symptoms

- Abdominal and pelvic pain ++++
- Vaginal bleeding ++++ (blood may be trapped between the placenta and uterus)

Signs

- Hypertonic and tender uterus ++++
- Vaginal bleeding ++++
- Back pain +++
- Fetal distress (tachycardia, bradycardia)
- Preterm labor ++
- Maternal shock
- Fetus demise
- Disseminated intravascular coagulation (DIC)

Workup

- Diagnosis is clinical.
- PT/PTT and DIC panel
- Ultrasound is often nondiagnostic even in critical cases +++.
- Hematocrit is frequently normal +++.
- Type and crossmatch blood
- Rh status

Comments and Treatment Considerations

Oxygen, two large-bore intravenous lines, hemodynamic support, and fetal monitoring should be initiated. Cessation of contraction, a rapidly enlarging uterus, or boardlike rigidity may be suggestive of increasing severity of abruption. RhoGAM should be given for mothers who are Rh negative. Emergent obstetric consultation is required.

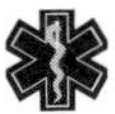

PLACENTA PREVIA

Placenta previa should be considered in all patients with vaginal bleeding in the third trimester, and an ultrasound should be obtained before an invasive pelvic examination is performed.

Symptoms

- Vaginal bleeding, often sudden, painless, and profuse

Signs

- Vaginal bleeding

Workup

- Ultrasound is diagnostic +++++.
- Hematocrit
- Type and crossmatch blood

Comments and Treatment Considerations

Oxygen, two large-bore intravenous lines, hemodynamic support, and fetal monitoring should be initiated. Emergent obstetric consultation is required. RhoGAM should be given to mothers who are Rh negative.

REFERENCES

Clark SL, Koonings PP, Phelan JP: Placenta previa/accreta and prior cesarean section, *Obstet Gynecol* 66:89, 1985.

Combs CA, Nyberg DA, Mack LA et al: Expectant management after sonographic diagnosis of placental abruption, *Am J Perinatol* 9:170, 1992.

Lowe TW, Cunningham FG: Placental abruption, *Clin Obstet Gynecol* 33:406, 1990.

NONPREGNANT PATIENTS

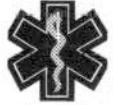

DYSFUNCTIONAL UTERINE BLEEDING

Anovulation is the most frequent cause of dysfunctional vaginal bleeding and, by definition, is unrelated to organic or anatomic lesions of the uterus. A pregnancy test is required to rule out complications of pregnancy.

Symptoms

- Vaginal bleeding +++++

Signs

- Vaginal bleeding +++++
- Normal pelvic examination

Workup

- Pregnancy test
- Hematocrit, type and crossmatch if unstable
- Endometrial biopsy to rule out endometrial cancer if patient is older than 35 to 40 years of age or is otherwise at high risk

Comments and Treatment Considerations

Dysfunctional uterine bleeding is a diagnosis of exclusion. For severe bleeding, patients may require intravenous hormonal treatment, curettage, or occasionally hysterectomy. Stable patients are generally treated with outpatient hormonal therapy, such as medroxyprogesterone (Provera) 10 mg po for 7 to 10 days. Patients should be counseled that they will have a withdrawal bleed after completing the course of treatment. Obstetric and gynecologic follow-up is suggested.

REFERENCES

Bayer SR, DeCherney AH: Clinical manifestation and treatment of dysfunctional uterine bleeding, *JAMA* 269:1823, 1993.

Choung CJ, Brenner PF: Management of abnormal uterine bleeding, *Am J Obstet Gynecol* 175:787, 1996.

Wathen PI, Henderson MC, Witz CA: Abnormal uterine bleeding, *Med Clin North Am* 79:329, 1995.

CHAPTER 35

Vision, Change in

JOSEPH ENGLANOFF

The precise etiology of nontraumatic loss of vision is diverse and includes anatomic, vascular, infectious, toxicologic, autoimmune, and psychogenic causes. The key decision for the emergency physician is to determine which patients with acute loss of vision have true emergencies. It is important to obtain a history that focuses on the extent and time interval of the loss, as well as any associated symptoms. The physical examination should include visual acuity check, evaluation for foreign body, pupillary, funduscopic, and slit-lamp evaluations, as well as intraocular pressure measurement. Finally, with many ophthalmologic emergencies, particularly central retinal artery occlusion, retinal detachment, and temporal arteritis, time is of the essence. Immediate action needs to be taken to correct the current loss of vision and to prevent further loss of vision.

The characteristics of visual field loss help to localize the causative lesion. Lesions in front of the optic chiasm (optic nerve and retina) cause monocular symptoms. Lesions behind the chiasm produce homonymous hemianopias (loss of right or left visual field in both eyes). Chiasm lesions affect both eyes in different ways, such as bitemporal hemianopia (loss of temporal visual fields in both eyes).

An afferent pupillary defect (APD) is present when direct pupillary constriction to light in the affected eye is less than the consensual response when light is shined in the unaffected eye. Moving the light from the unaffected to the affected eye therefore leads to pupillary dilation. An APD suggests pathology of an afferent structure of vision (e.g., retina or optic nerve) in the affected eye.

Ophthalmologic consultation is required for all patients with loss of vision. In addition to a routine examination, indirect funduscopic examination (usually done by an ophthalmologist) is required in most cases.

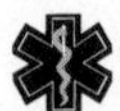

AMAUROSIS FUGAX

Amaurosis fugax is unilateral loss of vision usually caused by an atheromatous plaque at the carotid bifurcation that either embolizes or causes a temporary reduction in retinal circulation.

Symptoms

- Completely painless process (unless associated with a migraine)
- Monocular complete or partial loss of vision that may last seconds to (occasionally) 1 to 2 hours
- Visual loss may be described as a "curtain lowering" in eye

Signs

- Normal eye and funduscopic examination (except if coexisting disease)
- Occasionally, signs of central retinal artery occlusion are seen on funduscopic examination.
- Concomitant contralateral arm or leg weakness or numbness may be present if this is an embolic phenomenon.

Workup

- Complete history, detailing the event and determining if the visual loss is truly monocular or possibly binocular. Previous episodes, transient ischemic attacks (TIA), cerebrovascular accidents, heart or valvular disease, and intravenous drug abuse should be investigated.
- Complete ophthalmologic evaluation including visual field tests and dilated funduscopic examination
- Depending on the history and clinical findings, other tests may be appropriate.
- A CBC with platelet count may be helpful to rule out polycythemia or thrombocytosis.
- Carotid duplex may be helpful to determine origination of embolus.

- Cardiac echocardiogram may be helpful to determine origination of embolus.
- CT or MRI may be helpful if a postchiasmic lesion is suspected or if other neurologic signs or symptoms accompany monocular visual loss.

Comments and Treatment Considerations

Since amaurosis fugax is a form of TIA, it should be investigated and treated as such, with emphasis on rapid detection of extracranial arterial disease, cardiac abnormalities, and hematologic disorders. In one study, 16% of patients with amaurosis fugax eventually suffered a stroke or permanent loss of vision in the affected eye, or both.

See Chapter 36, Weakness and Fatigue.

REFERENCES

Burde RM: Amaurosis fugax: an overview, *J Clin Neuro Ophthalmol* 9:185, 1989.

Lord RS: Transient monocular blindness, *Aust N Z J Ophthalmol* 18:299, 1990.

The Amaurosis Fugax Study Group: Current management of amaurosis fugax, *Stroke* 21:201, 1990.

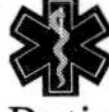

RETINAL DETACHMENT

Retinal detachment is separation of the inner neuronal layer of the retina from the outer pigment epithelial layer. It is more common in patients with diabetes, the elderly (average age of onset is in the fifth decade), trauma patients, and in individuals with previous retinal detachment.

Symptoms

- Painless event
- Monocular complaints of flashes of light, floaters (specks of pigment or blood), or a "curtain" moving over the field of vision
- Loss of vision or a visual field defect varies and may be gradual or sudden in onset.
- Visual acuity remains normal until the macula is involved.

Signs

- Normal anterior chamber
- Afferent pupillary defect may be present.
- Blood in the vitreous may occur, since bleeding is common with retinal detachment.
- Retina may appear to have an elevation, flap, hole, or an undulatory appearance; direct ophthalmoscopy demonstrates that portions of the retina are in focus while other portions are not.

Workup

- Indirect ophthalmoscopy by an ophthalmologist is mandatory.
- Ultrasound is frequently used to evaluate the retina, since a concomitant vitreous hemorrhage may prevent visualization of the retina.

Comments and Treatment Considerations

Retinal detachment is a true emergency requiring immediate ophthalmologic intervention, which aims to reattach the detached portion, thereby restoring retinal blood supply, and to prevent further undermining and detachment. If left untreated, it may progress to complete loss of vision, especially if the macula becomes separated. Treatment consists of air or silicon oil injections, cryotherapy, photocoagulation, diathermy, and scleral buckling.

REFERENCES

Cavallerano AA: Retinal detachment, *Optom Clin* 2:25, 1992.

Classe JG: Clinicolegal aspects of vitreous and retinal detachment, *Optom Clin* 2:113, 1992.

Reichel E: Vitreoretinal emergencies, *Am Fam Physician* 52:1415, 1995.

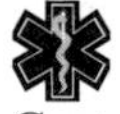

CENTRAL RETINAL ARTERY OCCLUSION

Central retinal artery occlusion is frequently caused by an embolism from carotid artery disease and primarily affects the elderly, with an increased incidence in men.

Symptoms

- Monocular
- Painless
- Sudden and complete or partial loss of vision

Signs

- Pale fundus (compared with the other eye) with a cherry red spot in the center of the macula (Fig. 35-1)
- Afferent pupillary defect to some degree is almost always present.
- Retinal arterioles may have a "boxcar" appearance, that is, segmentation of the blood column in the arterioles.

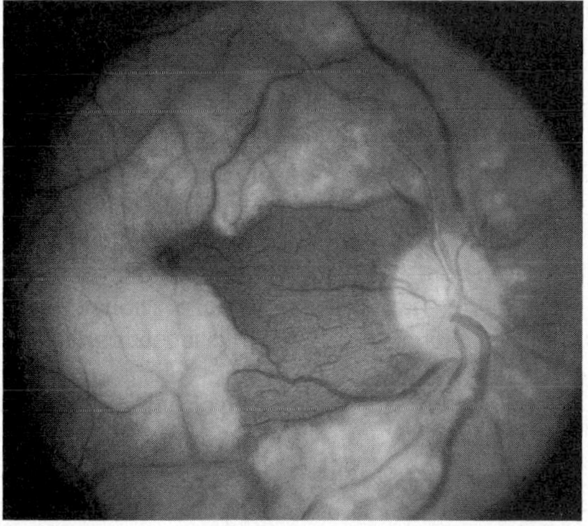

Fig. 35-1 Central retinal artery obstruction with a patent cilioretinal artery *(1)* sparing the fovea. Diffuse retinal whitening from retinal ischemia appears several hours after the arterial occlusion. The normal-appearing retina between the optic nerve and fovea is perfused by the centrally located cilioretinal arteriole. (From Palay DA, Krachmer JH: *Ophthalmology for the primary care physician,* St Louis, 1997, Mosby.)

Workup

- Full dilated funduscopic examination (including indirect by an ophthalmologist), which should exclude other causes of painless, monocular loss of vision such as retinal detachment and vitreous hemorrhage.
- Orbit or brain CT, ESR, and WBC counts are of no benefit.

Comments and Treatment Considerations

Early intervention and treatment may relieve the occlusion; vision is permanently lost if the process persists for more than 2 hours. Immediate ophthalmologic consultation is critical.

While awaiting the ophthalmologist's arrival, the emergency physician should attempt to dislodge the embolus by applying

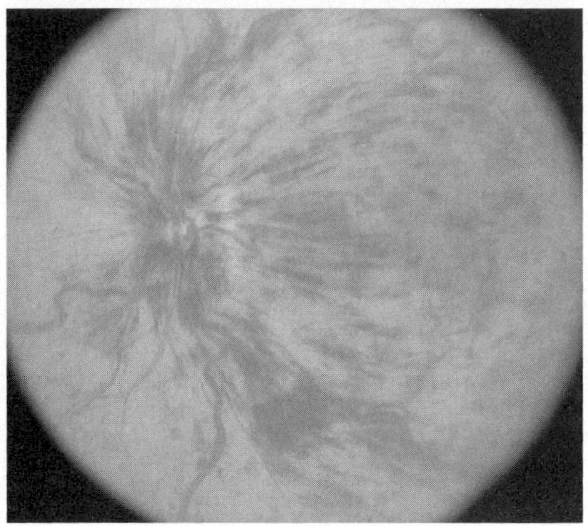

Fig. 35-2 Central retinal vein occlusion in a patient with 20/400 visual acuity. Note the dramatic retinal hemorrhages in all four quadrants. Significant venous dilation and tortuosity are present. Mild to moderate ischemia is seen with diffuse cotton-wool spots. The optic disc is blurred with peripapillary hemorrhage. (From Palay DA, Krachmer JH: *Ophthalmology for the primary care physician,* St Louis, 1997, Mosby.)

digital pressure to the globe repeatedly for 5 seconds and releasing for 5 seconds.

Increasing P_{CO_2} by having the patient breathe into a brown paper bag for 10 minutes each hour may relieve vasospasm. Acetazolamide (Diamox) 500 mg po may be given in addition to timolol 0.5% eye drops. Sublingual nitroglycerin may cause vascular dilation. The ophthalmologist may attempt an anterior chamber paracentesis to decompress the globe and dislodge the embolus.

Retinal vein occlusion can also occur and cause visual impairment or loss (Fig. 35-2).

REFERENCES

Atebara NH, Brown GC, Cater J: Efficacy of anterior chamber paracentesis and Carbogen in treating acute nonarteritic central retinal artery occlusion, *Ophthalmology* 102:2029, 1995.

Henkind P, Chambers JK: Arterial occlusive disease of the retina. In Duane TD, Jaeger EA, editors: *Clinical ophthalmology*, Philadelphia, 1986, Harper & Row.

Stern WH, Archer DB: Retinal occlusion, *Ann Rev Med* 32:101, 1981.

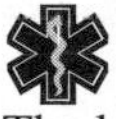

TEMPORAL (GIANT CELL) ARTERITIS

The loss of vision itself is a painless process; i.e., the eye is not painful, but the surrounding structures may be painful. It is usually a sudden, near complete, monocular loss of vision that may become bilateral.

See Chapter 15, Headache.

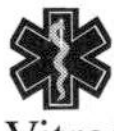

VITREOUS HEMORRHAGE

Vitreous hemorrhage should be considered in patients with diabetes mellitus, hypertension, and trauma.

Symptoms

- Painless event
- Gradual or sudden loss of vision that may vary from normal vision to only light perception.

- Black spots with flashing lights that move with eye movement is a common complaint. Some patients report seeing a red haze.
- Usually a unilateral process, but bilateral involvement has been reported.

Signs

- Anterior chamber, usually normal
- Mild afferent pupillary defect may be present (possibly associated with retinal detachment).
- Red light reflex may be decreased or absent.
- Inability to visualize the fundus is common with large vitreous hemorrhages.

Workup

- Clinical diagnosis can be confirmed by performing a full dilated posterior pole examination.
- Indirect ophthalmoscopy or ultrasound is used to rule out retinal detachment.

Comments and Treatment Considerations

Vitreous hemorrhage may be easily discovered, yet the cause of the hemorrhage must be ascertained. Treatment depends on the cause. Retinal detachment must be definitively ruled out, and ED ophthalmologic consultation is essential.

If no cause can be found and the area of hemorrhage is large, then the patient may be admitted to the hospital. Aspirin, NSAIDs, and other anticlotting agents are avoided. Bed rest with the head of the bed elevated for 2 to 3 days is recommended. Some patients require cryotherapy, laser photocoagulation, or vitrectomy.

REFERENCES

Benson WE, Spalter HF: Vitreous hemorrhage, *Surv Ophthalmol* 15:297, 1971.

Dana MR, Werner MS, Viana MA, et al: Spontaneous and traumatic vitreous hemorrhage, *Ophthalmology* 100:1377, 1993.

Spraul CW, Grossniklaus HE: Vitreous hemorrhage, *Surv Ophthalmol* 42:3, 1997.

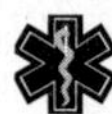

OPTIC NEURITIS

Optic neuritis causes loss of vision that is usually unilateral (more common in adults) but is sometimes bilateral (more common in children). It is caused by demyelination of the optic nerve and has a gradual onset (hours to days). Optic neuritis is a common finding in multiple sclerosis (MS). In some patients it is related to a previous (4 to 6 weeks), nonspecific viral illness. Other possible causes should be investigated, including sarcoidosis, SLE, toxoplasmosis, Lyme disease, HIV, CMV, and syphilis.

Symptoms

- Loss of vision can range from minimal loss to no light perception.
- Loss of vision is usually associated with decreased color vision and light intensity perception.
- Pain with eye movement is very common.

Signs

- Afferent pupillary defect (varying degrees)
- Central scotoma or arcuate visual field defects are possible.
- Optic nerve head may appear swollen with edema and possible retinal hemorrhages.
- Optic nerve head may appear normal if retrobulbar optic neuritis is present (more common in adults)

Workup

- Diagnosis is clinically based and often is one of exclusion. A history confirming the course of vision loss and occurrence of any previous episodes is useful. A list of past and current medication use may be helpful (ethambutol and tamoxifen use should be solicited).
- Complete ophthalmologic evaluation including a dilated funduscopic examination and visual field test
- Complete and thorough neurologic examination is essential.
- MRI may assist in diagnosing MS and in ruling out an intracranial or orbital tumor that is compressing the optic nerve.

Comments and Treatment Considerations

The treatment of optic neuritis is controversial. Many suggest observation only; others recommend systemic steroids. The association between monocular optic neuritis and the development of MS in many patients is well established, with MS developing in the majority within 4 years. Information concerning steroid use is conflicting, but steroids may diminish the chance for subsequent development of MS. Consultation with a neurologist or ophthalmologist who will follow the patient is an essential part of management. Recovery ensues within 4 to 6 weeks for approximately 90% of patients.

REFERENCES

Beck RW, Cleary PA, Anderson MM, et al: A randomized, controlled trial of corticosteroids in the treatment of acute optic neuritis. The Optic Neuritis Study Group, *N Engl J Med* 326:581, 1992.

Beck RW, Cleary PA, Trobe JD, et al: The effect of corticosteroids for acute optic neuritis on the subsequent development of multiple sclerosis, *N Engl J Med* 329:1764, 1993.

McDonald WI: Optic neuritis and its significance, *Clin Exp Neurol* 26:1, 1989.

Wray SH: Optic neuritis: guidelines, *Curr Opin Neurol* 8:72, 1995.

CHAPTER 36

Weakness and Fatigue

JORGE VOURNAS
JONATHAN EDLOW (STROKE)
MYLES GREENBERG (HYPOVOLEMIA, SEPSIS, and TOXIC SHOCK SYNDROME)

Patients can mean very different things when they complain of weakness. The first step in creating a differential diagnosis focuses on distinguishing a generalized, subjective sense of fatigue or energy loss (which can occur in a multitude of systemic processes, such as infection, metabolic abnormality, or myocardial infarction) from decreased motor strength, typically due to abnormalities of muscle, nerve, or neuromuscular junction. Although the pattern of weakness (diffuse, localized, or in a particular distribution) does not have an absolute relation to the underlying cause, it provides some of the most important clues to help direct further evaluation.

When weakness is due to a *cortical lesion,* symptoms and signs are typically contralateral to the lesion and thus localized to one side of the body; they are also frequently associated with other concordant neurologic deficits. Alterations in the quality or coordination of muscle movements can result from *cerebellar dysfunction* and also typically occur along with other cerebellar and posterior fossa findings. Lesions in the *spinal cord* typically produce a motor or sensory "level" below which neurologic deficits are pronounced, with normal function above the lesion. Some spinal cord diseases are characterized by changing levels over a variable period of time. *Nerve root* lesions produce findings limited to the distribution served by the involved roots, but because of significant overlap in the innervation of individual muscles, motor findings are typically subtle if only a single root is involved. Some diseases involve multiple nerve roots, which also occurs with processes that involve an anatomic area containing multiple roots, such as the brachial plexus or the cauda equina.

Peripheral nerve damage eventually leads to lower motor neuron signs (atrophy, flaccid paralysis, fasciculations, and depressed reflexes), as well as weakness isolated to the muscles served by the involved nerve.

Muscle disease, whether primary or due to some other underlying cause (hypothyroidism or hyperthyroidism, toxic myopathy, hypokalemia, systemic vasculitis, and so forth) commonly produces weakness that is most pronounced in proximal muscles; patients complain of difficulty getting out of a chair or raising their arms to brush their hair or put on a shirt. Weakness of *neurologic* origin is classically most pronounced in distal muscles (e.g., interfering with fine movements of the hand).

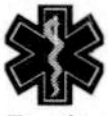

ACUTE MYOCARDIAL INFARCTION

It is well known that elderly patients who have an acute myocardial infarction (AMI) may not have chest pain. Between 20% and 30% of patients over the age of 70 who have an AMI have no chest pain and present with weakness alone.

See Chapter 7, Chest Pain.

REFERENCES

Calle P, Jordaens L, De Buyzere M, et al: Age-related differences in presentation, treatment, and outcome of acute myocardial infarction, *Cardiology* 85:111, 1994.

Presentation of myocardial infarction in the elderly, *Lancet* 2:1077, 1986.

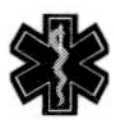

HYPOVOLEMIA

Hypovolemia is a condition of decreased intravascular volume that may be caused by acute blood loss or dehydration. It is primarily a clinical diagnosis. In acute blood loss, hematocrit will be normal until there is time for fluid equilibration, which dilutes the intravascular compartment. Symptoms and signs vary according to the cause of hypovolemia.

Symptoms

- Symptoms of disorders that lead to hypovolemia (e.g., bleeding, vomiting, diarrhea, fever)
- Generalized weakness
- Dizziness (may be exaggerated by standing)

Signs

- Dry mucous membranes
- Poor skin turgor
- Tachycardia (may be blunted by beta-blockers)
- Orthostatic vital signs/tilt test; the sensitivity and specificity of orthostatic vital signs are poor. Patients who report feeling dizzy with position change should be considered to have orthostatic hypotension even if their vital signs do not meet the classic criteria. Specificity is high if pulse change >30; unnecessary to test in the presence of symptoms or tachycardia.
- End-organ hypoperfusion (e.g., low urinary output, abnormal mental status, chest pain)
- Decreased jugular venous pressure

Workup

- Hypovolemia is a clinical diagnosis.
- Hematocrit: repeat after hydration to check for occult blood loss
- Thorough search of all areas for potential blood loss (chest, abdomen, pelvis, retroperitoneum, and gastrointestinal tract)
- Ultrasonographic, nuclear medicine, or radiographic workup for sources of bleeding may sometimes be required. Certain adjunctive laboratory tests are sometimes helpful.
- BUN, creatinine: provides information on renal perfusion and function

Comments and Treatment Considerations

Large-bore intravenous access and administration of isotonic fluids should generally be initiated as the source of dehydration is investigated. Placement of a Foley catheter to record ongoing urinary output can be helpful.

See Chapter 33, Trauma, Approach to, and Chapter 6, Bleeding.

REFERENCES

Fuchs SM, Jaffe DM: Evaluation of the tilt test in children, *Ann Emerg Med* 16:386,1987.

Knopp R, Claypool R, Leonardi D: Use of the tilt test in measuring acute blood loss, *Ann Emerg Med* 9:72, 1980.

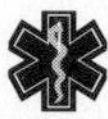

SEPSIS AND TOXIC SHOCK SYNDROME

Many types of infection can cause hypotension and a sepsis syndrome. The elderly and immunocompromised are particularly susceptible to infectious insults and may show early compromise. Common sources for infection should be considered, including genitourinary, abdominal for CNS, and pulmonary. Toxic shock syndrome (TSS) is mediated by *Staphylococcus aureus* exotoxins causing multiorgan system dysfunction. Although it is widely known to occur in women using tampons, TSS can occur in males and children, and in nonmenstrual females. Fever, rash, and hypotension are the most prominent features of TSS.

Symptoms

- Symptoms specific to focus of infection
- Weakness
- Fever
- Rash (desquamation in TSS; petechial rash may occur in meningococcemia)
- Diarrhea (++++ in TSS)
- Myalgias (+++++ in TSS)
- Vomiting (++++ in TSS)
- Headache (++++ in TSS)
- Sore throat (+++ in TSS)
- Vaginal discharge (++ in TSS)
- Rigors (++ in TSS)

Signs

- Signs specific to site of infection
- Toxic shock: rash (diffuse macular erythroderma +++++)
- Fever >38.5° C (may be hypothermic in some septic patients)

Workup

- Tests are directed at finding the source of overwhelming infection and evidence of multiorgan involvement.

- Urinalysis
- Chest x-ray
- Blood and urine cultures
- Lumbar puncture when indicated
- Electrolytes, BUN, creatinine
- CT scanning or occasionally exploratory laparotomy may be indicated when the abdomen is the likely source.

Comments and Treatment Considerations

The mainstays of the treatment of sepsis and toxic shock are fluid resuscitation and intravenous antibiotics (although antibiotics are likely only marginally useful in TSS). In TSS, tampons or nasal packing still in place should be removed. Antibiotic treatment should initially consist of broad-spectrum coverage (including *Pseudomonas*) or be directed at the causative organism(s), if known (e.g., in TSS, antistaphylococcal penicillins or cephalosporins). A Foley catheter should be placed to monitor urine output. Patients who have multisystem or cardiovascular compromise may require pressors or invasive hemodynamic monitoring.

REFERENCES

Chesney PJ, Davis JP, Purdy WK, et al: Clinical manifestations of toxic shock syndrome, *JAMA* 256:741, 1981.

Chow AW, Wong CK, MacFarlane AMG, Bartlett KH: Toxic shock syndrome: clinical and laboratory findings in 30 patients, *Can Med Assoc J* 130:425, 1984.

Shands KN, Schmid GP, Dan BB, et al: Toxic shock syndrome in menstruating women: association with tampon use and *Staphylococcus aureus* and clinical features in 52 cases, *N Engl J Med* 303:1436, 1980.

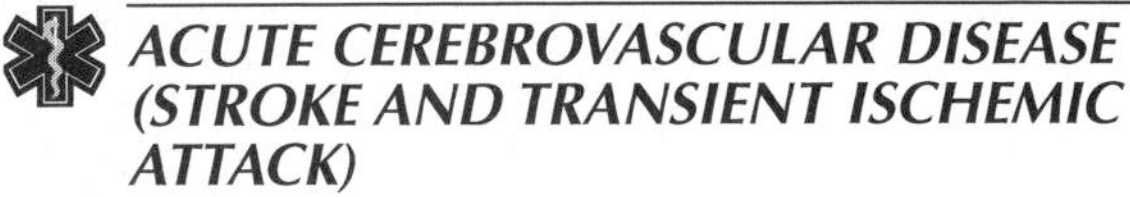

ACUTE CEREBROVASCULAR DISEASE (STROKE AND TRANSIENT ISCHEMIC ATTACK)

Acute cerebrovascular disease refers to conditions that either transiently (transient ischemic attack) or permanently (stroke) cause CNS dysfunction. The working criteria for establishing a diagnosis of stroke generally include the abrupt onset of focal neurologic symptoms that are attributable to one vascular territory and that have been present for at least 24 hours. Strokes can be ischemic or hemorrhagic. Ischemic strokes are caused by embolism or thrombosis and may become hemorrhagic. TIA is distinguished from stroke by resolution of ischemic symptoms within 24 hours, with the vast majority of cases resolving within a few hours. Careful neurologic examination is the key to diagnosis of stroke. Immediate neuroimaging may confirm a stroke, its type, and other significant pathologic conditions requiring care. However, CT scans within 24 to 48 hours of a nonhemorrhagic stroke may be normal. "Stroke mimics," such as Todd's paralysis secondary to seizure, tumor, metabolic derangements, infections, migraine headache, and Bell's palsy account for a significant minority of patients with neurologic deficits.

Symptoms

- Focal neurologic symptoms (weakness is dominant, sensory accompanies) ++++; specific symptoms vary according to vascular territory involved.
- Headache +++
- In posterior circulation stroke, motor loss may be unilateral, bilateral, or absent depending on the lesion. Nausea, vomiting, dizziness, and occipital headache are common.

Signs

- Focal neurologic signs ++++ ; specific signs are a function of which vascular territory is involved.
- Atrial fibrillation is associated with increased incidence of stroke
- In posterior circulation stroke, cranial nerve and cerebellar findings may be subtle.

Workup

- CT scan to differentiate hemorrhagic versus ischemic stroke, also to exclude other diagnoses (e.g., brain tumor, subdural hematoma)
- ECG to detect atrial fibrillation

- Specific tests and observation to detect stroke mimics, such as hypoglycemia or hyperglycemia, hyponatremia, (rarely) hepatic encephalopathy, infectious diseases, or postictal state
- Carotid noninvasive tests, MR angiography for TIA
- Transesophageal cardiac echocardiography to investigate possible source for embolic stroke

Comments and Treatment Considerations

Airway, breathing, and circulation must be vigilantly monitored. Anticoagulation drugs and aspirin may be considered, especially for TIA. Thrombolytic treatment should be considered for nonhemorrhagic stroke patients who seek treatment within 3 hours of symptom onset, although actual benefit is controversial.

REFERENCES

Hacke W, Kaste Markku, Fieschi et. al: Intravenous thrombolysis with recombinant tissue plasminogen activator for acute hemispheric stroke: The European Cooperative Acute Stroke Study (ECASS), *JAMA* 274:1017, 1995.

Leys D, et al: Misdiagnoses in 1250 consecutive patients admitted to an acute stroke unit, *Cerebrovasc Dis* 7(suppl 5):284, 1997.

The National Institute of Neurological Disorders and Stroke rt-PA Stroke Study Group: Tissue plasminogen activator for acute ischemic stroke, *N Engl J Med* 333:1581, 1995.

Wardlaw JM, Warlow CP, Counsell C: Systematic review of evidence on thrombolytic therapy for acute ischaemic stroke, *Lancet* 350:607, 1997.

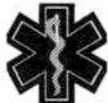

RENAL FAILURE AND UREMIA

Uremia is caused by renal failure. General weakness with evidence of fluid overload on physical examination is common, but uremia may occur in nonoliguric renal failure and normal volume status. Seizures can also be associated with the dialysis dysequilibrium syndrome (includes headache, nausea, muscle cramps, agitation, delirium, and convulsions), which usually occurs near the end of or after a rapid dialysis or ultrafiltration procedure.

Symptoms

- Neurologic symptoms: confusion, tremor, and generalized weakness
- Symptoms of renal failure: oliguria, anuria, nausea, vomiting, fatigue, edema, and shortness of breath

Signs

- Neurologic findings: tremor, weakness, myoclonus, tetany, asterixis, and encephalopathy
- Signs of fluid overload: edema, hepatosplenomegaly, rales, increased jugular venous distention, and an S3
- AV grafts and dialysis catheters in unconscious patients
- Seizures are usually generalized; however, focal motor seizures are not uncommon. Status epilepticus is rare.

Workup

- Patients with renal failure often exhibit multiple laboratory abnormalities (CBC, electrolytes, calcium, phosphorus, magnesium, BUN, creatinine, and glucose)
- ECG
- Chest x-ray to evaluate for fluid overload

Comments and Treatment Considerations

Dialysis is required for the treatment of uremia and should be done immediately in cases of life-threatening hyperkalemia after temporizing measures are initiated (e.g., calcium chloride 5 ml of 10% solution IV or calcium gluconate 10 ml of 10% solution IV given over 2 minutes; insulin 10 units regular IV with 1 ampule of D50; sodium bicarbonate 1 to 2 ampules). Sodium polystyrene sulfonate (Kayexalate) may also be used to lower potassium levels pending dialysis.

REFERENCES[www]

Rosenthal, RH, Heim, ML, Waeckerle JF: First time major motor seizures in an emergency department, *Ann Emerg Med* 9:242, 1980.

Wijdicks EFM, Sharbrough FW: New-onset seizures in critically ill patients, *Neurology* 43:1042, 1993.

[www]Additional references are available on the following web site: www.signsandsymptoms.com.

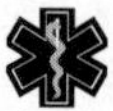 *ADRENAL INSUFFICIENCY*

Adrenal insufficiency is a rare condition that occurs most commonly as a result of chronic treatment with glucocorticoids. Rapid discontinuation of chronic glucocorticoid treatment, as well as stressors such as infection or surgery, can precipitate acute adrenal insufficiency. Primary adrenal insufficiency (Addison's disease) and secondary adrenal insufficiency (failure of the hypothalamic-pituitary axis leading to decreased ACTH) is infrequently diagnosed in the ED. Patients who are receiving ongoing steroid treatment and who are acutely ill (often hypovolemic and hypotensive, and possibly hypoglycemic) are generally treated with "stress-dose steroids" because of adrenal suppression caused by the exogenous glucocorticoids. This therapy is in addition to therapy designed to address a primary medical or surgical condition that is often present.

Symptoms

- Symptoms of primary illness when secondary to physiologic stressor
- Weakness +++++
- Fatigue +++++
- Anorexia +++++
- Weight loss +++++ (when chronic)
- Nausea and vomiting +++
- Abdominal pain +++
- Diarrhea or constipation ++

Signs

- Lethargy
- Hypotension ++++
- Hyperpigmentation +++++ (when chronic)

Workup

- ED diagnosis in clinical.
- Electrolytes: hypoglycemia, hyponatremia, and hyperkalemia are frequently seen, particularly in chronic adrenal insufficiency. Hypercalcemia may also occur.

- Evaluation for a primary process (urinalysis, chest x-ray, ECG, CBC, and other tests as clinically indicated)
- ACTH stimulation test: serum cortisol levels are drawn before ACTH and at predetermined intervals after treatment if cause is uncertain. Treat with dexamethasone phosphate 4 mg IV q6-8h.

Comments and Treatment Considerations

Adrenal insufficiency is most frequently a consideration in clinically ill ED patients taking steroids. In these patients, hydrocortisone hemisuccinate 100 mg IV should be given. IVF and IV glucose should be administered as needed. Diagnosis and treatment of any primary disease process are necessary.

REFERENCES[www]

Dunlop D: Eighty-six cases of Addison's disease, *Br Med J* 2:887, 1963.

Streck WF, Lockwood DH: Pituitary adrenal recovery following short-term suppression with corticosteroids, *Am J Med* 66:910, 1979.

Tzagournis M: Acute adrenal insufficiency, *Heart Lung* 7:603, 1978.

Vesely DL: Hypoglycemic coma: don't overlook adrenal crisis, *Geriatrics* 37:71, 1982.

[www]Additional references are available on the following web site: www.signsandsymptoms.com.

BOTULISM

Botulism is a neurotoxin-mediated paralysis affecting acetylcholine release at the neuromuscular junction (NMJ) and autonomic ganglion. *Clostridium botulinum*, a gram-positive, rod-shaped, spore-forming anaerobic bacterium that is ubiquitous in soil and water, produces the toxin. The spores germinate in an anaerobic media such as home-canned goods.

Symptoms and signs differ somewhat depending on the type of botulism: foodborne, wound, or infant. With foodborne botulism, patients classically present 12 to 36 hours after ingestion with a descending symmetric motor paralysis, autonomic instability, no sensory component, and normal mental status. In infantile botulism, spores are ingested and germinate in the infant's immature intestines and slowly release toxin.

The diagnosis should be considered in patients with autonomic and cranial nerve (e.g., diplopia, dysarthria, and dysphagia) dysfunction. Descending flaccid paralysis is common and may rapidly progress to ventilatory failure.

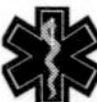

FOODBORNE BOTULISM

Symptoms

- Nonspecific early: nausea, vomiting, weakness, malaise, constipation
- Dysphagia +++++
- Fatigue +++
- Descending paralysis beginning with cranial nerves: dry mouth ++++ , diplopia ++++ , dysarthria ++++ , upper extremity weakness +++ , lower extremity weakness +++
- Respiratory failure (late)

Signs

- Descending paralysis: cranial nerve dysfunction (ptosis ++++, extraocular muscle weakness +++, miosis +++), descending muscle weakness or paralysis
- Reflexes, normal +++ or decreased +++
- Sensation and sensorium are usually intact.

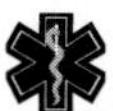

WOUND BOTULISM

Symptoms

- Similar to foodborne except GI complaints are less prominent and the onset is over days instead of hours.
- May occur in patients who use intravenous drugs.

Signs

- Abscess or other wound. The spores germinate in the anaerobic environment of the abscess and release toxin into the bloodstream.

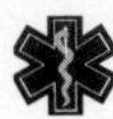

INFANT BOTULISM

Median age of onset is 2 to 4 months of age but may occur up to 1 year of age. The most commonly identified source of botulism spores is honey or corn syrup, but these account for less than 50% of cases. Botulism may also occur in breastfed babies. Approximately half of all cases in the United States occur in California, Pennsylvania, and Utah, presumably because of the high spore counts in the soil of these states. Most infants do not have respiratory difficulty, but many eventually require mechanical ventilation. The presentation of infant botulism is similar to that for sepsis, meningitis, and dehydration. Botulism should be considered, but only after a complete septic workup has been done and the patient has received antibiotics.

Symptoms

- Poor feeding/sucking +++++
- Constipation over 3 days ++++
- Lethargy +++

Signs

- Poor head control +++++
- Hypotonia ++++
- Weak cry ++++
- Expressionless face +++
- Depressed reflexes
- Decreased gag

FOODBORNE, WOUND, AND INFANT BOTULISM

Workup

- The diagnosis of botulism is purely clinical. Confirmatory tests should be done, but treatment must be started before the results become available.
- Serum, stool, wound, or food samples should be sent to the CDC for toxin testing.

Comments and Treatment Considerations

Patients with botulism should be admitted to the ICU, since most ultimately require respiratory support and respiratory failure may occur quickly. Decontamination of the GI tract (gastric lavage, cathartic agents, or enemas) or wound site should be considered. The CDC recommends intravenous infusion of one vial of trivalent equine antitoxin. Guanidine may be useful. Infants are given supportive care only. Antitoxin is available from the CDC. The CDC Botulism weekday phone number is (404) 639-2206 or 639-3311; nights and weekends (404) 639-2888.

If botulism is strongly suspected, aminoglycosides are contraindicated because they potentiate the neuromuscular blockade of the toxin.

REFERENCES

Hatheway CL: Botulism: the present status of the disease, *Curr Top Microbiol Immunol* 195:55, 1995.

Hughes JM, Blumenthal JR, Merson MH, et al: Clinical features of types A and B food-borne botulism, *Ann Intern Med* 95:442, 1981.

Shapiro RL, Hatheway C, Swerdlow DL: Botulism in the United States: a clinical and epidemiologic review, *Ann Intern Med* 129:221, 1998.

Wigginton JM, Thill P: Infant botulism: a review of the literature, *Clin Pediatr* 32:669, 1993.

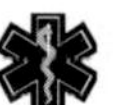

MYASTHENIA GRAVIS

Myasthenia gravis (MG) is an autoimmune disease in which antibodies against nicotinic acetylcholine receptors (Ach-R) both decrease the number of receptors and change the morphology of the neuromuscular junction (NMJ). The trigger for the autoimmune response is unknown, but a drug-induced form is reversible. Incidence follows a bimodal distribution occurring in women in their second and third decades and in men in their sixth and seventh decades.

Symptoms

- Blurry vision and eyelid weakness ++++
- Generalized weakness ++++
- Other bulbar muscles become affected resulting in dysarthria, dysphagia, weakness in the muscles of mastication, and a characteristic nasal-sounding voice. The muscles of the neck, diaphragm, and proximal extremity muscles then become involved in a descending fashion.

Signs

- Weakness of bulbar muscles, particularly eyelid weakness
- Reflexes are usually normal.
- Sensation and mental status are intact.
- Affected muscles are easily fatigable.

Workup

The Tensilon test (edrophonium) is the primary diagnostic test. Atropine should be available in case of severe bradycardia or other severe cholinergic effect induced by edrophonium. A predetermined muscle should be tested using both a placebo and edrophonium. Onset of improved strength begins within 30 seconds and lasts 5 minutes. A test is considered positive if there is unequivocal increase in strength.

Immunodiagnosis can be made in many patients by testing for Ach-R antibody. EMGs have been used to help confirm the diagnosis.

Comments and Treatment Considerations

Treatment of MG begins with pyridostigmine (Mestinon), a cholinesterase inhibitor. Thymectomy is also considered, as is immunosuppressive therapy (steroids, azathioprine [Imuran], and cyclosporine) for severe cases.

Patients with known MG may have weakness that could represent myasthenic crisis or cholinergic crisis from overtreatment with Mestinon. Patients with cholinergic crisis should also have other muscarinic symptoms, such as hypersecretion and tachycardia. Further treatment with Mestinon in cholinergic crisis can be dangerous.

Plasma exchange or intravenous IgG may achieve short-term control during a crisis or before surgery. A crisis is defined as a life-threatening impairment of respiration. A vital capacity of less than 1 L is indicative of impending respiratory failure and is more sensitive than the development of hypercapnia.

REFERENCES

Drachman DB: Myasthenia gravis, *N Engl J Med* 330:1797, 1994.

Hopkins LC: Clinical features of myasthenia gravis, *Neurol Clin* 12:243, 1994.

LAMBERT-EATON MYASTHENIC SYNDROME

Lambert-Eaton myasthenic syndrome (LEMS) is an autoimmune disease, often paraneoplastic, in which antibodies develop to the presynaptic acetylcholine-releasing terminal of the neuromuscular junction and parasympathetic effector junction resulting in decreased acetylcholine release. Age of onset is 40 to 80 years old.

Symptoms

- Presents insidiously as proximal muscle weakness, especially the thighs and hips, and autonomic dysfunction
- Ptosis has been reported in up to 25% of patients.
- Autonomic dysfunction includes dry mouth, impotence, and postural hypotension.
- Respiratory weakness may be seen but is generally neither common nor severe. Prolonged paralysis may develop in some patients postoperatively with the use of neuromuscular blocking agents.

Signs

- Proximal muscle weakness
- Hyporeflexia, which follows the weakness
- Waddling gait due to hip weakness
- Sensation and sensorium are normal.
- Dry mouth, postural hypotension, and ptosis may be found.

Workup

Because LEMS is associated with cancer in 40% of cases, an extensive search for cancer must be done.

- Chest x-ray
- CBC
- Chem panel, since patients may have other paraneoplastic syndromes such as SIADH.
- A Tensilon test should be done in equivocal cases, along with acetylcholine receptor antibody titer, since LEMS is often difficult to distinguish from myasthenia gravis. There is an LEMS antibody test as well.

Comments and Treatment Considerations

Patients without respiratory compromise or obvious cancer should be referred to a neurologist for EMG studies and to a primary care physician for a more extensive search for malignancy. CT scanning, bronchoscopy, and other diagnostic tests should be considered. Patients should be followed closely for at least 4 years after diagnosis.

REFERENCES

McEvoy KM: Diagnosis and treatment of Lambert-Eaton myasthenic syndrome, *Neurol Clin* 12:387, 1994.

Sanders DB: Lambert-Eaton myasthenic syndrome: clinical diagnosis, immune-mediated mechanisms, and update on therapies, *Ann Neurol* 37(suppl):63, 1995.

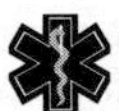

GUILLAIN-BARRÉ SYNDROME

Guillain-Barré syndrome (GBS) is an acute autoimmune demyelinating peripheral neuropathy. Viral illness precedes symptoms by several weeks in about two thirds of cases. *Campylobacter enteritis* is responsible for 10% to 25% of cases and is associated with a more severe and permanent form of GBS. In this subset of patients, the axon itself is affected as well as the myelin sheath. Classical GBS presents with an acute symmetric ascending paralysis over several days. Weakness progresses over 1 to 3 weeks and then slowly improves over the next 6 months.

Symptoms

- Weakness begins in the distal legs, but proximal muscles may appear more affected.
- Possible progression of weakness to trunk and arms
- Bulbar muscle weakness (primarily ocular and facial) less common ++
- Facial involvement, possibly asymmetric
- Sensory complaints are less prominent but common and include paresthesias and numbness

Signs

- Distal muscle weakness
- Diminished or absent reflexes in the affected muscles
- Sensorium remains intact.
- 30% require mechanical ventilation.
- Autonomic dysfunction may be prominent. It manifests in 50% of patients as labile blood pressure, heart rate, and urinary retention.
- A Miller-Fischer variant starts with ophthalmoplegia and ataxia and is followed by a descending paralysis.
- Loss of position and vibratory sense may occur.

Workup

- The ED diagnosis of GBS is largely clinical.
- Assessment of respiratory status is paramount. Patients must be adequately ventilated and the airway protected. Respiratory status should be evaluated both clinically and by pulmonary function tests. Forced vital capacity and pulse oximetry are most often followed. A forced vital capacity <12 to 15 ml/kg or <1 L in an adult may be considered an indication for intubation, although most ED airway decisions are made on a clinical basis.
- A lumbar puncture may show albuminocytologic dissociation. Protein content of >400 mg/L and a cell count of <10 cells/ml (all mononuclear) would be confirmatory. LP is often normal early in the disease but eventually shows this profile.

Comments and Treatment Considerations

All patients should be admitted. Those with severe weakness, rapid progression, or respiratory compromise should be admitted to an ICU setting. Depolarizing agents for intubation (e.g., succinylcholine) should be avoided. GBS patients are also exquisitely sensitive to vasoactive substances. Only short-acting medicines should be used to treat high or low blood pressure and should be avoided if possible.

Plasma exchange and IV immunoglobulin may be considered. Steroids have been shown to be of no benefit and may possibly be detrimental.

REFERENCES

Fulgham JR, Wijdicks EF: Guillain-Barré syndrome, *Crit Care Clin* 13:1, 1997.

Kohn MS: Weakness. In Rosen P, Barkin RM, Hockberger RS, et al, editors: *Emergency medicine: concepts and clinical practice*, ed 4, St Louis, 1997, Mosby.

Pascuzzi RM, Fleck JD: Acute peripheral neuropathy in adults: Guillain-Barré syndrome and related disorders, *Neurol Clin* 15:529, 1997.

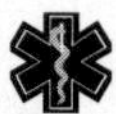

HYPOKALEMIC PERIODIC PARALYSIS

Hypokalemic periodic paralysis (HPP) is an autosomal dominant inherited disorder with imperfect penetration. Attacks are characterized by weakness or paralysis of the limbs and trunk and usually occur after a large carbohydrate meal, with rest after strenuous exercise, or after sleep. A family history is common, but sporadic cases do occur. First attacks occur at a median age of 15 years old, but patients may be as old as 30 years. Attacks may recur frequently.

Symptoms

- Episodic periods of weakness or paralysis affecting the limbs and trunk but sparing the bulbar and diaphragm muscles

Signs

- Limb and trunk weakness
- Diminished reflexes
- Sensation and sensorium are intact, but patients have been known to become agitated during attacks.

Workup

- Chem 7 shows hypokalemia and excludes other electrolyte disorders.
- ECG may show evidence of hypokalemia: flat or inverted T waves, U waves, prolonged PR interval, or sagging ST segments.

Comments and Treatment Considerations

Patients are easily treated with oral potassium replacement (bulbar muscles and the ability to swallow remain intact).

Because there is not a body deficit of potassium, and hypokalemia results from intracellular shifts, it is easy to overcorrect the potassium and cause hyperkalemia. Treatment is started with 60 to 120 mEq of oral potassium.

Acetazolamide is used to prevent attacks but is poorly tolerated. Daily potassium does not prevent attacks.

REFERENCES

Cannon L, Bradford J: Hypokalemic periodic paralysis, *J Emerg Med* 4:287, 1986.

Links TP, Smit AJ, Molenaar WM, et al: Familial hypokalemic periodic paralysis: clinical, diagnostic, and therapeutic aspects, *J Neurol Sci* 122:33, 1994.

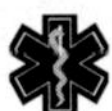

THYROTOXIC PERIODIC PARALYSIS

Thyrotoxic periodic paralysis is hypokalemic weakness similar to HPP. Patients are usually male (95%), Asian (90%), and between 20 to 39 years old (80%). Weakness usually precedes other manifestations of thyrotoxicosis. The exact mechanism causing paralysis is unknown.

Symptoms

- Similar to HPP. It presents as episodic weakness progressing over hours, typically after awakening from sleep. It affects the extremities (legs > arms) and the trunk.
- Sensation and sensorium are intact.
- Tremulousness (from hyperthyroidism) may be present.

Signs

- Similar to HPP. Reflexes are absent or diminished. Bulbar muscles and diaphragm are spared. The patient may also show signs of thyroid hormone excess: tachycardia, goiter, exophthalmos, or lid lag.

Workup

- See HPP
- Thyroid function studies (TSH, free T4)

Comments and Treatment Considerations

Treatment is the same as for HPP. Potassium replacement should be done orally and slowly to avoid hyperkalemia. Once the hyperthyroidism is controlled, these patients will not have any further problems with weakness.

See Thyrotoxicosis in Chapter 24, Palpitation and Tachycardia.

REFERENCES

Bergeron L, Sternback GL: Thyrotoxic periodic paralysis, *Ann Emerg Med* 17:843, 1988.

Miller D, delCastillo J, Tsang TK: Severe hypokalemia in thyrotoxic periodic paralysis, *Am J Emerg Med* 7:584, 1989.

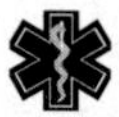

TICK PARALYSIS

Tick paralysis occurs most often in Australia, South Africa, and North America. Although primarily a veterinary problem, it also affects humans. In North America, the pregnant female tick *Dermacentor andersoni* is largely responsible for cases of paralysis. The toxin resides in the salivary gland of the tick and blocks the peripheral motor neuron release of acetylcholine at the NMJ. Children are most often affected, girls more than boys, and dark-haired people more than light-haired people. Bites occur in the spring and summer months. The diagnosis should be considered in patients with symptoms and signs consistent with the disease who have recently traveled to a tick-infested area.

Symptoms

- Begin after several days of tick attachment
- Ataxia, irritability, and lethargy are the first symptoms.

Signs

- Ascending flaccid paralysis ensues shortly after initial symptoms and progresses from hours to days. Affected muscles are areflexic.

- Paralysis eventually reaches the cranial nerves and respiratory muscles if not diagnosed and the tick removed.
- Patients may have paresthesias, but sensation remains intact.
- Sensorium is intact.
- Pupils are reactive.
- An attached tick is found.

Workup

- Search for the tick. They are most often found in the scalp but also may reside in the axilla, pubic/perianal area, popliteal fossa, or ear canal.
- No other studies are necessary if a tick is found.

Comments and Treatment Considerations

Tick removal is curative in ticks found in the United States. The tick is grasped with forceps as close to the site of attachment as possible and is removed carefully to avoid leaving the head in the skin. Symptoms generally improve within several hours but may not completely resolve for several days. Death may occur (more common in children) if the tick is not located and removed.

REFERENCES

Kincaid JC: Tick bite paralysis *Semin Neurol* 10:32, 1990.

Tick paralysis—Washington, 1995, *Morb Mortal Wkly Rep* 45:325, 1996.

APPENDIX A

World Wide Web Resources and Decision Support

JOHN D. HALAMKA

www.signsandsymptoms.com offers:

- Up-to-date electronic resources
- Links to free Medline searching
- Links to the best Internet sites for emergency in the areas of knowledge bases
- Educational resources
- Intelligent agents to search for emergency medicine topics
- Full reference list for *Signs and Symptoms in Emergency Medicine*

Several decision support features are also available, including clinical formulas that will automatically calculate answers from the data input by users. The following are included on the web site:

- Alveolar-arterial oxygen gradient (sea level) = $P(A\text{-}a)O_2 = (FiO_2 \times 713) - (PaCO_2/0.8) - PO_2$
- Anion gap = Serum Na− (Serum CL+ Serum HCO_3)
- Creatinine clearance (ml/min estimate) = (140 − age) (wt in kg)/(72 × serum Cr)
- Fractional excretion of sodium = (urine Na × serum Cr)/(serum Na × urine Cr) × 100
- Serum osmolality = [(2 × Na) + (glucose/18) + (BUN/2.8) + (Mannitol/18) + (EtOH (mg/dl)/4.6)]
- Osmolar gap = Serum osmolality measured − [(2 × Na) + (glucose/18) + (BUN/2.8) + (Mannitol/18)+ (EtOH (mg/dl)/4.6)]
- QTc = QT / Square root (RR)
- Temperature conversion
  — °C = 5(F − 32)/9
  — °F = (C × 9)/5 + 32

APPENDIX B

Emergency Drug Reference

KENNETH R. LAWRENCE

Drug	Dose
Adenosine	6 mg rapid IV; may repeat with 12 mg rapid IV; 12 mg may be repeated once
Pediatric	0.1-0.2 mg/kg rapid IV; maximum single dose 12 mg
Atropine*	
Arrest	1 mg IV; may repeat q3-5 min; maximum 0.04 mg/kg
Bradyrhythmia	0.5 mg IV; may repeat q3-5 min to total 0.04 mg/kg
Pediatric	0.02 mg/kg IV; minimum 0.1 mg; maximum single dose 0.5 mg for child, 1 mg for adolescent; may be repeated once
Bretylium	
Arrest	5 mg/kg IV; followed if needed by 10 mg/kg to maximum of 30 mg/kg
Stable	5-10 mg/kg over 10 min; may repeat in 10-30 min; maximum 30 mg/kg/24 hr
Diltiazem	0.25 mg/kg IV (consider 10-20 mg initial adult dose); may repeat in 5-10 min as 0.35 mg/kg dose; maintenance drip 5-15 mg/hr
Dobutamine	2-20 μg/kg/min IV; titrate to effect
Dopamine	2-20 μg/kg/min IV; titrate to effect
Epinephrine*	
Arrest	1 mg IV (10 ml 1:10,000) q3-5 min; may consider increasing dosages
Bradyrhythmia	2-10 μg/min
Anaphylaxis	0.3 mg (0.3 ml of 1:1000) SQ; may repeat
Anaphylaxis	0.1 mg (1 ml of 1:10,000 or 10 ml 1:100,000) slow IV; may repeat

*Medications that may be given by endotracheal tube. Dose should be 2 to 2.5 × IV dose.

Drug	Dose
Pediatric arrest	0.01 mg/kg IV of 1:10,000 q3-5 min; 0.1 mg/kg per ETT; infusion 0.1 μg/kg/min; titrate to effect
Pediatric anaphylaxis	0.01 mg/kg (1:1000) SQ; maximum single dose 0.3 mg; may repeat
Pediatric anaphylaxis	0.01 mg/kg (1:10,000 or 1:100,000) slow IV; maximum single dose 0.1 mg; may repeat
Furosemide	0.5-1.0 mg/kg IV
Isoproterenol	2-10 μg/min; titrate to heart rate; use with caution
Lidocaine*	
Arrest	1.5 mg/kg q3-5 min; maximum 3 mg/kg
Drip	2-4 mg/min
Pediatric	1 mg/kg IV; infusion 20-50 μg/kg/min
Magnesium SO4	1-2 g IV over 2 min
Morphine SO4	1-3 mg slow IV; may repeat to desired response
Naloxone*	0.4-4.0 mg IV
Nitroglycerine	0.3 mg SL; may repeat q3-5 min IV: begin 10-20 μg/min; watch blood pressure
Nitroprusside	0.1-5.0 μg/kg/min; titrate to blood pressure
Norepinephrine	0.5-30 μg/min IV; titrate to blood pressure
Procainamide	Arrest dose: 20-30 mg/min IV; maximum 17 mg/kg
Sodium bicarbonate	0.5-1.0 mEq/kg IV
Verapamil	2.5-5.0 mg IV; may repeat 15-30 min 5-10 mg IV; consider pretreatment with calcium gluconate, 5 ml IV 10% solution

*Medications that may be given by endotracheal tube. Dose should be 2 to 2.5 × IV dose.

APPENDIX C

Pediatric Emergency References and Defibrillation and Cardioversion

KENNETH R. LAWRENCE

Pediatric Emergency References

Fluid bolus: 20 ml/kg normal saline rapid IV
Glucose 0.5-1.0 mg/kg (2-4 ml/kg D25)

	Age		
	Premature	**Newborn**	**6 mo**
Weight	2.5 kg	3 kg	7 kg
Laryngoscope	0	1	1
Endotracheal tube	2.5-3.0	3.0-3.5	3.5-4.5
Chest tube	10-14 Fr	12-18 Fr	14-20 Fr
Nasogastric tube	5 feed	5-8 feed	8 Fr
Foley catheter	5 feed	5-8 feed	8 Fr

Defibrillation and Cardioversion

Defibrillation	Adult: 200 J, 200-300 J, 360 J *Pediatric:* 2 J/kg, 4 J/kg, 4 J/kg
Cardioversion	*Pediatric:* Begin at 0.5 J/kg
Ventricular tachycardia or atrial fibrillation	Adult: 100 J, 200 J, 300 J, 360 J
Paroxysmal supraventricular tachycardia of atrial flutter	Adult: 50 J, 100 J, 200 J, 300 J, 360 J
Polymorphic ventricular tachycardia	Adult: 200 J, 360 J

Pediatric Emergency References—cont'd

	Age	
1-2 yr	**5 yr**	**8-10 yr**
10-12 kg	16-18 kg	24-30 kg
1	2	2 or 3
4.0-4.5	5.0-5.5	5.5-6.5
14-24 Fr	20-32 Fr	28-34 Fr
10 Fr	10-12 Fr	14-18 Fr
10 Fr	10-12 Fr	12 Fr

INDEX

C

T